DATE DUE

OCT - 2 1996	
Oct. 17	
29	
Nov 23	
Dec 6	
FEB 2 6 1997	
SEP 3 0 1997	
OCT 2 1 1997	
Reg # 35F1066E6	
JUL 1 0 1998	
Reg 35F01064	
due Oct 6/98	
OCT 2 1 1998	
JAN 2 4 2000	
DEC 1 5 2003	

BRODART   Cat. No. 23-221

Sexual Pharmacology

Sexual Pharmacology

Edited by

ALAN J. RILEY,
MALCOLM PEET,
and
CATHERINE WILSON

CLARENDON PRESS · OXFORD
1993

Oxford University Press, Walton Street, Oxford OX2 6DP
Oxford New York Toronto
Delhi Bombay Calcutta Madras Karachi
Kuala Lumpur Singapore Hong Kong Tokyo
Nairobi Dar es Salaam Cape Town
Melbourne Auckland Madrid
and associated companies in
Berlin Ibadan

Oxford is a trade mark of Oxford University Press

Published in the United States
by Oxford University Press Inc., New York

A catalogue record for this book is available from the British Library

Library of Congress Cataloging in Publication Data
Sexual pharmacology / edited by Alan J. Riley, Malcolm Peet, and
Catherine Wilson.
Includes bibliographical references and index.
1. Sexual disorders—Chemotherapy.   2. Psychosexual disorders—
Chemotherapy.   3. Drugs and sex.   4. Psychotropic drugs—Side
effects.   I. Riley, A.   II. Peet, Malcolm.   III. Wilson, Catherine, Dr.
[DNLM: 1. Sex Behavior—drug effects.   2. Sex Disorders—drug
therapy.   WM 611 S5127 1994]
RC556.S487 1994   616.85'83061—dc20   93-15874
ISBN 0-19-262283-8

Typeset by Downdell, Oxford
Printed and bound in
Great Britain by Bookcraft Ltd,
Midsomer Norton, Bath

Preface

The past decade has seen a growing interest in the sexual effects of drugs, but the literature is spread across an enormous number of journals and symposia reports relating to a variety of medical, psychological, and biological disciplines. This book brings together much of the current knowledge of the subject. The idea for the book came out of two symposia. In 1990 the Society for Drug Research convened a meeting at St George's Hospital Medical School, London, organized by Catherine Wilson and Alan Riley, on *Drugs and sexuality* and in the following year Malcolm Peet organized a symposium on *Human sexuality and psychopharmacology* which was held in the University of Sheffield. Both symposia were well attended, emphasizing the great interest in the sexual effects of drugs.

There are two components to sexual pharmacology: appreciating which drugs are associated with sexual difficulties and developing or using drugs to treat sexual dysfunction. Both are covered in this book.

As an ever increasing number of people now find themselves on a variety of therapeutic drugs, it is essential to appreciate the liability of such drugs to impair sexual function. Adverse sexual effects are an important cause of non-compliance with drug regimens. Changes in sexual expectation has confounded this problem—many people now wish to continue sexual activity in to elderly life which is the time of most frequent use of therapeutic drugs.

The sexual effects of antihypertensive medication is reviewed by Huws, while Barnes and Harvey provide a comprehensive account of psychiatric drugs and sexuality. The sexual effects of anticonvulsants, antiparkinsonian, and miscellaneous drugs are capably covered by Peet and Gillow. No account of the effects of drugs on sexual function would be complete without considering recreational drugs; these are discussed by Huws and Sampson.

For many years sexual side effects of some drugs, developed for other purposes, have been used in the management of sexual dysfunction. There is now increasing activity in the pharmaceutical industry to develop drugs specifically for this indication. Wilson discusses pharmacological targets for the control of male and female sexual behaviour; particular focus on the effects of dopaminergic and serotinergic agents on sexual behaviour in the female rat is provided by Ahlenius; while Foreman and Doherty describe experimental approaches for the pharmacological management of erectile dysfunction. Early drug development generally requires studies conducted in animal models and the relevance of these to human sexual behaviour is discussed by Barfield. Reduced sexual desire might be considered the sexual dysfunction of the 1990s and for this reason a chapter, written by Kellett, is devoted to human sexual desire and its modification by drugs. As pharmacological agents for sexual dysfunction are developed it is essential that they are appropriately evaluated in the human. Issues concerning the evaluation of drugs on human sexual function are discussed by Riley and Riley, who, in a second chapter also describe the current status of pharmacotherapy for sexual dysfunction.

With multi-author books there is always the risk of repetition and we are aware that this has occurred in *Sexual pharmacology*. We make no apology for this because much can be lost by overzealous editing. We also make no apology for the few inconsistencies of meaning between chapters. These were deliberately not removed as they serve to demonstrate the difficulties that are encountered in interpreting data.

We thank the authors for producing first class manuscripts and Oxford University Press for their patience. We believe *Sexual pharmacology* will prove helpful to those who are involved in drug development and to all prescribing doctors.

1993   A.J.R.
                                                                                                    M.P.
                                                                                                    C.W.

Contents

Contributors

Sven Ahlenius, Department of Neuropharmacology, Astra Research Centre, S-151 85 Södertälje, Sweden.

Ronald J. Barfield, Department of Biological Sciences, Rutgers University, New Brunswick, NJ 08903, USA.

Thomas R.E. Barnes, Charing Cross and Westminster Medical School, St Dunstan's Road, London W6 8RP, UK.

Paul C. Doherty, Lilly Research Laboratories, Eli Lilly and Company, Lilly Corporate Center, Indianapolis, IN 46285, USA.

Mark M. Foreman, Lilly Research Laboratories, Eli Lilly and Company, Lilly Corporate Center, Indianapolis, IN 46285, USA.

Janice Gillow, Department of Psychiatry, Northern General Hospital, Sheffield S5 7AU, UK.

Carol A. Harvey, Charing Cross and Westminster Medical School, St Dunstan's Road, London W6 8RP, UK.

Rhodri Huws, Marital and Sexual Difficulties Clinic, Whiteley Wood Clinic, Sheffield, UK.

John Kellett, Department of Geriatrics, St George's Hospital Medical School, London, UK.

Malcolm Peet, Department of Psychiatry, Northern General Hospital, Sheffield S5 7AU, UK.

Alan J. Riley, SMC Research, Field Place, Dunsmore, Aylesbury, Buckinghamshire HP22 6QH, UK.

Elizabeth J. Riley, SMC Research, Field Place, Dunsmore, Aylesbury, Buckinghamshire HP22 6QH, UK.

Gwyneth Sampson, Marital and Sexual Difficulties Clinic, Whiteley Wood Clinic, Sheffield, UK.

Catherine A. Wilson, Roberts Barnes Laboratory, Department of Obstetrics and Gynaecology, St George's Hospital Medical School, London SW17 0RE, UK.

Abbreviations

αMSH	α-melanocyte stimulating hormone (α-melanotrophin)
A9,A10	dopamine cell body groups in the VTA
AII	angiotensin II
ACE	angiotensin-converting enzyme
ACTH	adrenocorticotrophic hormone
AMPT	α-methyl-p-tyrosine
ARC/ME	arcuate/median eminence
AVP	arg-vasopressin
CGRP	calcitonin gene-related peptide
CNS	central nervous system
CRF	corticotrophin-releasing factor
CRH	corticotrophin-releasing hormone
D_1-D_4	dopamine receptors
DA	dopamine
5,7-DHT	5,7-dihydroxytryptamine
DOI	(±)-1-(2,5-dimethoxy-4-iodophenyl)-2-amino-propane
DOPA	3,4-dihydroxyphenylalanine
DOPAC	dihydroxyphenyl acetic acid
EL	ejaculatory latency
EOP	endogenous opioid peptides
FSH	follicle-stimulating hormone
GABA	γ-aminobutyric acid
GAG	gamma-acetylenic-gaba
GnRH	gonadotrophin-releasing hormone
HSD	hypoactive sexual desire
5-HT	5-hydroxytryptamine (sub-types 1A, 1B, 1C, 1D, 2, 3, 4 are indicated by 5-HT_{1A}, 5-HT_{1B}, etc.)
5-HTP	5-hydroxytryptophan
I	intromission
IL	intromission latency
LH	luteinizing hormone
LTH	luteotrophic hormone (prolactin)
LQ	lordosis quotient
M	mounts
MAO	monoamine oxidase
MCG	midbrain central grey
MCPP	*meta*-chlorophenylpiperazine

ML	mount latency
MPOA	medial preoptic area
MPTP	N-methyl-4-phenyl-1,2,5,6-tetrahydropyridine-HCL
NPY	neuropeptide Y
OB	oestradiol benzoate
6OHDA	6-hydroxydopamine
8-OHDPAT	8-hydroxy-2-(di-*n*-propylamino) tetralin
PEI	post-ejaculatory interval
PGC	paragigantocellular
PGE_1	prostaglandin E_1
POA	preoptic area
POMC	pro-opiomelanocorticotrophin
PCPA	*para*-chlorophenylalanine
(+)PPP	(+)-3-(3 hydroxyphenyl)-N-propylpiperidine HCL
(−)PPP	(−)-3-(3 hydroxyphenyl)-N-propylpiperidine HCL
RP	refractory period
THIP	4,5,6,7-tetrahydroisoxazolo[5,4-C] pyridin-3-ol HCL. Also gabaoxadol HCL
TLE	temporal lobe epilepsy
TMCPP	M-trifluoromethylphenylpiperazine HCL
VIP	vasoactive intestinal peptide
VMN	ventromedial nucleus
VTA	ventral tegmentum area

1

Pharmacological targets for the control of male and female sexual behaviour

Catherine A. Wilson

INTRODUCTION

Mammalian sexual behaviour is controlled by gonadal steroids acting at the level of the central nervous system (CNS). The extent of hormonal control varies with sex and species. In both male rodents and primates, testosterone is essential for copulatory behaviour and in the female rodent, sexual behaviour is completely dependent on the presence of oestrogen, with progesterone acting synergistically. In primates, certain aspects of sexual activity, namely arousal and proceptive behaviour, may also be dependent on steroids, but copulatory behaviour is thought to be independent of them.

Within the brain, the steroid hormones have a two-fold action: (1) they act on membrane receptors to increase the excitability of neurones; and (2) they act genomically within the cell nucleus to increase neurotransmitter synthesis, either directly (in the case of peptide neurotransmitters) or in-directly, by increasing production of the enzymes responsible for synthesis of the non-peptide transmitters. It is assumed that these transmitters mediate the action of the hormones which control sexual activity, and so by manipulating neurotransmitter activity with pharmacological agents, the action of steroids on sexual activity can be mimicked or antagonized. In rodents, however, alteration of neurotransmitter activity in the absence of steroids has never been shown to stimulate female sexual activity, and only a transient and temporary effect has been seen in males. This indicates that lowering the threshold of activation of neuronal tracts, by steroid action, is essential before any increase in neurotransmitter turnover rate can take effect.

Most drugs affect CNS function by altering neurotransmitter activity, and so pharmacological targets for the control of sexual behaviour are those drugs which manipulate the neurotransmitters known to be involved in this control. Clearly it is necessary to investigate which neurotransmitters are of prime importance, their sites of action, and, if possible, their receptor type so that drugs can be devised which will affect a particular neurotransmitter, at a specific site, and will act selectively on a receptor type.

Components of sexual behaviour can be categorized in all mammals as follows.

In the male

(1) arousal,

(2) copulatory activity,

(3) penile reflexes.

In the female

(1) attractiveness,

(2) proceptive behaviour,

(3) receptive behaviour.

Each aspect has its own neuronal control and so can be selectively affected. Laboratory tests for the effects of drugs on sexual activity are usually carried out on rodents, in particular the rat. Whether the changes in sexual activity noted in the animals after drug treatment are really due to a specific action on sexual behaviour/response or due to other factors that do not particularly reflect sexuality, for instance general arousal, cannot easily be elucidated. In addition, these changes cannot be equated with similar effects which might be observed in non-human primates and humans. For example, the time taken for a male rat to initiate sexual activity in the presence of a receptive female might be considered a measure of sexual arousal or motivation. It might, on the other hand, indicate a change in perception of the external environment. In reality, changes in various components of sexual behaviour are scored and assumptions are made which can then be investigated further, either by comparing the effect of the drugs on other behavioural tests, or by testing in other species.

This review summarizes the findings, from the literature, of the effect of a number of neurotransmitters on sexual activity in the rodent. Although the terms 'stimulatory' and 'inhibitory' effect on sexual activity are used, they are only meant to convey the operational changes noted, after administration of pharmacological agents, on the components of sexual behaviour. It is interesting, however, to note that the drug effects on arousal/desire (see Chapter 6) and on sexual activity in the rat often change in parallel (see Baum 1983; Pfaff and Schwartz-Giblin 1988; Sachs and Meisel 1988; Wallen 1990).

MALE SEXUAL BEHAVIOUR

(For further references see Johnson and Everitt 1988; Sachs and Meisel 1988; Everitt 1990; Hughes *et al.* 1990.)

Male behavioural components

Male sexual behaviour can be divided into three components.

1. Arousal or motivation—this represents the ability of the male to initiate sexual activity. It includes locating the female and investigating her, which in the rat involves sniffing and licking the anogenital region and pursuing her in order to mount.
2. Copulatory behaviour—in the rat, this consists of mounting the female. If mounting is accompanied by penile penetration of the vagina, this is designated intromission.
3. Penile reflexes—this can be subdivided into erection and emission. Erection is due to venous occlusion between the corporal venous spaces and deeper veins of the penis concomitantly with arterial engorgement of the corpus cavernosum. This involves vasoconstrictor and dilator changes controlled by the autonomic nervous system and local peptide transmitters such as vasoactive intestinal peptide (VIP).

Rats are nocturnal, so when they are used for behavioural testing, they are kept under reversed lighting and observed by red illumination. Male sexual activity is tested by placing the rat in an observation arena of approximately 50 cm diameter. After a period of acclimatization (approximately 3–5 min), a receptive female is introduced. The following parameters are then scored:

(1) the time taken between introduction of the female and the first mount (mount latency, ML) and first intromission (intromission latency, IL);
(2) number of mounts (M) and intromissions (I) to reach ejaculation;
(3) the time taken from first mount to ejaculation (ejaculatory latency, EL);
(4) the time taken between ejaculation and the first mount of the next series of sexual activity (refractory period, RP; or post-ejaculatory interval, PEI). During approximately three-quarters of this period, the rat emits a 22 kHz vocalization which can be recorded with the aid of a bat detector. Its function is not understood—it may be a signal to the female informing her to keep away during the post-ejaculatory interval (PEI), or a signal to other males preventing them from associating with the female. During the PEI, the electroencephalogram (EEG) shows sleep-like patterns and the rat is relatively immobile.

Sachs has taken the components of this test and grouped them to form three measures of copulatory activity:

(a) copulatory rate factor (ML, IL, EL, and PEI);

(b) a hit rate factor (percentage of attempts in which the male achieves intromission, i.e. $I/M \times 100$ per cent) which measures the theoretical copulatory efficiency;

(c) intromission count factor (number of I per ejaculation). The threshold to ejaculation is defined by the intromission count factor and EL.

In a normal sexually active rat, 8 to 12 intromissions are required to reach ejaculation, the hit rate factor being 50 to 80 per cent. The EL is 4–6 min followed by a PEI of approximately 5 min.

Drugs which facilitate behaviour

(a) increase the proportion of rats engaging in copulatory activity;

(b) increase the number of rats achieving ejaculation;

(c) increase the number of ejaculations in a given time before sexual satiation;

(d) reduce the number of mounts and intromissions required to achieve ejaculation, and reduce the EL.

An inhibitory effect on sexual behaviour may occur indirectly due to impairment of motor activity or an enhancement of competing behaviours. Thus it is important to assess the effect of a drug on other behavioural activities, especially motor activity.

The type of sexual behavioural test described above provides an assessment of copulatory (consummatory) behaviour with only the latencies to initiation of copulation (ML and IL) providing a measure of arousal. Sexual arousal and/or reward (appetitive behaviour) can be separated from potency by noting mount frequency following penile anaesthesia. Other tests of arousal can involve operant methods used to measure reinforcing (rewarding) properties of the stimuli (the female). Everitt and Stacey (1987) have devised a test using second-order schedules with a female as a primary reward obtained only after bar-pressing often enough to switch on a light at least ten times (secondary reward). Other tests include conditioned place-preference paradigms associated with an ejaculation-induced reward state or associated with a receptive female (see Everitt 1990; Agmo and Berenfeld 1990).

Testing of pharmacological agents on male sexual behaviour is normally carried out on intact males that have been observed for their baseline sexual activity several times (at 2–3 day or even weekly intervals) before the drug test. Males can usually be subdivided into sexually 'vigorous' and 'sluggish' or even non-copulators (rarely more than 5 per cent of a group). The first subgroup can be used for testing potential inhibitory agents and the latter two for potential stimulators. Another way of obtaining a low baseline activity is to use a castrated rat given a low level of replacement testosterone.

Hormonal control of male sexual behaviour

In all mammals, male sexual behaviour is maintained by the testicular steroid hormone, testosterone. Thus, after castration, there is a gradual decline in sexual activity. In the rat this takes six to eight weeks, in man it takes between one and two years. The reason for this slow reduction is not understood and may be due to residual testosterone bound to its receptors or to a prolonged response once the receptors are activated, which may involve an action of arg-vasopressin (see p. 25). If testosterone replacement is provided at the time of castration, sexual activity is fully maintained: Fig. 1.1(a) shows the decline in number of rats reaching ejaculation in the 40 days after castration and the continuation of sexual activity if at the time of castration a subcutaneous implant of testosterone was put in place. If the testosterone implant is placed in the animal some weeks after castration, then sexual activity is reinstated, but in parallel with the slow decline after removal of endogenous testosterone, the increase is equally gradual (see Fig. 1.1(b)).

The sites and mechanisms of action of testosterone in its maintenance of male sexual activity has not been elucidated fully. Based on experiments in which testosterone implants were placed into discrete nuclear areas in the brain of castrated rats, it is agreed that it probably acts at multiple sites within the CNS, particularly in the preoptic area and anterior hypothalamus, to stimulate copulatory behaviour, but also at sites in the midbrain interacting with opioid and dopaminergic systems in the ventral tegmentum area and ventral striatum, enhancing recognition of the incentive cues emitted by the female. A large body of evidence supports the hypothesis that testosterone only affects male sexual activity after aromatization to oestradiol and that its other metabolite, dihydrotestosterone (which cannot be aromatized), either has no effect or a minor CNS effect and is only important for maintenance of the peripheral sex organs. However, some reports have shown that dihydrotestosterone can maintain copulatory behaviour in some species, including man, and will enhance the action of sub-threshold doses of oestradiol in rats.

Neuronal control of male sexual behaviour

Figure 1.2 depicts the pathways thought to link the areas concerned with the control of male sexual activity. The medial preoptic area (POA) appears to be the centre of this control concerned particularly with the organization of copulatory responses to the female (consummatory behaviour) rather than sexual arousal (appetitive responses) (Hughes *et al.* 1990). It is at the POA that implants of testosterone are most effective. Other parts of the CNS are more directly involved in the appetitive responses to unconditional and conditional incentives associated with a female and/or sexual interaction.

Catherine A. Wilson

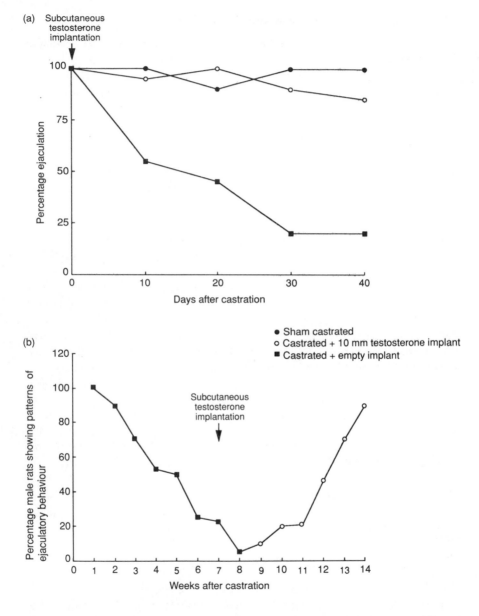

Fig. 1.1 Effect of castration and testosterone replacement on male sexual behaviour. (a) Percentage rats showing ejaculatory behaviour after castration with and without 10 mm testosterone silastic implant placed subcutaneously on the day of castration; (b) percentage rats showing ejaculatory behaviour after castration and subcutaneous placement of a testosterone implant seven weeks after castration (adapted from Johnson and Everitt 1988).

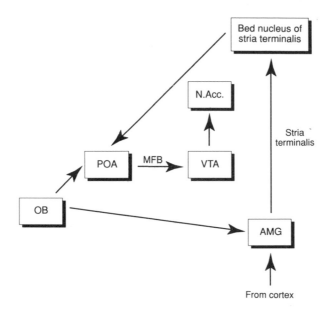

Fig. 1.2 Male neuronal circuit controlling sexual activity. Sites of neurotransmitter activity shown as POA, preoptic area; VTA, ventral tegmentum area; N.Acc., nucleus accumbens; OB, olfactory bulb; AMG, amygdala; MFB, medial forebrain bundle.

Lesion studies indicate that the animal perceives the outside environment (the presence of a female) via the olfactory bulbs, which then pass impulses directly to the preoptic area and also indirectly via the basolateral amygdala. The amygdala also conveys information from the external world received from cortical afferents (these could include auditory and sensory stimuli) to the POA via the stria terminalis to the bed nucleus of the stria terminalis. These tracts are particularly involved in control of the appetitive or arousal aspects of sexual activity and lesions in these areas have no affect on con-summatory or copulatory aspects.

Male copulatory behaviour involves the transformation of sexual motivation into non-stereotypic volitional approach to the female followed by mounting, and so on. The preoptic area integrates the information from the external environment with the internal endocrine environment and sends impulses to the ventral tegmentum area (VTA) in the midbrain to stimulate the reward centres sited there. This area also receives information from the basolateral amygdala. Dopamine cell body groups (A9, A10) in the VTA project via the ventral striatum to the nucleus accumbens and to the brain-stem and thence to the spinal cord (not shown in Fig. 1.2). This is thought to be the reward system translating arousal (desire) into movement (sexual activity) (Agmo and Fernandez 1989). Administration of a dopamine agonist into the nucleus accumbens stimulates male sexual activity, presumably mimicking endogenous dopamine activity, while the same agonist acting on the autoreceptors on cell bodies in the VTA is inhibitory (Hull *et al.* 1990). Thus the basolateral amygdala mediates the stimulus–reward associations of behaviour via an action on the dopamine-dependent system of the ventral striatum (Everitt *et al.* 1989). There is also evidence that an endogenous opioid system acts in the nucleus accumbens to enhance appreciation of a reward stimulus directly and/or interacts with the mesencephalic dopaminergic neuronal activity (Mehrara and Baum 1990). These systems may be modulated by 5-hydroxytryptamine (5-HT) since when this is injected into the nucleus accumbens it inhibits sexual activity, while stimulation of the autoreceptors on the serotonergic cell bodies situated in the midbrain raphes enhances behaviour (Hillegaart *et al.* 1991).

There are also tracts from the forebrain (i.e. POA) descending via the brainstem to the spinal cord which control penile reflexes. Normally the forebrain exerts a tonic inhibition on penile reflexes, in part via the paragigantocellular reticular nucleus in the ventral medulla which sends projections to the pelvic afferent neurones and interneurones (Marson and McKenna 1990). Arousing stimuli from the sexual partner serve to disinhibit the penile reflexes via this pathway which is polysynaptic and therefore 'allows' a great deal of opportunity for complex neural processing and integration to occur within the reflex system (see Stern 1990).

FEMALE SEXUAL BEHAVIOUR

(See Pfaff and Schwartz-Giblin (1988) for further references.)

Female behavioural components

Female sexual behaviour can be divided into three components.

1. Attractiveness, which is mediated by production of pheromones and changes in the vascularity of the perineum, usually a dilatation, causing flushing. This is under hormonal control both in rodents and primates.
2. Proceptive behaviour, which occurs in both rodents and primates although the behavioural characteristics vary with species. Female rats, for instance, perform a 'hopping and darting' movement with rapid vibration of the ears (which is actually the only visible manifestation of a rapid vibration of the head), designated as 'ear-wiggling'. The purpose of these activities, together with 'attractiveness', is to increase the likelihood of male-initiated copulation (Baum 1983; Wallen 1990). The

female also paces copulation through a pattern of approaches and with-drawals to and from the male. This solicitation determines the type and amount of coital stimuli received by the female, which is important for neuroendocrine reflexes (Erskine 1989).

3. Receptive behaviour, which is the acceptance of the pursuit and mount-ing and eventually ejaculation by the male. In response to mounting, a receptive female rat assumes a lordotic position, that is on mounting the male exerts pressure with his forepaws on the flanks of the female and also applies pressure to the perineal area. Stimulation of pressure receptors in these areas induces the female to become immobile, arch her back, raise her rump, and deflect the tail to expose the vagina.

In order to test the effect of agents or manipulations on female rat behaviour, it is usual to carry out the tests during the dark period and observe the rats under red illumination. The female is introduced to a series of observation arenas, each containing a sexually vigorous male. The number of times the female rat responds to a male mount and/or intro-mission with a lordotic response is then noted and expressed as a percentage of the mounts, called the lordosis quotient, LQ (LQ = number of lordoses/number of mounts × 100 per cent). It is usual to submit the female to 10 or 20 mounts in order to obtain an LQ which is only a measure of receptivity. More detailed measurements of lordosis can be scored, such as the degree of arching of the back and the duration for which the lordotic position is maintained. Proceptive behaviour is assessed by scoring the number of 'hopping and darting' movements performed and the frequency and in-tensity of 'ear-wiggling'.

Other tests can be devised in which the female must gain access to either a tethered male or one in a separate compartment. Similarly, attractiveness can be estimated by noting the interest shown by a male in gaining access or investigating a female either tethered or separated from him.

Hormonal control of female sexual behaviour

In primates there is evidence that attractiveness is controlled mainly by oestrogen (which stimulates pheromonal secretions and induces vasodilata-tion of the perineum). The evidence for the hormonal control of proceptive behaviour in primates is conflicting and probably differs with species, but on the whole oestrogens and/or androgens appear to enhance proceptive behaviour in both human and non-human primates. Receptivity appears to be independent of hormonal control although in some primates progester-one has an inhibitory effect, as seen over the luteal phase of the menstrual cycle and in pregnancy (see Baum 1983; Johnson and Everitt 1988).

In rodents, all aspects of female sexual activity are under hormonal regulation and ovariectomy causes an immediate cessation of all sexual activity. Replacement with either oestrogen alone or oestrogen followed by progesterone will reinstate sexual behaviour. The oestrogen acts on specific receptors located in various areas of the hypothalamus, midbrain, and limbic system, such as the ventromedial nucleus (VMN), preoptic area (POA), midbrain central grey (MCG), and amygdala. Stimulation of these receptors will enhance lordotic activity approximately 48 h later. The receptors must be occupied for the first 12 h, although this need not be continuous and two pulses of oestradiol (each lasting 1 h) given at an interval of not less than 4 h and not more than 13 h will be sufficient to induce lordosis. The oestrogen induces the appearance of progesterone receptors in the hypothalamus (although not the midbrain) and if progesterone is given at least 23 h after the oestrogen, it will synergize with it, such that a significantly lower concentration of an oestrogen priming dose is effective.

Progesterone has little or no effect when given alone and so acts mainly to enhance the action of oestrogen. However, the presence of progesterone is essential for induction of proceptive behaviour and so in the intact animal the action of the two hormones are closely interrelated. Again, in rodents, progesterone has a biphasic effect and after enhancing the action of oestrogen it then antagonizes it and so terminates the period of receptivity. These two effects are exerted at the same site in the hypothalamus, and the mechanism of the reversal is not understood, but it seems to be physiologically important as a refractory period does not occur after a dose of oestrogen alone.

Experiments using steroid implants placed into discrete areas of the brain show that the main site of action of both steroids is the VMN, in particular the latero-ventral part where steroid receptors are situated.

There are three models which can be used when testing for the effects of pharmacological agents on female sexual activity in the rat:

1. The intact rat, on the afternoon of proestrus when steroid levels are high and the animal undergoes a period of receptivity ('heat'). The advantage of this model is that it is physiologically normal. Its disadvantages are that the cyclicity of the animal must be followed for some days by vaginal smearing in order to ascertain the day of proestrus, and once copulation has occurred, the animal will become either pseudopregnant or pregnant and therefore will not be receptive for two weeks or three weeks, respectively.

2. The ovariectomized rat, with steroid replacement. This is the usual model and the hormone treatments can be varied in order to induce a low or high state of receptivity suitable for testing putative stimulatory or inhibitory agents, respectively.

As mentioned earlier (p. 1), no agent has ever been shown to stimulate female sexual activity in the absence of a background of oestrogen, so that a low dose of oestradiol benzoate (OB)—for instance 1–2 µg per rat OB subcutaneously—will induce little or no sexual activity, but with this priming a potential stimulatory agent will be able to exert an effect. A high state of activity can be produced by treating the rats with 1–2 µg per rat OB followed by 0.2–0.5 mg per rat progesterone, usually given 48 h later. The period of onset of action after giving progesterone subcutaneously is 3 h and so testing usually takes place 4–6 h after the injection. When progesterone is given intravenously, its effects can be seen 40–60 min later. High receptivity can be induced by OB alone, a suitable dose being 20–50 µg; but these rats will show little proceptive behaviour. Other regimes include daily administration of very low concentrations of oestradiol for 3 or 4 days with progesterone (if given) added on the last day 4 h before testing takes place.

3. Since progesterone has such a marked synergistic effect with oestrogen, it is important to avoid the possibility that some pharmacological agents may act by stimulating endogenous secretion of adrenal progesterone, so a third model—and perhaps the most suitable—is the ovariectomized plus adrenalectomized rat. The steroid priming is the same as after ovariectomy only, and the animals remain healthy if maintained on 0.9 per cent w/v saline instead of drinking water.

Neuronal control of female sexual behaviour

The main sites of activation of female sexual behaviour are the ventromedial nucleus (VMN) and the midbrain central grey (MCG) as shown by lesion studies, electrochemical stimulation, and implantation of steroids. Similar studies have shown that the preoptic area (POA) and septal area are sites of inhibition of female activity.

Oestrogen has a dual effect on neuronal activity: firstly a membrane effect altering electrical activity, and secondly and following the membrane effect a genomic effect stimulating protein synthesis. Application of oestrogen into the VMN either *in vitro* or *in vivo* can increase the discharge rates of slowfiring neurones and induce firing in previously silent neurones, but it only affects those VMN neurones with axons passing to the MCG. The threshold of arousal of neurones in the MCG is also reduced by oestrogen. Conversely oestrogen can exert inhibitory effects in the POA, reducing excitation of the neurones in this site.

Oestrogen treatment also induces changes in the intracellular appearance of the neurones in the latero-ventral portion of the VMN (a site of oestrogen receptors), with increases in stacked rough endoplasmic reticulum and in dense-core vesicles in the Golgi, indicating an increase in protein synthesis. In particular, oestrogen increases the production of preproenkephalin and a 70 kDa protein, the latter (designated E170) being a member of the heat-shock protein 70 family which have a role in intracellular processing and secretion. E170 may act to facilitate the processing, axonal transport, and secretion of a number of neuroactive substances including met-enkephalin, processed from preproenkephalin, in the VMN neurones, which project to the MCG. The met-enkephalin released at this site stimulates lordosis, perhaps by disinhibiting a system that is normally under an inhibitory (GABAergic perhaps) control (Mobbs *et al.* 1989). It is clear that the increase in protein synthesis in the VMN and the transport of the proteins to the MCG are essential for inducing receptivity, as the effects of both oestrogen and progesterone can be prevented by protein-synthesis inhibitors and colchicine, which blocks axonal transport.

Thus the VMN appears to be the most important forebrain centre of control for stimulation of lordosis. It seems to exert a tonic effect which is constantly under inhibitory control from other forebrain centres. Lesion studies show that these centres include the POA, septum, and olfactory bulbs. A variety of neurotransmitters can alter neuronal activity in the VMN and POA, and their effect is related directly to their effect on lordosis. Thus acetylcholine, oxytocin, and gonadotrophin-releasing hormone (GnRH), which all stimulate lordosis, all increase neuronal firing in the VMN.

Figure 1.3 depicts the neuronal pathways linking the hypothalamic and midbrain areas involved in female sexual control. The cell bodies in the VMN project to the MCG and the reticular field lateral to the MCG via a lateral hypothalamic pathway. Neurones in the POA also pass via a medial pathway to the MCG, with GnRH as the transmitter. Although the POA normally exerts an inhibitory effect on behaviour, GnRH is stimulatory.

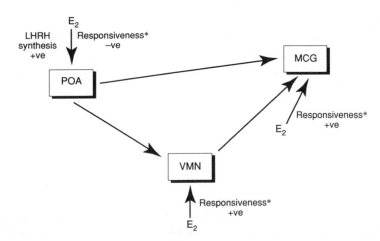

Fig. 1.3 Female neuronal circuit controlling sexual activity. Sites of neurotransmitter activity shown as VMN, ventromedial nucleus; POA, preoptic area; MCG, midbrain central grey. The asterisks show where oestrogen (E_2) increases (+ ve) or decreases (− ve) the resting discharge rate of silent or slowly firing neurones.

Under the influence of oestrogen the electrical discharge rate of the POA neurones are reduced (thus attenuating the normal inhibitory effect of the POA) and at the same time oestrogen enhances GnRH synthesis. These various hypothalamic systems stimulate the neurones in the MCG and in the reticular field surrounding it which have already been made more responsive by a direct action of oestrogen. The neurones from the MCG and its surrounding areas descend to the ventral medial medullary reticular formation. At this site, they meet ascending reticulo-spinal neurones arriving via the antero-lateral column of the spinal cord from dorsal roots L1, L2, L5, and S1. The reticulospinal neurones together with the lateral vestibular spinal tract control the deep back muscles important for lordosis; they integrate postural adaptation across segmental levels of the cord to induce the vertebral dorsiflexion of lordosis. Thus in the receptive female, lordosis occurs after stimulation of the pressure receptors on the flanks (L1 and L2) and rump (L5 and S1) which affect the deep back muscles via the reticulo-spinal neurones which have been sensitized or stimulated by the neurones descending from the MCG, at the level of the medullary reticular formation (see Fig. 1.4).

NEUROTRANSMITTERS AS PHARMACOLOGICAL TARGETS FOR THE CONTROL OF SEXUAL BEHAVIOUR

This review has so far given a brief précis of our understanding of the control of male and female sexual activity and some of the ways it can be quantified so that the significance of any behavioural alteration after pharmacological manipulation can be assessed.

There are two possible targets for pharmacological control of sexual behaviour—one involves mimicking or antagonizing the action of steroid hormones with agents acting on steroid receptors; the other involves mimicking or manipulating the activity of endogenous neurotransmitters which mediate the effects of the steroids and induce the relevant changes in response to information from both the internal and external environments. Thus it is important to know what role the neurotransmitters play in the circuitry controlling sexual behaviour, including their sites of action and the receptor subtypes involved. There is a vast amount of literature on this subject, which can be separated into (a) the correlation of changes in the endogenous transmitter activity with changes in sexual activity, and (b) the effect on sexual activity of manipulating neurotransmitter activity. In reality, very little work has been done on subgroup (a) and so this review concentrates on the effect of drugs which alter the neurotransmitter activity or the effect of administration of the neurotransmitters themselves on sexual behaviour, with endogenous neurotransmitter changes mentioned when known.

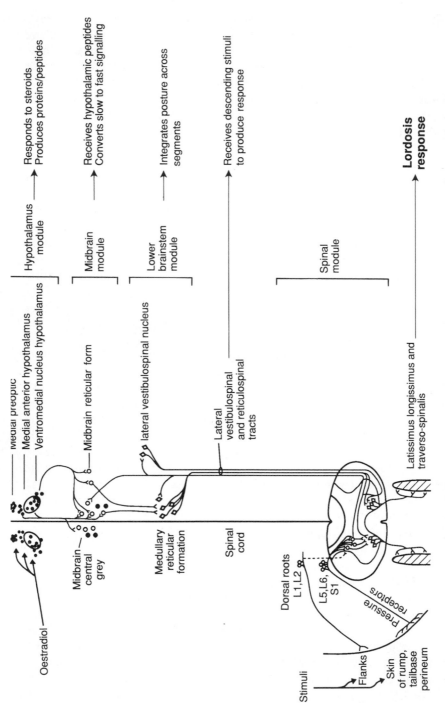

Fig. 1.4 Summary diagram of the neuronal circuit for activating lordosis behaviour (adapted from Pfaff 1980).

The problem with some of the older literature is that pharmacologists have not understood what comprises sexual activity and have measured less meaningful behavioural components such as, for example, male to male mounting. Similarly, behaviourists have not always realized that all pharmacological agents act on more than one receptor and a variety of drugs acting on a common receptor type must be tested to control for each others' 'side-effects' (for example, pirenperone was considered to act selectively on $5\text{-}HT_2$ receptors, but may actually exert its effect on male behaviour via α_1-adrenergic receptors (Mendelson and Gorzalka 1984*a*; Foreman *et al.* 1989)).

There are more difficult and basic problems of interpretation and understanding of the results. For instance two or more systems with a common neurotransmitter may have opposing effects on sexual behaviour, and so the effect of a given agent will depend on its access to one or other of the systems, which in turn will be controlled by its site of administration and/or its pharmacodynamic properties. Thus αMSH, 5-HT, and naloxone have different effects depending on whether they are injected into the third ventricle or lateral ventricle (see Sirinathsinghji and Herbert 1981; Thody *et al.* 1981; Wilson and Hunter 1985*a*; Raible and Gorzalka 1986). The physiological state of the animal may influence which of the two opposing systems has a predominant effect. For example, the opioid systems in the forebrain and spinal cord appear to have differential importance as inhibitory controls over female receptivity—in the lactating rat, the forebrain system exerts the major effect, since intracerebral but not intrathecal naloxone stimulates behaviour. Conversely in the steroid-primed-ovariectomized rat it is the spinal cord system that predominates as only intrathecal naloxone is effective (Forsberg *et al.* 1987*a*). Dopaminergic agents have stimulatory or inhibitory effects at the same dose depending on whether the recipient animal is in a receptive or non-receptive state (Grierson *et al.* 1988). Although in these experiments the two groups had the same steroid milieu, it is possible that the former group was more sensitive to oestrogen. Gonadal steroids alter neurotransmitter receptor density and endogenous neurotransmitter synthesis, release, and uptake and so may well alter the effect of exogenous agents that mimic or manipulate endogenous neurotransmitter activity.

THE EFFECT OF NEUROTRANSMITTERS ON MALE SEXUAL BEHAVIOUR

(For further references see Bitran and Hull 1987.)

Non-peptide neurotransmitters

Dopamine

Dopamine (DA) appears to be involved in all three components of male sexual behaviour, that is, arousal, copulatory activity, and penile reflexes.

Arousal DA is an important neurotransmitter in the midbrain system controlling emotionally motivated behaviour and general aspects of behaviour and general aspects of arousal. The A9 and A10 DA cell body groups in the substantia nigra and ventral tegmentum pass to the ventral striatum and nucleus accumbens respectively, and these tracts are thought to be the centre of the motivational process in sexual activity. Reduction of DA activity by lesions (using 6-hydroxydopamine, 6OHDA) or DA antagonists (both selective D_2 and mixed D_1/D_2 antagonists) in these areas reduce arousal without affecting copulatory activity as assessed by increased ML, IL, PEI, post-ejaculatory vocalization, and time taken to gain access to females in both first- and second-order schedules. DA agonists have the opposite effect. (McIntosh and Barfield 1984b; Brackett *et al.* 1986; Agmo and Fernandez 1989; Cagiano *et al.* 1989; Pfaus and Phillips 1989; Agmo and Picker 1990; Everitt 1990; Hull *et al.* 1990.)

It has been suggested that the stimulatory effect of DA on copulatory activity (see below) is an indirect effect and due to its stimulation of arousal. As mentioned previously (p. 5), testosterone acts on the POA to send impulses to the midbrain to stimulate the reward centres sited there. This is mediated via the A9 and A10 cell body groups projecting into the striatum and brainstem and thence to the spinal cord to translate arousal (desire) into movement (sexual activity) (Brackett *et al.* 1986; Agmo and Fernandez 1989). Recent measurements of endogenous DA support this hypothesis as copulatory activity enhances DA release in the nucleus accumbens which lasts until ejaculation and then falls during the PEI to rise again at the beginning of the next cycle of sexual activity (Ahlenius *et al.* 1987; Mas *et al.* 1990; Pfaus *et al.* 1990; Pleim *et al.* 1990). Testosterone appears to be important in maintaining DA activity in the nucleus accumbens as levels of DA and DOPAC (dihydroxyphenylacetic acid chief metabolite of DA) fall after castration and rise with testosterone replacement (Alderson and Baum 1981; Mitchell and Stewart 1989). Both D_2 and D_1 receptors may be involved in the arousal effects of DA as both selective D_2 and D_2/D_1 agents are effective and D_1 sites are involved in reward stimulation (Nakajima and McKenzie 1986).

Copulatory activity Taking the parameters of mount and intromission frequencies (MF and IF) and EL as measures of copulatory activity, most reports in the literature indicate that DA has a stimulatory effect which is exerted via D_2 receptors. This has been shown extensively in rodents, and also in man by administration of a variety of DA agonists followed by D_2 antagonists which reverse their effects. A D_1 agonist (SKF82526) has no effect on male sexual behaviour, although a D_1 antagonist (Sch23390) reduces the ejaculatory threshold. The ratio of D_2 to D_1 activity may be important in the control of several aspects of sexual activity, in particular an increase in $D_2:D_1$ may reduce ejaculatory latency, but at the same time it appears to impair penile reflexes (Hull *et al.* 1989). Examples of the DA agonists are DOPA (Da Prada *et al.* 1973; Gray *et al.* 1974; Tagliamonte *et al.* 1974; Malmnas 1976), apomorphine (Ahlenius and Larsson 1984*a*; Dallo *et al.* 1986; Hull *et al.* 1986, 1989; Pehek *et al.* 1988), lisuride (Ahlenius *et al.* 1980*a*; Baggio and Ferrari 1983; Hlinak *et al.* 1983; Ahlenius and Larsson 1984*b*), bromocryptine (Ahlenius *et al.* 1982; Dallo *et al.* 1986), RDS 127 (Clark *et al.* 1982, 1983; Clark and Smith 1986), quinelorane, LY163502 (Foreman and Hall 1987). Antagonists that have been used to reverse the effect of the agonists include pimozide (Malmnas 1973; Pfaus and Phillips 1989; Agmo and Picker 1990), haloperidol (Tagliamonte *et al.* 1974; Agmo and Fernandez 1989; Pfaus and Phillips 1989), metoclopramide, sulpiride, and clozapine (Pfaus and Phillips 1989), spiperidone and cisflupenthixol (Pehek *et al.* 1988; Agmo and Fernandez 1989; Agmo and Picker 1990; Hull *et al.* 1990; Warner *et al.* 1991). Some of these antagonists reduced copulatory activity when given alone, but this may have been due to motor disturbances (Baum and Starr 1980; Ahlenius and Larsson 1990).

The only site of action identified so far for the stimulatory effect of DA on copulatory activity is the POA (Hull *et al.* 1986, 1989; Bitran *et al.* 1988*a*; Warner *et al.* 1991). Supporting the concept that DA may mediate the action of testosterone at this site, DA turnover in the POA falls after castration and is raised by administration of testosterone (Gunnett *et al.* 1986). Another site of action may be the substantia nigra (A9 cell body group which project to the neostriatum) since lesions in this area reduce mount and ejaculatory frequency (Brackett *et al.* 1986).

Recently the DA agonist apomorphine, given either systemically or into the POA, was shown to restore mounting and intromission activity even in the absence of testosterone in long-term castrates in which this behaviour had been virtually eliminated (Scaletta and Hull 1990). This emphasizes the important role of the dopaminergic systems in the control of male copulatory activity.

Penile reflexes   DA agonists such as apomorphine, RSD 127, quinperole, R(+)-3-(3-hydroxyphenyl)-N-propylpiperidine HCL (R-(+)PPP) and lisuride have a dual effect on penile erection and a solely stimulatory effect on emission; their effects are reversed by DA antagonists. The stimulatory effect on erection requires the presence of testosterone (Baggio and Ferrari 1983; Berendsen and Gower 1986; Clark and Smith 1986) and is probably exerted within the forebrain on postsynaptic DA receptors (Pehek *et al.* 1988). BH920 (a presynaptic DA agent) also stimulates erection but this may be due to an action on α_2-adrenergic receptors (Ferrari *et al.* 1985) since S(−)-3-(3-hydroxyphenyl)-N-propylpiperidine HCL (S-(−)PPP), another autoreceptor agonist, is ineffective (Gower *et al.* 1986). The DA agonists can also exert an inhibitory effect on erection (in the case of apomorphine at a higher concentration), but at the same time still stimulating emission. This may be a direct effect at the penile level as it can occur in spinally transected rats (Stefanick *et al.* 1982; Bitran *et al.* 1989).

Returning to the stimulation of penile erection, the site of action may be the paraventricular nucleus, since injections of dopaminergic agonists induced the yawning–penile-erection syndrome specifically in this area (Melis *et al.* 1987). It has been suggested that DA exerts this effect by inhibiting an opioid system (Berendson and Gower 1986), or by stimulating the release of ACTH and αMSH which are known to cause the yawning-penile-erection syndrome in several species (Holmgren *et al.* 1985) or by inhibiting the release of noradrenaline in the corpora cavernosa (see Foreman and Wernicke 1990).

Noradrenaline

The forebrain is innervated by a noradrenergic system originating in the locus coeruleus. Based on results obtained after administration of pharmacological agents or lesions of the noradrenergic system, it appears that noradrenaline (NA) acting on α_1-adrenergic receptors stimulates arousal (Clark 1980; Clark *et al.* 1984, 1985*a*). NA also inhibits penile reflexes and although it is clear that this is a peripheral effect, it is not clear whether this is exerted via α_1 or α_2 receptors (Stefanick *et al.* 1983). Any effect on copulatory behaviour is probably indirect and a result of the effects on arousal or reflexes.

These conclusions are based on the fact that lesions of the locus coeruleus, inhibition of NA synthesis, and inhibition of NA release (using α_2 agonists, which are thought to act presynaptically, inhibiting the release of endogenous NA) all increase ML, IL, and PEI. On the other hand, NA agonists and agents that enhance release of endogenous NA (using, for example, the α_2 antagonist, yohimbine) have the reverse effect (Hansen and Ross 1983; Segal *et al.* 1983; McIntosh and Barfield 1984*c*; Clark *et al.* 1985*a*, 1985*b*; Smith and Davidson 1990; Clark 1991). Yohimbine is particularly effective in stimulating arousal and this may be because the noradrenergic cell bodies in the locus coeruleus are normally under tonic α_2-adrenergic inhibition (Quintin *et al.* 1986). Yohimbine has an inverted U-shaped dose response curve presumably because it acts on other sites in higher concentrations (Sala *et al.* 1990). Unusually, it has a stimulatory effect in rats in the absence of testosterone and it is also still effective after penile anaesthesia of sexually naïve rats, indicating that its action is directed on arousal and not the ascending stimuli from the genitalia (Clark *et al.* 1984, 1985*b*).

The effect of β-adrenergic agents on male behaviour has only recently been investigated and the results are inconclusive. Clenbuterol (a β_2 agonist) is inhibitory in active rats, but in sluggish rats both a single injection and chronic treatment increases the number of rats ejaculating and speeds up activity with a reduction in ML, EL, and PEI (Benelli *et al.* 1990). On the other hand, the selective β_2 antagonists artenolol and labetalol had no effect. Propranolol (a non-selective β antagonist) is inhibitory (Smith *et al.* 1990) but this may be due to an action on 5-HT_{1A} receptors and/or a membrane-stabilizing effect.

5-Hydroxytryptamine

The serotonergic tracts innervating the forebrain originate in the medial and dorsal raphe. The major target for the cell bodies in the dorsal raphe is the striatum, while those in the medial raphe project to nucleus accumbens, hippocampus, and cortex. Both systems innervate the hypothalamus and there may also be 5-HT pericarya within the hypothalamus in the dorso-medial nucleus. The multiple effects of 5-HT on physiological and behavioural parameters are due to the existence of multiple receptors, that is 5-HT_{1A}, 5-HT_{1B}, 5-HT_{1C}, 5-HT_{1D}, 5-HT_2, 5-HT_3, and 5-HT_4. 5-HT_{1D} and 5-HT_4 receptors have not been detected in the CNS as yet and sub-types 1C and 2 are thought to be closely related (Schmidt and Peroutka 1989).

5-HT has an inhibitory effect on most aspects of male sexual activity, particularly copulatory behaviour. The action is mediated via 5-HT_2 receptors and the stimulatory actions seen after agents acting on other receptors (e.g. 5-HT_{1A}) is probably due to inhibition of the release of endogenous 5-HT. 5-HT also exerts an effect on penile reflexes via several classes of 5-HT_1 receptors, and this action may be closely interrelated with the dopaminergic control of penile reflexes.

All treatments which reduce endogenous 5-HT activity including lesioning of 5-HT neuronal tracts with 5,7-dihydroxytryptamine (5,7-DHT), inhibition of 5-HT synthesis using *para*-chlorophenylalanine (PCPA), or administration of selective 5-HT_2 antagonists stimulate sexual activity. This effect can only be demonstrated significantly in rats that are not fully active, that is sluggish rats, non-copulators, or castrated rats soon after the operation, but not long-term castrates (indicating that some background testosterone is required) (see Sachs and Meisel 1988 and Wilson and Hunter 1985*a*, for early references; McIntosh and Barfield 1984*a*; Rodriguez *et al.* 1984; Mendenez-Abraham *et al.* 1988; Foreman *et al.* 1989). The effect of PCPA can be reversed by systemic 5-hydroxytryptophan (5-HTP; the precursor to 5-HT) treatment which itself, in the presence of a decarboxylase inhibitor and an uptake inhibitor, can inhibit copulatory activity (Ahlenius and Larsson 1985*a*, 1991). Quipazine, a non-selective agonist and 1-(2,5-dimethoxy-4-iodophenyl)-2-aminopropane (DOI), a selective 5-HT_2 agonist, also inhibit behaviour and the effect of these agents can also be reversed by antagonists acting on 5-HT_2 receptors (Ahlenius *et al.* 1980*b*; Mendelson and Gorzalka 1984*a*; Foreman *et al.* 1989; Watson and Gorzalka 1990). Central administration of 5-HT itself inhibits sexual activity when injected into the POA and nucleus accumbens (Hillegaart *et al.* 1989; Verma *et al.* 1989) and stimulates sexual behaviour when injected into the dorsal and medial raphe, where it probably exerts an effect on autoreceptors on the

5-HT cell bodies and so inhibits endogenous 5-HT release (Hillegaart *et al.* 1989). The 5-HT$_{1A}$ agonist, 8-OHDPAT, acts similarly to 5-HT in the raphe area but is also stimulatory in the nucleus accumbens; perhaps it is acting on autoreceptors at both sites (Hillegaart *et al.* 1991). The 5-HT tract originating in the median raphe and terminating in the nucleus accumbens may have some physiological importance, since 5-HT turnover is increased in the nucleus accumbens at times of sexual activity (Ahlenius *et al.* 1987). The evidence seems clear that 5-HT has an inhibitory effect via 5-HT$_2$ receptors and perhaps the site of this action is in the POA, since 5-HT concentrations in this area are raised at times of sexual refractoriness (Hoffman *et al.* 1987). No changes, however, are seen in 5-HT and other indole compounds in the cerebral spinal fluid associated with the refractory period (Qureshi *et al.* 1989).

More recent reports show that 5-HT$_{1B}$ agonists, that is RU 24969, MCPP (1-(m-chlorophenyl)piperazine HCl) and TFMPP (m-trifluoromethylphenylpiperazine HCl) are also inhibitory and this is not due to any motor impairment (Fernandez-Guasti *et al.* 1989). However, selective 5-HT$_{1A}$ agonists, including 8-OHDPAT, isaperone, buspirone, indorenate, and 5-methoxy-N,N-dimethyltryptamine all stimulate male sexual behaviour and their effects (with the exception of indorenate) can be prevented by 5-HT$_{1A}$ antagonists such as pindolol. Whether the 5-HT$_{1A}$ agonists are acting on presynaptic neurones, preventing release of endogenous 5-HT which normally exerts an inhibitory effect, or whether they act on postsynaptic 5-HT$_{1A}$ receptors, opposing the 5-HT$_2$ effect, is not known (Ahlenius and Larsson 1989, 1991; Ahlenius *et al.* 1989*b*; Fernandez-Guasti *et al.* 1989, 1990*a*; Lee *et al.* 1990; Mathes *et al.* 1990).

5-HT has a complex effect on penile reflexes—acting on 5-HT$_{1A}$ receptors, it is inhibitory, as indicated by the effects of intrathecal administration of 8-OHDPAT and busperone. It is also inhibitory via 5-HT$_{1D}$ receptors and since this can be seen in pithed rats, this must be a peripheral effect (Finberg and Vardi 1990). On the other hand, acting on 5-HT$_{1C}$ receptors it is stimulatory, and this effect can be antagonized by 5-HT$_{1A}$ and 5-HT$_2$ agonists (Berendsen *et al.* 1990). It is thought that the 5-HT$_{1C}$ system may mediate the stimulatory effects of a dopaminergic system on penile reflexes, as non-selective 5-HT antagonists can inhibit the effect of dopaminergic agonists as do selective 5-HT$_2$ agonists (Gower *et al.* 1986; Berendsen and Broekkamp 1987).

Acetylcholine

A cholinergic system acting via muscarinic receptors appears to have a dual effect on male sexual activity. Firstly it reduces the threshold to ejaculation, since muscarinic agonists such as carbachol and oxytremorine injected into the lateral ventricle, POA, or substantia nigra reduce the number of intromissions to reach ejaculation, while muscarinic antagonists such as scopolamine and atropine reduce the percentage of rats ejaculating. At the same time, stimulation of a muscarinic system reduces arousal as the ML and IL are prolonged and sometimes copulation is not initiated. This effect is more marked after administration into the lateral ventricle than POA, indicating that the latter may be the site of stimulation of copulatory behaviour while another site adjacent to the ventricles controls arousal (Agmo 1976; Ahlenius and Larsson 1985*b*; Bitran and Hull 1987; Hull *et al*. 1988*a*, *b*; Winn 1991).

GABA

Based on the effect of drugs which raise GABA activity in the POA or lumbo-sacral region, GABA seems to have an inhibitory effect on intro-mission patterns of male sexual behaviour. This is independent of its other inhibitory effects on motor activity and is not due to any disturbance in the motor patterns underlying pelvic thrusting. Its effect is probably exerted via both GABA-A and -B receptors (Agmo and Paredes 1985; Fernandez-Guasti *et al*. 1986*a*, *b*; Agmo and Contreras 1990) although its effect on penile reflexes may only be exerted by GABA-B receptors (Leipheimer and Sachs 1988; Bitran *et al*. 1988*b*).

GABA concentrations rise in the cerebral spinal fluid during the PEI and the GABA-A antagonist, bicuculline, infused into the POA reduces the PEI and the ultrasonic vocalization (22 kHZ) that is normally emitted over this period. It is possible that GABA is particularly involved in the control of the PEI (Fernandez-Guasti *et al*. 1985*c*, 1986*a*, *b*, *c*; Qureshi and Södersten 1986).

Benzodiazepine agonists (diazepam and chlordiazepoxide) and the inverse agonist FG7142 reduce male sexual activity, which is distinct from their effects on motor activity. Benzodiazepine antagonists reverse the effect of the benzodiazepines but have no effect on behaviour themselves. Bicuculline and picrotoxin do not reverse the action of the benzodiazepines indicating that GABA is not involved in their behavioural effects (Fernandez-Guasti *et al*. 1990*b*; Agmo and Fernandez 1991).

Peptide neurotransmitters

Opioids

The effect of opiate drugs and endogenous opioid peptides on sexual behaviour has been studied extensively, due to the marked effects seen after chronic intake of narcotics and the interest in remedial therapy during withdrawal. In humans, heroin and morphine suppress all aspects of sexual behaviour and this continues over the withdrawal period (see Pfaus and Gorzalka 1987).

There are three main endogenous opioid transmitters within the CNS: β-endorphin, met-enkephalin, and dynorphin, which are roughly selective for μ, δ, and $\varkappa$ receptors, respectively. Most experiments in rats have invest-igated the action of morphine and β-endorphin (both mainly μ-agonists) and the non-selective opiate antagonists, naloxone and naltrexone. Even limit-ing investigations to these agents has produced puzzling and conflicting results.

The results so far indicate that an endogenous opioid system acting in the mesencephalic area, perhaps in the ventral tegmentum area, stimulates recognition and appreciation of a reward stimulus, in this case, a female. At the same time, however, the opioid system disturbs the ability of the animal to match the information that induces sexual arousal with the correct output, that is the copulatory or consummatory behaviour, and this site of transition is probably within the POA. Thus although many reports indicate that the opiates and endogenous opioid peptides (EOP) act in the POA to inhibit copulatory behaviour, it is rather the initiation of consummatory activity that is inhibited. Perhaps the reward stimuli provided by the opiates substitutes for the other reward stimulus of copulatory activity. In the physiological state, therefore, the EOP system in the ventral tegmentum area is involved in recognition of the female and stimulates arousal, this then modulates activity in the POA, where an opioid system must be 'switched off' in order to allow expression of copulatory or consummatory behaviour. Testosterone, which is essential for both motivation and copu-latory activity, presumably acts at the amygdala, ventral tegmentum area, and ventral striatum to enhance the opioid and also dopaminergic reward system and at the same time acts at the POA to reduce opioid activity. The evidence for all this is provided in numerous reports detailed in the next section.

Copulatory behaviour When morphine and β-endorphin are applied systematically, into the lateral ventricle or into the POA, they exert an inhibitory effect on copulatory behaviour while the non-specific antagonists naloxone and naltrexone reverse the opiate effects and/or have a stimu-latory action on most parameters of sexual behaviour when given by them-selves (Meyerson 1981; Hughes *et al.* 1987*a*; Miller and Baum 1987; for other early references see Pfaus and Gorzalka 1987). The fact that the two opiate antagonists and also a δ-receptor antagonist have stimulatory effects indicates that sexual behaviour is under a tonic opioid inhibition and that possibly met-enkephalin is the primary mediator (Myers and Baum 1978, 1980; Pfaus and Gorzalka 1987). Some reports show that naloxone has no effect in sexually active rats, but it is effective in naïve, sluggish, and sexually exhausted rats (Gessa *et al.* 1979; McIntosh *et al.* 1980; Pfaus and Gorzalka 1987). Perhaps in these latter groups of animals endogenous opioid levels are raised. Levels of β-endorphin are higher over periods of sexual quiescence in seasonal breeders (hamsters) and in socially subordinate primates (talapoin monkeys) in which sexual behaviour is reduced (Herbert 1989).

However, as mentioned above, this opioid inhibition is not due to suppression of copulatory activity itself, but rather the initiation of copulatory behaviour since if β-endorphin is placed in the POA after the first intromission, it has no effect, even if the next intromission is delayed by one hour (by removal of the female), as long as it is the same female. If a different female is placed with the male after the first intromission the inhibitory effect of β-endorphin reappears (Stavy and Herbert 1989; Herbert and McGregor 1990).

Penile reflexes Intrathecal administration of morphine also has a naloxone-reversible suppressant effect on copulatory behaviour and morphine blocks spontaneous and dopamine-induced penile erections, while naloxone potentiates dopamine agonists. So there may be a separate inhibitory opioid system interacting with a dopaminergic control of penile erections within the spinal cord (Ferrari and Baggio 1982; Berendsen and Gower 1986).

Arousal In circumstances where the opiates appear to prevent copulatory activity, no inhibitory effect on arousal is ever observed, and as indicated above they may, in fact, be involved in enhancing appreciation of a reward stimuli, such as a receptive female. This has been shown by the normal investigatory behaviour of males treated with β-endorphin in conditioned place preference for a receptive female (Herbert 1989). When morphine and dynorphin are injected into the ventral tegmentum area they increase arousal and copulatory behaviour. The μ agonist may act via the dopaminergic mesolimbic system as morphine increases DA turnover in the nucleus accumbens (Agmo and Paredes 1988; Clark *et al.* 1988; Band and Hull 1990; Mitchell and Stewart 1990). Naloxone, on the other hand, has an inhibitory effect on arousal behaviour in castrated and sexually exhausted rats (Miller and Baum 1987) and in normal rats inhibits conditioned place preference associated with a receptive female (Baum 1989; Agmo and Berenfeld 1990; Hughes *et al.* 1990; Mehrara and Baum 1990). It is suggested that the endogenous opiate peptides are involved in appreciation of reward (sex, food, and so on) and naloxone attenuates the recognition of the incentive and motivational cues and so, in fact, can increase ML and PEI and has even been shown to inhibit copulatory activity (at low dose and injected into the third ventricle) (Myers and Baum 1979; Sirinathsinghji and Herbert 1981; Agmo *et al.* 1989*a*). The lengthening of the PEI by naloxone indicates that it reduces the reward engendered by continuing mating (Sachs *et al.* 1981; Agmo and Paredes 1988; Baum 1989).

In summary, the endogenous opioids appear to enhance arousal at the level of the mesencephalon and inhibit initiation of copulatory behaviour at the POA and also suppress penile reflexes within a spinal cord circuitry. β-endorphin has been utilized in most of the experiments and the involvement of the enkephalins, which also inhibit male copulatory activity, and dynorphin has yet to be elucidated (Pfaus and Gorzalka 1987). There are close interactions between testosterone and EOP and DA and EOP which also needs further investigation.

Other POMC peptides

β-endorphin, ACTH, and α-melanotrophin (α-melanocyte-stimulating hormone, αMSH) are all products of a common precursor, pro-opiomelano-corticotrophin (POMC) which in turn is stimulated by the hypothalamic peptide corticotrophin-releasing factor (CRF) present in neurones in the paraventricular nucleus.

Central, but not peripheral, injections of ACTH and αMSH induce penile erections in rats and rabbits (Bertolini *et al.* 1975) and αMSH injected into the POA of rats also enhances sexual arousal as indicated by a reduction in the ML and EL and an increase in number of responses under a second-order schedule of sexual reinforcement and number of responses required to earn a receptive female (Hughes *et al.* 1988, 1990).

It has been suggested that ACTH and αMSH act as endogenous antagonists to the opioids, since morphine reverses the effects of both hormones on penile reflexes and αMSH antagonizes the action of β-endorphin in the POA (Bertolini and Gessa 1981; Hughes *et al.* 1988).

Prolactin

In man and rats hyperprolactinaemia depresses all aspects of sexual behaviour, that is arousal, copulatory activity, and penile reflexes, the latter being inhibited at a supraspinal level since transection of the spinal cord allows reflexes to return to normal. The effect is not due to reduction of steroid secretion either by the gonads or adrenals since testosterone levels do not alter in hyperprolactinaemia and exogenous prolactin still has an inhibitory effect in castrated, steroid-treated animals (Bailey and Herbert 1982; Doherty *et al.* 1981, 1982, 1985, 1986; Shrenker and Bartke 1985).

Mild oestrogen-induced hyperprolactinaemia in male rats causes a reduction in DA turnover in the POA (Lookingland and Moore 1984) and since the dopaminergic system at this site is thought to stimulate behaviour, this may be the cause of the suppression of behaviour by prolactin. In extreme hyperprolactinaemia (a thousand-fold higher than in the previous report), DA turnover in the POA was enhanced, but this may induce desensitization of the DA receptors and so again result in reduced DA activity (Kalra *et al.* 1983). More recently, however, Doherty *et al.* (1989) have shown that hyperprolactinaemia does not alter motor activity, nor does it alter the response to DA agonists, so it seems unlikely that the DA system is involved in suppression of sexual behaviour by prolactin. Other possibilities are that prolactin enhances GABA and/or opioid systems, since prolactin increases GABA concentrations in the striatum and can be antagonized by naloxone (Drago and Scapagnini 1983).

In contrast to chronic high levels of prolactin, acute administration of prolactin or short-term hyperprolactinaemia (five days) stimulates copulatory activity and reduces ML and IL. This may be due to an acute stimulation of endogenous DA activity (Drago *et al.* 1981; Drago and Scapagnini 1983).

Oxytocin

Oxytocin stimulates male copulatory activity and grooming behaviour. The former is seen after systemic and intraventricular administration, especially in sluggish (aged) males, but it does not stimulate non-copulators (Arletti *et al.* 1985, 1990). The effect on grooming is probably mediated via a stimulatory dopaminergic system (Drago *et al.* 1986). Oxytocin concentration rises in the cerebro-spinal fluid after ejaculation, indicating that it may be physiologically important (Hughes *et al.* 1987*b*).

Arg-vasopressin

Arg-vasopressin (AVP) has been shown to inhibit copulation in rabbits, but has no effect in rats whether given systemically or intraventricularly (Kihlstrom and Agmo 1974; Bohus 1977). However, a vasopressin agonist (desglycinamide lys-VP) delays the decline in behaviour normally noted after castration (Bohus 1977). AVP-containing neurones in the bed nucleus stria terminalis and medial amygdala projecting to the lateral habenular nucleus and lateral septum are sensitive to steroids. AVP content in these tracts falls after castration and is reinstated with testosterone replacement. The time course of the changes is slow, in parallel with the slow changes in sexual activity. In Brattleboro rats, which do not possess vasopressin, sexual behaviour disappears almost immediately after castration. Based on these findings De Vries (1990) suggests that AVP may have a physiological role in delaying the post-castration decrease in intromission and ejaculatory patterns.

Angiotensin II

Angiotensin II (AII) inhibits male sexual activity and when given intraventricularly it increases ML, IF, and PEI. This is not associated with its effect on drinking (Clark 1989).

Gonadotrophin-releasing hormone

Gonadotrophin-releasing hormone (GnRH) is thought to have an important physiological role in the stimulation of female sexual behaviour. In males, it is also stimulatory, but its physiological significance is not known and although it is known to act centrally, the site within the CNS is not unknown (Dorsa *et al.* 1985). Its stimulatory effect can be seen in intact animals that are not fully active—it has no effect in highly vigorous rats nor in castrated rats even if they are maintained on a low level of testosterone (Moss *et al.* 1975; Myers and Baum 1990).

Substance P

Substance P stimulates male behaviour, reducing ML and EL in intact (but not castrated) rats and antiserum to substance P has the opposite effect (Dornan and Malsbury 1984, 1989).

Neuropeptide Y

Neuropeptide Y (NPY) inhibits male sexual behaviour, reducing the percentage of rats copulating and worsening all parameters of sexual behaviour (ML, IL, EL, M and I frequency, and PEI). This is seen after intraventricular injections or administration into the POA. The reduction in sexual activity is noted in rats deprived of food during the behavioural test and so this inhibition is not due to a shift toward increased feeding (another component of the behavioural effects of NPY). NPY has no effect on penile reflexes (Clark *et al.* 1985*c*; Kalra *et al.* 1988; Poggioli *et al.* 1990).

Cholecystokinin-8

Cholecystokinin-8 (CCK-8) has no effect on male sexual behaviour (Dornan and Malsbury 1989). In suitably primed males, CCK-8 injected into the POA can stimulate female behaviour (Bloch *et al.* 1988, 1989).

THE EFFECT OF NEUROTRANSMITTERS ON FEMALE SEXUAL BEHAVIOUR

Non-peptide neurotransmitters

Dopamine

It is suggested that DA enhances proceptive behaviour and arousal in females, but at the same time inhibits receptive behaviour and so any manipulation that reduces endogenous DA activity invariably increases lordotic activity. These manipulations include electrolytic and neurotoxic lesions of DA cell bodies and nerve terminals, inhibition of DA synthesis, and administration of DA antagonists (Ahlenius *et al.* 1972*a*; Caggiula *et al.* 1978; Herndon *et al.* 1978; Sirinathsinghji *et al.* 1986). In the physiological situation there is a significant reduction in DA turnover in the arcuate/median eminence (ARC/ME) area associated with increased receptivity (Clark *et al.* 1986; Wilson *et al.* 1991*a*).

The interpretation of the effects of raising dopamine activity has been more difficult. Some reports indicate that DA agonists exert an inhibitory effect via D_2-postsynaptic receptors. It is suggested that the stimulatory effects, usually noted at lower concentrations, are probably due to a pre-synaptic effect inhibiting release of endogenous DA. D_1 receptors are not involved at all (Everitt *et al.* 1975*a*; Everitt and Fuxe 1977; Michanek and Meyerson 1982; Fernandez-Guasti *et al.* 1987; Grierson *et al.* 1988).

Other reports show that DA agonists are mainly stimulatory and in contrast to the above it is suggested that this effect is a postsynaptic one, and any inhibitory effect seen at higher concentrations may be due to induc-tion of stereotypic behaviour which disrupts the directed sexual activity (Hamberger-Bar and Rigter 1975; Foreman and Moss 1979; Foreman and Hall 1987). If DA is a stimulatory agent, it may act at the VMN since direct injection of DA into this area is stimulatory (Foreman and Moss 1979) and pergolide (a DA agonist) can maintain lordosis after lesioning of the VMN (Mathews *et al.* 1983).

Perhaps like some of the other transmitters, DA has opposing effects at different sites, and is inhibitory in the ARC/ME, where DA activity is inversely related to receptivity, and stimulatory in the VMN.

Noradrenaline

It is hypothesized that the ascending noradrenergic system supplies the somatosensory information from the vagina necessary for the initiation of lordosis and that while DA is important for arousal, NA acting at the VMN switches systems, suppressing the DA system (which normally enhances proceptive behaviour), and enhancing a passive immobile receptive be-haviour. This suggestion is based on the fact that lesions of the ventral noradrenergic bundles inhibit lordosis without affecting proceptivity, while DA antagonists have the opposite effect (Caggiula *et al.* 1978; Hansen *et al.* 1980).

Administration of noradrenaline (NA) itself has a stimulatory effect on lordotic activity when injected into the VMN/ARC area (Foreman and Moss 1978*a*; Wilson unpublished results). It is possible that NA mediates the effects of both oestrogen and progesterone in inducing receptivity. NA release in the VMN is enhanced by both oestrogen alone and progesterone in oestrogen-primed animals. The latter effect was shown by *in vivo* dialysis sampling in the VMN, the rise in NA release occurring at the same time as the increase in lordotic activity (Varthy and Etgen 1989). *In vitro* studies have shown that there is an enhanced release of NA from medial basal hypothalamic fragments taken from oestrogen-primed receptive animals compared with untreated and non-receptive primed animals and this was accompanied by a fall in NA content. Measurements of NA turnover in the VMN show it is not greater in receptive animals than in the other groups. The increase in release without apparent change in synthesis will eventually result in depletion of stores and so perhaps provide a mechanism for termin-ating oestrous behaviour (Celis *et al.* 1989; Wilson *et al.* 1991*a*). In addition to mediating steroid effects, it has also been suggested that NA mediates the stimulatory effects of GnRH on lordosis, since the action of this peptide is inhibited by adrenergic antagonists (Mora and Diaz-Veliz 1986; Gonzalez-Mariscal and Beyer 1989). The noradrenergic system may also sensitize the hypothalamus towards the ovarian steroids and so enhance receptivity in this way—α_1-adrenergic activation increases hypothalamic oestrogen-receptor density in rats (Montemayor *et al.* 1990) and progesterone receptor density in guinea-pigs (Nock and Feder 1981, 1984).

There is controversy over the receptor sub-types involved in mediating the effects of NA, mainly because the drugs used to elucidate this problem are not sufficiently selective for particular receptor sub-types or in their mode of action. More recent evidence suggests that the stimulatory effect of NA in the VMN is exerted via α_1-adrenergic receptors, particularly because the specific α_1-antagonist, prazosin, has a marked inhibitory effect on lordosis (Etgen 1990). This is contrary to findings in an earlier report using other pharmacological agents such as phenoxybenzamine and phentolamine (Foreman and Moss 1978*a*).

There is conflict over the role of the β-adrenergic receptor in mediating the action of NA. Some reports suggest that the β-receptors also stimulate behaviour, since isoprenaline (a β-agonist) infused into the VMN stimulates lordosis and propranolol is inhibitory (Foreman and Moss 1978*a*; Fernandez-Guasti *et al.* 1985*b*). Fernandez-Guasti *et al.* (1985*a*) have suggested that concomitant α_1 and β activation is required for full stimulation of cAMP which mediates the effect of NA. However, this is based on the use of propranolol, which has a marked membrane-stabilizing effect which may be responsible for its inhibitory effects. When a pure β-antagonist, metoprolol, was placed in the VMN or POA, it had no effect, while a β-agonist, salbutamol, and a partial agonist, pindolol, were inhibitory. This suggests that β-adrenergic activation inhibits sexual behaviour (Mendelson and Gorzalka 1988; Etgen 1990) and correlates with the functional desensitization of β-receptors which occurs over the period of sexual receptivity after an injection of oestradiol benzoate (Etgen and Petitti 1987). NA itself has been shown to exert an inhibitory effect on lordosis when infused into the POA (Caldwell and Clemens 1986) and so an inhibitory β-adrenergic system may be important at this site. Alternatively, the inhibitory effect may be exerted via α_2-adrenergic receptors. This is suggested by earlier reports showing that systemic clonidine (an α_2-agonist) inhibits sexual behaviour in rats (NB: it is stimulatory in guinea-pigs) and both clonidine and NA in the POA are reversed by yohimbine (α_2-antagonist). However, neither yohimbine nor a more selective α_2-antagonist, idazoxan, have any effect themselves when placed in the POA (Etgen 1990).

Many publications are concerned with the effects of NA in female guinea-pigs and these conclude that both α_1 and α_2 adrenergic agonists are stimulatory and both are needed for full activation. α_1-adrenergic activity mediates the hormone priming process, while α_2-adrenergic activity is necessary for an ongoing lordotic response (Crowley *et al.* 1976; Nock and Feder 1979, 1984; Vincent *et al.* 1987; Vincent and Feder 1988).

In summary, NA has a stimulatory effect on female sexual activity in the VMN, possibly mediated via α_1- and/or β-adrenergic receptors. It is inhibitory in the POA and in the rat this effect may be exerted via β- and/or α_2-adrenergic receptors.

5-Hydroxytryptamine

Early investigations into the role of 5-HT on female sexual behaviour employed a variety of pharmacological agents that were not sufficiently selective toward the 5-HT system, nor was the possibility investigated that dual effects might be elicited by 5-HT agents. Thus up to 1982, most reports concluded that 5-HT was inhibitory to female sexual activity. Inhibitors of 5-HT synthesis (*p*-chlorophenylalanine (PCPA) and *para*-chloramphetamine), neurotoxic agents (5,7-DHT), and two 5-HT antagonists (methysergide and cinanserin) all stimulated sexual behaviour in non-receptive rats illustrating the inhibitory effect of endogenous 5-HT (see Wilson and Hunter 1985*a* for early references). Confirming this, administration of 5-HTP systemically or 5-HT itself into the POA and VMN inhibited behaviour in receptive animals (Ward *et al.* 1975; Foreman and Moss 1978*b*; Sietnieks and Meyerson 1982).

A few of the early reports did not support this conclusion. Chronic administration of PCPA, which induced severe depletion of 5-HT, either had no stimulatory effect (Södersten *et al.* 1976; Eliasson and Meyerson 1977) or even inhibited lordosis when given to receptive animals (Segal and Whalen 1970; Singer 1972; Gorzalka and Whalen 1975; Al Satli and Aron 1981). Conversely, raising endogenous 5-HT activity with uptake inhibitors enhanced receptivity (Hamberger-Bar *et al.* 1978).

Since the conflict was mainly concerned with the results obtained after PCPA administration, a careful analysis was made of the effects of PCPA on lordosis and 5-HT activity. There was no correlation between reduction in endogenous 5-HT levels and stimulation of lordosis seen four hours after a single injection of PCPA, while there was a good correlation between the inhibitory effect of PCPA on lordosis and depletion of endogenous 5-HT seen 24 h after administration of the drug. The inhibitory effect was reversed by 5-HTP which significantly raised the depleted levels of 5-HT, while the stimulatory effect of PCPA was not reversed by 5-HTP (Wilson *et al.* 1982). It is suggested that this stimulation was either due to a transitory reduction in hypothalamic catecholamines or a transitory release of 5-HT from nerve terminals (Ahlenius *et al.* 1972*b*; Wilson *et al.* 1982).

The potential stimulatory effect of 5-HT on sexual behaviour was supported by the inhibitory effects of a wide variety of 5-HT antagonists, many of them not very selective for the 5-HT receptor sub-types, but all having a common antagonist action at 5-HT$_2$ receptors (e.g. cyproheptadine, metitepine, cinanserin, mianserin, metergoline, pizotefin, betanserin, and pirenperone). The early findings on the stimulatory effects of methysergide and cinanserin were still found, although cinanserin had a dual effect and was inhibitory in receptive animals. Conversely, 5-HT agonists could be shown to stimulate behaviour in non-receptive animals and again all had a common effect at $5-HT_2$ receptors (e.g. 5-HTP, MK212, harmine, quipazine, and DOI) (Hunter *et al.* 1985; Wilson and Hunter 1985*b*; Mendelson and Gorzalka 1985*a*, *b*, 1986*a*, *b*; James *et al.* 1989*a*). Thus the more recent reports indicate that 5-HT is stimulatory, acting on $5-HT_2$ receptors.

However, it is clear that 5-HT exerts an inhibitory effect as well—the earlier findings that destruction of 5-HT neurones by 5,7-DHT enhances lordotic activity (Everitt *et al.* 1975*b*; Zemplan *et al.* 1977) have been confirmed more recently after administration of 5,7-DHT into the lateral ventricle and VMN in particular. The destruction of 5-HT nerve terminals and depletion of 5-HT levels in the VMN correlated more significantly than other areas with an increase in lordotic activity suggesting that this is the site of an inhibitory effect of 5-HT (Luine *et al.* 1983; Frankfurt and Azmitia 1984; Frankfurt *et al.* 1985; Moreines *et al.* 1988).

There are numerous reports showing that selective $5-HT_{1A}$ agonists such as 8-OHDPAT and isaperone, and $5-HT_{1B}$ agonists such as Ru 24969, MCPP, TMCPP, and gepirone inhibit female sexual activity and the effect of the $5-HT_{1A}$ agonists can be reversed by $5-HT_1$ antagonists, but not selective $5-HT_2$ or dopamine antagonists (Ahlenius *et al.* 1986; Mendelson and Gorzalka 1986*b*, *c*; Fernandez-Guasti *et al.* 1987). Although 5-HTP is stimulatory in non-receptive animals (Hunter *et al.* 1985) it is inhibitory in receptive rats and this effect can be reversed by $5-HT_1$ but not $5-HT_2$ antagonists (Ahlenius *et al.* 1989*a*). $5-HT_{1A}$ receptors are present on 5-HT cell bodies and dendrites as well as postsynaptically in various areas containing 5-HT nerve terminals. Whether stimulation of type 1A receptors inhibits sexual activity by an autoregulatory effect on presynaptic sites, inhibiting the release of endogenous 5-HT, or whether the inhibitory effect is a postsynaptic one mediating a separate 5-HT control over behaviour, is not known. Recent experiments have shown that administration of 8-OHDPAT directly into the VMN has a marked and immediate inhibitory effect on behaviour (Uphouse *et al.* 1991) and the authors suggest that this is a postsynaptic effect. $5-HT_3$ receptors may also mediate the inhibitory effects of 5-HT, since $5-HT_3$ antagonists (ondansetron, GR38032F; MDL7222; and granisetron, BRL 43694) stimulate receptivity (James *et al.* 1989*a*).

There is a close interrelationship between gonadal steroids and 5-HT. Both oestrogen alone and oestrogen plus progesterone can alter 5-HT turnover in specific areas of the brain (see James *et al.* 1989*b*) and they can also alter the density of $5-HT_1$ and $5-HT_2$ receptors (Biegon *et al.* 1982; Wilson *et al.* unpublished results). Correlating steroid-induced changes in receptivity with 5-HT activity, it seems that 5-HT may be the mediator of the stimulatory effect of progesterone on sexual activity since depletion of endogenous 5-HT prevents lordosis normally induced by oestrogen plus progesterone, but not lordosis induced by oestrogen alone (Wilson *et al.* 1982). In addition, administration of progesterone to oestrogen-primed rats enhances the action of 5-HT agonists on both sexual and myoclonus behaviour, again indicating that progesterone may act to enhance endogenous 5-HT activity (Sietnieks and Meyerson 1982; O'Connor and Feder 1985). The opposite relationship does not exist since 5-HT depletion (using 5,7-DHT) does not alter oestrogen or progesterone receptor density (Luine *et al.* 1987).

A comparison of 5-HT activity in specific hypothalamic nuclei in receptive and non-receptive rats shows that 5-HT turnover is significantly lower in the VMN and significantly higher in the ME of receptive than non-receptive animals (James *et al.* 1989*b*). It is possible that the 5-HT is inhibitory at the VMN, acting on 5-HT_{1A} receptors, and stimulatory at the ME, acting on 5-HT_2 receptors. Supporting evidence for the latter is the finding that 5-HT turnover rises in the ME on the evening of proestrus in intact female rats, at the time of increased receptivity (Vitale *et al.* 1984).

In summary, 5-HT has a dual effect on female sexual behaviour, stimulating activity via 5-HT_2 receptors (one possible site being the ME), and inhibiting activity at the VMN, perhaps via 5-HT_{1A} and/or 5-HT_3 receptors.

Acetylcholine

Both pharmacological experiments and noting changes in cholinergic activity in the forebrain indicate that acetylcholine has a stimulatory effect on lordosis, exerting its effect via M_2 receptors. Selective M_2 agonists (e.g. oxytremorine) but not M_1 agonists (e.g. McN-A343) are stimulatory after administration into the ventricles, the POA, VMN, MCG, and midbrain reticular formation, while mixed M_1 and M_2 antagonists (but not selective M_1 antagonists) have the opposite effect. The stimulatory effects have been noted in both ovariectomized steroid-primed rats and intact rats on the day of proestrus. The action of the cholinergic agents are independent of the adrenals and progesterone (Clemens and Dohanich 1980; Clemens *et al.* 1980, 1981; Dohanich *et al.* 1984, 1991; Richmond and Clemens 1986*a*, *b*; Kaufman *et al.* 1988; Dohanich and Cada 1989; Menard and Dohanich 1989, 1990).

Lesions in the VMN impair the stimulatory effects of muscarinic agonists suggesting either that VMN neurones stimulate a cholinergic system or cholinergic-sensitive neurones are present within the VMN. However, injection of agonists into the VMN or POA, which avoid the ventricles and therefore reduce diffusion, are ineffective. This suggests that while the VMN is important, muscarinic activity must be stimulated at multiple sites

(Dohanich *et al.* 1984; Dohanich and McEwen 1986; Richmond and Clemens 1988). Pfaff has suggested that cholinergic terminals in the VMN stimulate impulses descending to the MCG and oestrogen enhances the action of this system by increasing acetylcholine synthesis at the site of cholinergic cell bodies (in the diagonal band) and terminals (in the VMN) (Luine and McEwen 1983; Pfaff and Schwartz-Giblin 1988). Alternatively, or in addition, acetylcholine may act by sensitizing the hypothalamus to oestrogen, as a muscarinic agonist (bethanecol) increases oestrogen-binding sites (Lauber 1988). Earlier findings indicated that oestrogen increased muscarinic receptors in the VMN, but this has not been confirmed (Rainbow *et al.* 1984; Dohanich *et al.* 1991).

GABA

GABA has an inhibitory effect on female sexual behaviour and this effect is probably exerted at the POA via both GABA-A and -B receptors. The evidence for this is provided by reports showing that high concentrations of muscimol (a GABA-A agonist) and gamma acetylenic GABA (GAG; an inhibitor of GABA degradation) given systemically can inhibit lordosis (Masco *et al.* 1986; Qureshi *et al.* 1988), and that GABA-A (muscimol and THIP i.e. Gaboxadol) and GABA-B (baclofen) agonists are inhibitory in the POA, while ineffective in the VMN (Fernandez-Guasti *et al.* 1986*d*; Agmo *et al.* 1989*b*; McCarthy *et al.* 1990). Oestrogen reduces the number of high-affinity GABA-A receptors (O'Connor *et al.* 1985) and in this way remove an inhibitory influence on receptivity.

GABA concentrations rise in the cerebro-spinal fluid of females after ejaculation by the male and this may be associated with the suppression of female behaviour during the PEI. During this period, female sexual activity can be re-established by the GABA antagonist bicuculline, although in other studies bicuculline was not able to reverse the effect of GABA agonists (Qureshi *et al.* 1988; Agmo *et al.* 1989*b*; McCarthy *et al.* 1990).

Prostaglandins

Prostaglandin E_2 (Pgl E_2) stimulates receptivity in female rats and indomethacin (an inhibitor of Pgl synthesis) is inhibitory (Rodriguez-Sierra and Komisaruk 1977, 1982). However, in guinea-pigs, Pgl E_1 and Pgl $F_2\alpha$ are inhibitory and may act to overcome the stimulatory noradrenergic system. It is suggested that the Pgl may have a physiological role in terminating oestrus in this species (Irving *et al.* 1981).

Peptide neurotransmitters

Opioids

Chronic narcotic opiates inhibit sexual arousal in women. In female rats, systemic administration of morphine reduces both proceptive and receptive behaviour, in doses that do not affect motor activity and the action is reversed by naloxone (Pfaus and Gorzalka 1987).

Experimental findings in female rats indicate that the μ and δ opioids have opposite effects on sexual activity. Pfaff and his co-workers have shown that a pre-requisite for oestrogen-induced lordosis is an increase in protein synthesis in the VMN. One of the proteins produced is prepro-enkephalin, which is converted to proenkephalin and thence met-enkephalin and this is then released at the MCG to disinhibit neurones from an inhibitory control (Mobbs *et al.* 1989; Lauber *et al.* 1990). Some pharmacological evidence supports this, since a selective δ agonist peptide (D-Tyr-Ser-Gly-Phe-Leu-Thr) stimulates lordosis, and the stimulatory effects of β-endorphin and morphiceptin, seen only in high concentrations (in the μg range, intraventricularly), are reduced by a mixed μ- and δ-receptor antagonist (naloxone) and a selective δ antagonist (ICI 154129), but not by a selective μ antagonist (naloxozone) (Wiesner and Moss 1984; Pfaus *et al.* 1986; Pfaus and Gorzalka 1987; Forsberg *et al.* 1987*b*). However, these findings have not been replicated using met-enkephalin itself (even given with an inhibitor of its degradation), which after central administration either into the ventricles or MCG inhibited lordosis (Bednar *et al.* 1987; Södersten *et al.* 1989).

Opposing the possible stimulatory opioid system, there may be an inhibitory system originating in the arcuate nucleus (ARC) and also passing to the MCG with β-endorphin as the transmitter (Kerdehlue *et al.* 1982). While systemic administration of β-endorphin has no effect on female sexual activity in the rat, intraventricular injections in relatively low concentrations (100–200 ng) inhibit female behaviour, and this is reversed by naloxone which itself has a stimulatory effect (Allen *et al.* 1985; Wiesner and Moss 1986*a*, *b*). Similar effects are seen after infusion of β-endorphin and naloxone into the MCG and it is suggested that β-endorphin normally exerts a tonic inhibitory effect on the GnRH system in the MCG. Antibodies raised against β-endorphin reverse the effect of the opioid, while antibodies against met-enkephalin and dynorphin are ineffective (Sirinathsinghji *et al.* 1983; Sirinathsinghji 1983*a*). Intrathecal and intravaginal administration of β-endorphin is also inhibitory and reversible by intrathecal injection of naloxone. This suggests that opioid neurones in the dorsal horn of the spinal cord process sensory information on copulatory stimulation and normally exert an inhibitory effect (Wiesenfeld-Hallin and Södersten 1984).

As mentioned above, in the μg range, β-endorphin can have a stimulatory action and separate reports show that naloxone can be inhibitory (Wiesner and Moss 1984; Forsberg *et al.* 1987*b*; Pfaus and Gorzalka 1987). It seems likely that in normal physiological concentrations the inhibitory effect of β-endorphin is exerted via μ receptors, and only at higher concentrations do non-specific effects on the stimulatory δ-receptors come into play.

Södersten also has suggested that the endogenous opioid peptides have a dual effect on female behaviour, at first facilitating receptivity perhaps by inducing a degree of analgesia to aid intromission into the vagina. After ejaculation, however, the opioid system in the spinal cord exerts an inhibitory effect and is responsible for the depression in female sexual behaviour in parallel with the period of depression in the male, after ejaculation. He further hypothesizes that this effect is not necessarily due to raised levels of endogenous opioids as suggested by others, but rather due to opioids present in the seminal fluid entering the female reproductive tract (Forsberg *et al.* 1990).

Other POMC peptides, including corticotrophin-releasing hormone (CRH) and corticosterone

CRH stimulates secretion of POMC peptides which include β-endorphin, ACTH, and αMSH.

When CRH is administered centrally into the VMN/ARC or the MCG, it inhibits lordosis, and this can be overcome by naloxone and an antibody to β-endorphin but not an antibody to met-enkephalin. Thus it is clear that CRF is acting mainly by stimulating the release of β-endorphin. However, it may also exert an effect via ACTH and/or corticosterone, since both of these hormones inhibit lordosis when injected centrally (Sirinathsinghji *et al.* 1982; Sirinathsinghji 1985; de Catanzaro 1987). Systemic administration of ACTH can, however, stimulate sexual excitement in rabbits, including lordosis, and it has a dual effect in rats, stimulating non-receptive and inhibiting receptive females (Baldwin *et al.* 1974; Sawyer *et al.* 1975; Wilson *et al.* 1979; de Catanzaro *et al.* 1981). No further experiments have been done to explain these dual effects.

αMSH has been investigated in greater depth than the other POMC peptides and appears to have a dual effect too. Its inhibitory action can be seen after systemic injections and is completely dependent on the presence of the adrenals (Thody and Wilson 1983). It is also inhibitory when injected into the lateral ventricles, where it is suggested that it acts to inhibit a normally stimulatory 5-HT_2 system (Raible and Gorzalka 1986; Raible 1988). The stimulatory effect of αMSH can be seen after subcutaneous injections in non-receptive animals and after administration into the third ventricle and VMN, where it is as potent as GnRH (Thody *et al.* 1979, 1981; Thody and Wilson 1983; Gonzalez *et al.* in press). Although αMSH alters DA activity specifically and selectively in the VMN, the latter does not mediate its effect since a DA antagonist does not inhibit αMSH activity. The changes are more probably related to the dopaminergic regulation of αMSH synthesis and release within the CNS (Wilson *et al.* 1991*b*). The stimulatory action of αMSH may, however, be mediated by NA, since a β-adrenergic antagonist can block the stimulatory effects of αMSH, and αMSH can stimulate the release of NA from hypothalamic fragments *in vitro* (Celis *et al.* 1989).

Prolactin

Prolactin can both inhibit and stimulate receptivity in female rats. The stimulatory effect may be a physiological one, since oestrogen can induce neurones in the VMN and a site just lateral to it to produce prolactin. These neurones descend to the MCG and injection of prolactin at this latter site stimulates behaviour (Harlan *et al.* 1983; Shivers *et al.* 1989). The pre-ovulatory prolactin surge may also have a physiological stimulatory role since inhibition of its release reduces lordotic activity at oestrus (Witcher and Freeman 1985). On the other hand, hyperprolactinaemia and intra-ventricular injections of prolactin inhibit lordosis; perhaps there are several sites of action for prolactin where it can exert opposing effects (Dudley *et al.* 1982).

Oxytocin

Oxytocin stimulates female sexual behaviour and may be physiologically important in mediating the effects of progesterone in the oestrogen-primed animal. When administered to ovariectomized rats primed with both steroids, oxytocin stimulates lordosis frequency and duration after injection into the POA, but it only enhances duration if applied to the VMN and it has no effect in the MCG (Caldwell *et al.* 1986; Schultze and Gorzalka 1991). The effects of exogenous oxytocin can be blocked by antagonists that reduce its uterotonic effect (V_2-antagonists) but not those that inhibit its effect on blood pressure (V_1-antagonists) (Caldwell *et al.* 1990). More importantly, receptivity and proceptivity induced by oestrogen and progesterone, but not oestrogen alone, can be inhibited by a specific oxytocin antagonist (d-(CH_2) 5[Tyr(Me)2 Thr4,Tyr-NH_2-9-] ornithine vasotocin) (Witt and Insel 1991).

The C-terminal tripeptide fragment of oxytocin (i.e. prolyl-leucyl-glucin-amide) may be the active metabolite of oxytocin mediating its effect, since this agent also stimulates lordosis and is dependent on progesterone (Gorzalka *et al.* 1991).

The origin of the oxytocin system and its site of action is not completely clear as yet. There are oxytocin cell bodies in the POA and oxytocin concentrations within these neurones fall after initiation of male mounting, indicating enhanced oxytocin release (Caldwell *et al.* 1989). There are oxytocin receptors in the latero-ventral area of the VMN and oestrogen induces an increase in oxytocin receptor density over 24 to 48 h, in this area and the area lateral to the VMN itself. Progesterone enhances this increase further and this can occur within 30 min indicating a direct receptor or membrane effect (Schumacher *et al.* 1990). These findings suggest that the VMN is the site of interaction between progesterone and oxytocin, which are primarily concerned with the control of the duration of lordosis at this site.

Arg-vasopressin

When arg-vasopressin (AVP) is injected into the ventricles, it has a dual effect, stimulating lordosis at 15 min and inhibiting at 90 min post-injection (Södersten *et al*. 1983; Caldwell *et al*. 1986). Södersten *et al*. (1985) have shown an inverse relationship between the circadian rhythm of AVP in the suprachiasmatic nucleus and lordotic activity and that an AVP antagonist can stimulate lordosis over the period of raised AVP levels, and administration of AVP itself can inhibit behaviour when lordotic activity is high and endogenous AVP levels are low. Södersten suggests that AVP has an inhibitory control over receptivity and this is not associated with any cardiovascular effects of AVP.

Gonadotrophin-releasing hormone

Gonadotrophin-releasing hormone (GnRH) was the first peptide shown to have a potent effect on sexual behaviour (Pfaff 1973; Moss and McCann 1973). It is active whether given systemically or centrally into the ventricles, POA, VMN/ARC, MCG, or into the spinal subarachnoid space (Moss and Foreman 1976; Rodriguez-Sierra and Komisaruk 1982; Sakuma and Pfaff 1983; Sirinathsinghji 1983*a*, *b*; Moss and Dudley 1990) and centrally administered GnRH antagonists have the expected inhibitory effect (Dudley *et al*. 1981). The effect is independent of the action of GnRH on the pituitary as it can be demonstrated in hypophysectomized rats and structural modifications show that GnRH analogues can be synthesized with selective actions, that is selectively stimulating sexual behaviour without affecting LH (luteinizing hormone) release (Kastin *et al*. 1980; Zadina *et al*. 1981).

Most interestingly, the GnRH fragment consisting of the last six amino acids of the decapeptide (Ac-GnRH5-10) is equally as effective as the parent compound in stimulating lordosis but does not appear to act on the usual GnRH receptors, as potent receptor blockers which inhibit GnRH itself do not antagonize the fragment (Moss and Dudley 1990).

GnRH neurones in the POA project into the MCG and Pfaff suggests that the GnRH released at the latter site is the physiological stimulatory mediator for lordosis (see Pfaff and Schwartz-Giblin 1988). This system may be under a tonic β-endorphin inhibitory control, since adminstration of β-endorphin into the MCG inhibits GnRH release (Sirinathsinghji 1983*a*). A further GnRH system may have a role in the spinal cord, processing somatosensory information necessary for the lordotic posture (Sirinathsinghji 1983*b*).

Substance P

Cell bodies containing substance P are present near the VMN and probably project into the MCG since administration of substance P in this area stimulates lordosis (Dornan and Malsbury 1984). Pfaff suggests that this stimulatory effect is mediated by enhanced release of met-enkephalin since substance P has been shown to stimulate the release of the opioid from brain fragments *in vitro* and the analgesic effects of substance P can be antagonized by a met-enkephalin antibody (see Mobbs *et al.* 1989).

Neuropeptide Y
Injection of NPY into the third ventricle reduces receptivity and proceptivity in steroid primed ovariectomized rats (Kalra *et al.* 1988).

Cholecystokinin-8
CCK-8 has a dual effect on receptivity. When injected into the ventricles, POA, or nucleus accumbens, it is stimulatory and antiserum to CCK-8 is inhibitory. However, CCK-8 can also be inhibitory when it is injected into the VMN (Mendelson and Gorzalka 1984*b*; Babcock *et al.* 1988; Dornan *et al.* 1989). Oestrogen reduces CCK-8 binding sites in the VMN and so may act to reduce this inhibitory control at oestrus (Akesson *et al.* 1987).

CONCLUSION

The multitude of transmitters that affect reproductive behaviour indicate that a variety of neuronal systems must be involved in controlling the various aspects of sexual activity, some perhaps having a primary role with others acting as 'fail-safe', or modulators. Some investigations into the interrelationships between the neuronal systems have been carried out, for instance the possibility that the effect of GnRH in the female is mediated via the noradrenergic system (Gonzalez-Mariscal and Beyer 1989) as is the stimulatory action of αMSH. Similarly, in the male αMSH and β-endorphin, which coexist in certain neurones, can modulate each other's effects (Hughes *et al.* 1988). Noradrenaline and NPY also coexist and like αMSH and β-endorphin have opposite effects on sexual behaviour in both sexes; they too may act to modulate each other.

In spite of the variety of systems, each possessing different transmitters, which appear to be involved in sexual activity, several examples exist in which two systems with a common transmitter exert opposite effects. In some cases this must be due to actions on different receptor sub-types and it is these systems that are of particular interest as sites for pharmacological treatment of sexual disorder.

Some behaviourists are sceptical of the large number of agents affecting sexual activity and have intimated that most of the results obtained are due to non-specific changes in arousal. They may, of course, be correct and it is important in all future work to try and ensure the specificity of any effect

Table 1.1 Summary of the effects of neurotransmitters on male and female sexual activity.

Neurotransmitter	Male			Female
	Arousal	Copulatory activity	Penile reflexes	Receptivity
Dopamine	+ (D$_2$, D$_1$)	+ (POA on D$_2$)	+ (CNS effect)	− (D$_2$)
Noradrenaline	+ (α1) − (α2)		− (Peripheral effect)	+ (VMN on α1) − (POA on α2,β)
5-hydroxytryptamine	− (Nuc. acc.)	− (POA on 2,1B) + (1A)	− (1A,1D) + (1C)	+ (2) − (1A,1B,3)
Acetylcholine	− (Mus)	+ (Mus)		+ (Mus)
GABA		− (A,B)	− (B)	− (A,B)
Prostaglandins				+ (E$_2$) − (E$_1$, F$_2\alpha$)
Opioids	+ (VTA)	− (Initiation at POA)	− (SC)	− (High affinity μ) + (Low affinity μ and δ)
ACTH		+	+	+ and −
αMSH		+ (POA)	+	+ (Via NA) − (Via antag. 5-HT$_2$)
Prolactin	−	− (Chronic) + (Acute)	−	− and +
Oxytocin		+		+

Neurotransmitter	Male			Female
	Arousal	Copulatory activity	Penile reflexes	Receptivity
Arg-vasopressin		–		– and +
Angiotensin II		–		+
Gonadotrophin-releasing factor		+		+
Substance P		+		+
Neuropeptide Y		–		–
Cholecystokinin-8		No effect		+ (POA) – (VMN)

D$_1$, D$_2$: dopamine 1 and 2 receptors; α1, α2, and β indicate the adrenergic receptor sub-types; 1A, 1B, 1C, 2, and 3 indicate the 5-HT receptor sub-types; mus, muscarinic receptor; A, B indicate the GABA-receptor sub-types; E$_2$, E$_1$, F$_{2\alpha}$ indicate prostaglandin types; POA, preoptic area; VMN, ventromedial nucleus; Nuc. acc., nucleus accumbens; VTA, ventral tegmentum area; SC, spinal cord; NA, noradrenaline.

noted by carrying out tests for other behavioural parameters indicating the state of arousal and perception.

It is clear from this review that the precise role, site, and mechanism of action of each agent investigated has not been elucidated fully and much work remains to be done.

REFERENCES

Agmo, A. (1976). Cholinergic mechanism and sexual behavior in the male rabbit. *Psychopharmacology*, **51**, 43–5.

Agmo, A. and Berenfeld, R. (1990). Reinforcing properties of ejaculation in the male rat: role of opioids and dopamine. *Behavioral Neuroscience*, **104**, 177–82.

Agmo, A. and Contreras, J.L. (1990). Copulatory thrusting pattern in the male rat after acute treatment with GABA transaminase inhibitors. *Physiology and Behavior*, **47**, 311–14.

Agmo, A. and Fernandez, H. (1989). Dopamine and sexual behavior in the male rat: a reevaluation. *Journal of Neural Transmission*, **77**, 21–37.

Agmo, A. and Fernandez, H. (1991). Benzodiazepine receptor ligands and sexual behavior in the male rat: the role of GABAergic mechanisms. *Pharmacology, Biochemistry and Behavior*, **38**, 781–88.

Agmo, A. and Paredes, R. (1985). Gabaergic drugs and sexual behaviour in the male rat. *European Journal of Pharmacology*, **112**, 371–8.

Agmo, A. and Paredes, R. (1988). Opioids and sexual behavior in the male rat. *Pharmacology, Biochemistry and Behavior*, **30**, 1021–34.

Agmo, A. and Picker, Z. (1990). Catecholamines and the initiation of sexual behavior in male rats without sexual experience. *Pharmacology, Biochemistry and Behavior*, **35**, 327–34.

Agmo, A., Fernandez, H., and Picker, Z. (1989*a*). Naloxone inhibits the faciltatory effects of 8-OH-DPAT on male rat sexual behaviour. *European Journal of Pharmacology*, **166**, 115–16.

Agmo, A., Soria, P., and Paredes, R. (1989*b*). GABAergic drugs and lordosis behavior in the female rat. *Hormones and Behavior*, **23**, 368–80.

Ahlenius, S. and Larsson, K. (1984*a*). Apomorphine and haloperidol-induced effects on male rat sexual behavior: no evidence for actions due to stimulation of central dopamine autoreceptors. *Pharmacology, Biochemistry and Behavior*, **21**, 463–6.

Ahlenius, S. and Larsson, K. (1984*b*). Lisuride, LY-141865, and 8-OH-DPAT facilitate male rat sexual behavior via a non-dopaminergic mechanism. *Psychopharmacology*, **83**, 330–4.

Ahlenius, S. and Larsson, K. (1985*a*). Antagonism by lisuride and 8-OH-DPAT of 5HTP induced prolongation of the performance of male rat sexual behavior. *European Journal of Pharmacology*, **110**, 379–81.

Ahlenius, S. and Larsson, K. (1985*b*). Central muscarinic receptors and male rat sexual behaviour: facilitation by oxotremorine but not arecoline or pilocarpine in methscopolamine pretreated animals. *Psychopharmacology*, **87**, 127–9.

Ahlenius, S. and Larsson, K. (1989). Antagonism by pindolol, but not betanolol, of 8-OH-DPAT-induced facilitation of male rat sexual behavior. *Journal of Neural Transmission*, **77**, 163–70.

Ahlenius, S. and Larsson, K. (1990). Effects of selective dopamine D_1 and D_2 antagonists on male rat sexual behaviour. *Experientia*, **46**, 1026–8.

Ahlenius, S. and Larsson, K. (1991). Opposite effects of 5-methoxy-N,N-dimethyl-tryptamine and 5-hydroxytryptophan on male rat sexual behavior. *Pharmacology, Biochemistry and Behavior*, **38**, 201–5.

Ahlenius, S., Engel, J., Eriksson, H., and Södersten, P. (1972*a*). Effects of tetra-benazine on lordosis behaviour and on brain monoamines in the female rat. *Journal of Neural Transmission*, **33**, 155–62.

Ahlenius, S., Engel, J., Eriksson, H., Modigh, K., and Södersten, P. (1972*b*). Importance of central catecholamines in the mediation of lordosis behavior in ovariectomised rats treated with oestrogen and inhibitors of monoamine synthesis. *Journal of Neural Transmission*, **33**, 247–55.

Ahlenius, S., Larsson, K., and Svensson, L. (1980*a*). Stimulating effects of lisuride on masculine sexual behavior of rats. *European Journal of Pharmacology*, **64**, 47–51.

Ahlenius, S., Larsson, K., and Svensson, L. (1980*b*). Further evidence for an inhibitory role of central 5-HT in male rat sexual behavior. *Psychopharmacology*, **68**, 217–20.

Ahlenius, S., Engel, J., Larsson, K., and Svensson, L. (1982). Effects of pergolide and bromocriptine on male rat sexual behavior. *Journal of Neural Transmission*, **54**, 165–70.

Ahlenius, S., Fernandez-Guasti, A., Hjorth, S., and Larsson, K. (1986). Suppression of lordosis behavior by the putative 5-HT receptor agonist 8-OH-DPAT in the rat. *European Journal of Pharmacology*, **124**, 361–3.

Ahlenius, S., Hillegaart, V., Hjorth, S., and Larsson, K. (1987). Effects of sexual interactions on the *in vitro* rate of monoamine synthesis in forebrain regions of the male rat. *Neuroscience and Biobehavioral Reviews*, **11**, 365–89.

Ahlenius, S., Larsson, K., and Fernandez-Guasti, A. (1989*a*). Evidence for the involvement of central $5HT_{1A}$ receptors in the mediation of lordosis behavior in the female rat. *Psychopharmacology*, **98**, 440–4.

Ahlenius, S., Larsson, K., and Arvidsson, L.E. (1989*b*). Effects of stereoselective $5HT_{1A}$ agonists on male rat sexual behavior. *Pharmacology, Biochemistry and Behavior*, **33**, 691–5.

Akesson, T.R., Mantyh, P.W., Mantyn, C.R., Matt, D.W., and Micevych, P.E. (1987). Estrous cyclicity of ^{125}I-cholecystokinin octapeptide binding in the ventro-medial hypothalamic nucleus. *Neuroendocrinology*, **45**, 257–62.

Alderson, L.M. and Baum, M. (1981). Differential effects of gonadal steroids on dopamine metabolism in mesolimbic and nigro-striatal pathways of male rat brain. *Brain Research*, **218**, 189–206.

Allen, D.L., Renner, K.J., and Luine, V.N. (1985). Naltrexone facilitation of sexual receptivity in the rat. *Hormones and Behavior*, **19**, 98–103.

Al Satli, M. and Aron, C.L. (1981). Role played by serotonin in the control of estrous receptivity, ovarian activity and ovulation in the cyclic female rat. *Psycho-neuroendocrinology*, **6**, 121–9.

Arletti, R., Bazzani, C., Castelli, M., and Bertolini, A. (1985). Oxytocin improves male copulatory performance in rats. *Hormones and Behavior*, **19**, 14–20.

Arletti, R., Benelli, A., and Bertolini, A. (1990). Sexual behaviour of aging male rats is stimulated by oxytocin. *European Journal of Pharmacology*, **179**, 377–81.

Babcock, A.M., Block, G.J., and Micevych, P.E. (1988). Injections of cholecysto-kinin into the ventromedial hypothalamic nucleus inhibit lordosis behavior in the rat. *Physiology Behavior*, **43**, 195–9.

Baggio, G. and Ferrari, F. (1983). The role of dopaminergic receptors in the behavioral effects induced by lisuride in male rats. *Psychopharmacology*, **80**, 38–42.

Bailey, D.J. and Herbert, J. (1982). Impaired copulatory behaviour of male rats with hyper-prolactinaemia induced by domperidone or pituitary grafts. *Neuroendocrinology*, **35**, 186–93.

Baldwin, D.M., Haun, C.K., and Sawyer, C.H. (1974). Effects of intraventricular infusions of ACTH[1-24] and ACTH[4-10] on LH release, ovulation and behaviour in the rabbit. *Brain Research*, **80**, 291–301.

Band, L.C. and Hull, E.M. (1990). Morphine and dynorphin (1–13) microinjected into the medial preoptic area and nucleus accumbens: effects on sexual behavior in male rats. *Brain Research*, **524**, 77–84.

Baum, M.J. (1983). Hormonal modulation of sexuality in female primates. *Journal of Bioscience*, **33**, 578–82.

Baum, M.J. (1989). Brain opioids and sexual behaviour in the male rat. In *Brain opioid systems in reproduction* (ed. R. Dyer and J. Bicknell), pp. 216–28. Oxford University Press.

Baum, M.J. and Starr, M.S. (1980). Inhibition of sexual behaviour by dopamine antagonist or serotonin agonist drugs in castrated male rats given estradiol or dihydrotestosterone. *Pharmacology, Biochemistry and Behavior*, **13**, 57–67.

Bednar, I., Forsberg, G., and Södersten, P. (1987). Inhibition of sexual behavior in female rats by intracerebral injections of met-enkephalin in combination with an inhibitor of enkephalin degrading enzymes. *Neuroscience Letters*, **79**, 341–5.

Benelli, A., Zanoli, P., and Bertolini, A. (1990). Effect of clenbuterol on sexual behavior in male rats. *Physiology and Behavior*, **47**, 373–6.

Berendsen, H.H.G. and Broekkamp, C.L.E. (1987). Drug-induced penile erections in rats: indications of serotonin 1B receptor mediation. *European Journal of Pharmacology*, **135**, 279–87.

Berendsen, H.H.G. and Gower, A.J. (1986). Opiate–androgen interactions in drug-induced yawning and penile erections in the rat. *Neuroendocrinology*, **42**, 185–90.

Berendsen, H.H.G., Jenck, F., and Broekkamp, C.L.E. (1990). Involvement of $5-HT_{1C}$-receptors in drug-induced penile erections in rats. *Psychopharmacology*, **101**, 57–61.

Bertolini, A. and Gessa, G.L. (1981). Behavioral effects of ACTH and MSH peptides. *Journal of Endocrinological Investigation*, **4**, 241–51.

Bertolini, A., Gessa, G.L., and Ferrari, W. (1975). Penile erection and ejaculation: a central effect of ACTH-like peptides in mammals. In *Sexual behavior: pharmacology and biochemistry* (ed. M. Sandler and G.L. Gessa), pp. 247–57. Raven, New York.

Biegon, A., Fishette, C.T., Rainbow, T.C., and McEwen, B.S. (1982). Serotonin receptor modulation by estrogen in discrete brain nuclei. *Neuroendocrinology*, **35**, 287–91.

Bitran, D. and Hull, E.M. (1987). Pharmacological analysis of male rat sexual behavior. *Neuroscience and Biobehavioral Reviews*, **11**, 365–89.

Bitran, D., Hull, E.M., Holmes, G.M., and Lookingland, K.J. (1988a). Regulation of male rat copulatory behavior by preoptic incertohypothalamic dopamine neurons. *Brain Research Bulletin*, **20**, 323–31.

Bitran, D., Miller, S.A., McQuade, D.B., Leipheimer, R.E., and Sachs, B.D. (1988b). Inhibition of sexual reflexes by lumbosacral injection of a GABA B agonist in the male rat. *Pharmacology, Biochemistry and Behavior*, **31**, 657–66.

Bitran, D., Thompson, J.T., Hull, E.M., and Sachs, B.D. (1989). Quinelorane (LY163502), a D_2 dopamine receptor agonist, facilitates seminal emission, but inhibits penile erection in the rat. *Pharmacology, Biochemistry and Behavior*, **34**, 453–8.

Bloch, G.J., Babcock, A.M., Gorski, R.A., and Micevych, P.E. (1988). Effects of cholecystokinin on male copulatory behavior and lordosis behavior in male rats. *Physiology and Behavior*, **43**, 351–7.

Bloch, G.J., Dornan, W.A., Babcock, A.M., Gorski, R.A., and Micevych, P.E. (1989). Effects of site-specific CNS micro injection of cholecystokinin on lordosis behavior in the male rat. *Physiology and Behavior*, **46**, 725–30.

Bohus, B. (1977). Effect of desglycinamide-lysine vasopressin (DG-LVP) on sexually motivated T-maze behavior of the male rat. *Hormones and Behavior*, **8**, 52–61.

Brackett, N.L., Iuvone, P.M., and Edwards, D.A. (1986). Midbrain lesions, dopamine and male sexual behaviour. *Behavioural Brain Research*, **20**, 231–40.

Caggiula, A.R., Herndon, J.G. Jnr, Scanlon, R., Greenstone, D., Bradshaw, W., and Sharp, D. (1978). Dissociation of active from immobility components of sexual behavior and sensorimotor responsiveness. *Brain Research*, **172**, 505–20.

Cagiano, R., Barfield, R.J., White, N.R., Pleim, E.T., and Cuomo, V. (1989). Mediation of rat postejaculatory 22 kHz ultrasonic vocalization by dopamine D_2 receptors. *Pharmacology, Biochemistry and Behavior*, **34**, 53–8.

Caldwell, J.D. and Clemens, L.G. (1986). Norepinephrine infusions into the medial preoptic area inhibit lordosis behavior. *Pharmacology, Biochemistry and Behavior*, **24**, 1015–23.

Caldwell, J.D., Prange, A.J., and Pedersen, C.A. (1986). Oxytocin facilitates the sexual receptivity of estrogen-treated female rats. *Neuropeptides*, **7**, 175–89.

Caldwell, J.D., Jirikowski, G.F., Greer, E.R., and Pedersen, P.A. (1989). Medial preoptic area oxytocin and female sexual receptivity. *Behavioral Neurosciences*, **103**, 655–62.

Caldwell, J.D., Barakat, A.S., Smith, D.D., Hruby, V.J., and Pedersen, C.A. (1990). A uterotonic antagonist blocks the oxytocin-induced facilitation of female sexual receptivity. *Brain Research*, **512**, 291–6.

Celis, M.E., Bonney, R.M., Hole, D.R., and Wilson, C.A. (1989). The effect of αMSH on noradrenaline release from the ventromedial nucleus in sexually receptive female rats. *Journal of Endocrinology*, **119** (Suppl.), Abstract 110.

Clark, T.K. (1980). Male rat sexual behavior compared after 6-OHDA and electrolytic lesions in the dorsal NA bundle region of the midbrain. *Brain Research*, **202**, 429–43.

Clark, J.T. (1989). A possible role for angiotensin II in the regulation of male sexual behavior in rats. *Physiology and Behavior*, **45**, 221–4.

Clark, J.T. (1991). Suppression of copulatory behavior in male rats following central administration of clonidine. *Neuropharmacology*, **30**, 373–82.

Clark, J.T. and Smith, E.R. (1986). Failure of pimozide and metergoline to antagonize the RDS-127-induced facilitation of ejaculatory behavior. *Physiology and Behavior*, **37**, 47–52.

Clark, J.T., Smith, E.R., Stefanick, M.L., Aarneric, S.P., Long, J.P., and Davidson, J.M. (1982). Effects of a novel dopamine-receptor agonist RDS-127 (2-N,-N-di-n-propylamino-4,7-dimethoxyindane), on hormone levels and sexual behavior in the male rat. *Physiology and Behavior*, **29**, 1–6.

Clark, J.T., Stefanick, M.L., Smith, E.R., and Davidson, J.M. (1983). Further studies on alterations in male rat copulatory behavior induced by the dopamine-receptor agonist RDS-127. *Pharmacology, Biochemistry and Behavior*, **19**, 781–6.

Clark, J.T., Smith, E.R., and Davidson, J.M. (1984). Enhancement of sexual motivation in male rats by yohimbine. *Science*, **225**, 847–9.

Clark, J.T., Smith, E.R., and Davidson, J.M. (1985a). Evidence for the modulation of sexual behavior by α-adrenoceptors in male rats. *Neuroendocrinology*, **41**, 36–43.

Clark, J.T., Smith, E.R., and Davidson, J.M. (1985b). Testosterone is not required for the enhancement of sexual motivation by yohimbine. *Physiology and Behavior*, **35**, 517–21.

Clark, J.T., Kalra, P.S., and Kalra, S.P. (1985c). Neuropeptide Y stimulates feeding but inhibits sexual behavior in rats. *Endocrinology*, **117**, 2435–42.

Clark, J.T., Simpkins, J.W., and Kalra, S.P. (1986). Long-term weekly gonadal steroid treatment: effects on plasma prolactin, sexual behavior and hypothalamic-preoptic area catecholamines. *Neuroendocrinology*, **44**, 488–93.

Clark, J.T., Gabriel, S.M., Simkins, J.W., Kalra, S.P., and Kalra, P.S. (1988). Chronic morphine and testosterone treatment. Effects on sexual behavior and dopamine metabolism in male rats. *Neuroendocrinology*, **48**, 93–104.

Clemens, L.G. and Dohanich, G.P. (1980). Inhibition of lordotic behavior in female rats following intracerebral infusion of anticholinergic agents. *Pharmacology, Biochemistry and Behavior*, **13**, 89–95.

Clemens, L.G., Humphrys, R.R., and Dohanich, G.P. (1980). Cholinergic brain mechanisms and the hormonal regulation of female sexual behavior in the rat. *Pharmacology, Biochemistry and Behavior*, **13**, 81–8.

Clemens, L.G., Dohanich, G.P., and Witcher, J.A. (1981). Cholinergic influences on estrogen-dependent sexual behavior in female rats. *Journal of Comparative Physiological Psychology*, **95**, 763–70.

Crowley, W.R., Feder, H.H., and Morin, L.P. (1976). Role of monoamines in sexual behavior of the female guinea pig. *Pharmacology, Biochemistry and Behavior*, **4**, 67–71.

Dallo, J., Lekka, N., and Knoll, J. (1986). The ejaculatory behavior of sexually sluggish male rats with (−) deprenyl, apomorphine, bromocriptine and amphetamine. *Polish Journal of Pharmacology and Pharmacy*, **38**, 251–5.

Da Prada, M., Carruba, M., Saner, A., O'Brien, R.A., and Pletscher, A. (1973). The action of L-dopa on sexual behaviour of male rats. *Brain Research*, **55**, 383–9.

de Catanzaro, D. (1987). Alteration of estrogen-induced lordosis through central administration of corticosterone in adrenalectomized-ovariectomized rats. *Neuroendocrinology*, **46**, 468–74.

de Catanzaro, D., Gray, D.S., and Gorzalka, B.B. (1981). Effects of acute central and peripheral ACTH 1–24 administration on lordosis behavior. *Physiology and Behavior*, **26**, 207–13.

De Vries, G.J. (1990). Sex differences in neurotransmitter systems. *Journal of Neuroendocrinology*, **2**, 1–13.

Dohanich, G.P. and Cada, D.A. (1989). Reversal of androgen inhibition of estrogen-activated sexual behavior by cholinergic agents. *Hormones and Behavior*, **23**, 503–13.

Dohanich, G.P. and McEwen, B.S. (1986). Cholinergic limbic projections and behavioral role of basal forebrain nuclei in the rat. *Brain Research Bulletin*, **16**, 477–82.

Dohanich, G.P., Barr, P.J., Witcher, J.A., and Clemens, L.G. (1984). Pharmacological and anatomical aspects of cholinergic activation of female sexual behavior. *Physiology and Behavior*, **32**, 1021–6.

Dohanich, G.P., McMullan, D.M., Cada, D.A., and Mangum, K.A. (1991). Muscarinic receptor subtypes and sexual behavior in female rats. *Pharmacology, Biochemistry and Behavior*, **38**, 115–24.

Doherty, P.C., Bartke, A., and Smith, M.S. (1981). Differential effects of bromocriptine treatment on LH release and copulatory behavior in hyperprolactinaemic male rats. *Hormones and Behavior*, **15**, 4356–50.

Doherty, P.C., Bartke, A., Hogan, M.P., Klemcke, H., and Smith, M.S. (1982). Effects of hyperprolactinaemia on copulatory behavior and testicular human chorionic gonadotropin binding in adrenalectomized rats. *Endocrinology*, **111**, 820–6.

Doherty, P.C., Bartke, A., and Smith, M.S. (1985). Hyperprolactinemia and male sexual behavior: effects of steroid replacement with estrogen plus dihydrotestosterone. *Physiology and Behavior*, **35**, 99–104.

Doherty, P.C., Baum, M.J., and Todd, R.B. (1986). Effects of chronic hyperprolactinemia on sexual arousal and erectile function in male rats. *Neuroendocrinology*, **42**, 368–75.

Doherty, P.G., Lane, S.J., Pfeil, K.A., Morgan, W.W., Bartke, A., and Smith, M.S. (1989). Extra-hypothalamic dopamine is not involved in the effects of hyperprolactinaemia on male copulatory behavior. *Physiology and Behavior*, **45**, 1101–5.

Dornan, W.A. and Malsbury, C.W. (1984). Facilitation of lordosis by infusion of substance P in the midbrain central gray. *Neuroendocrinology*, **45**, 498–506.

Dornan, W.A. and Malsbury, G.V. (1989). Peptidergic control of male rat sexual behavior: the effects of intracerebral injections of substance P and cholecystokinin. *Physiology and Behavior*, **46**, 547–56.

Dornan, W.A., Block, G.J., Priest, C.A., and Micevych, P.E. (1989). Microinjection of cholecystokinin into the medial preoptic nucleus facilitates lordosis behavior in the female rat. *Physiology and Behavior*, **45**, 969–74.

Dorsa, D.M., Smith, E.R., and Davidson, J.M. (1981). Endocrine and behavioral effects of continuous exposure of male rats to a potent luteinizing hormone-releasing hormone (LHRH) agonist: evidence for central nervous system actions of LHRH. *Endocrinology*, **109**, 729–35.

Drago, F. and Scapagnini, U. (1983). Prolactin and behavior: a neurochemical susbtrate. In *Recent advances in male reproduction: molecular basis and clinical implications* (ed. R. D'Agata, M.B. Lipsett, P. Polosa, and H.J. van der Molen), pp. 299–303. Raven, New York.

Drago, F., Pellegrini-Quarantotti, B., Scapagnini, U., and Gessa, G.L. (1981). Short-term endogenous hyperprolactinaemia and sexual behavior of male rats. *Physiology and Behavior*, **26**, 277–9.

Drago, F., Caldwell, J.D., Pedersen, C.A., Continella, G., Scapagnini, U., and Prange, A.J. (1986). Dopamine neurotransmission in the nucleus accumbens may be involved in oxytocin-enhanced grooming behavior of the rat. *Pharmacology, Biochemistry and Behavior*, **24**, 1185–8.

Dudley, C.A., Vale, W., Rivier, J., and Moss, R.L. (1981). The effect of LHRH antagonist analogs and an antibody to LHRH on mating behavior in female rats. *Peptides*, **2**, 393–6.

Dudley, C.A., Jamison, T.S., and Moss, R.L. (1982). Inhibition of lordosis behavior in the female rat by intraventricular infusion of prolactin and by chronic hyperprolactinaemia. *Endocrinology*, **110**, 667–79.

Eliasson, M. and Meyerson, B.J. (1977). The effects of lysergic acid diethylamide on copulatory behaviour in the female rat. *Neuropharmacology*, **16**, 37–44.

Erskine, M.S. (1989). Solicitation behavior in the estrous female rat: a review. *Hormones and Behavior*, **23**, 473–502.

Etgen, A.M. (1990). Intrahypothalamic implants of noradrenergic antagonists disrupt lordosis behavior in female rats. *Physiology and Behavior*, **48**, 31–6.

Etgen, A.M. and Petitti, N. (1987). Mediation of norepinephrine-stimulated cyclic AMP accumulation by adrenergic receptors in hypothalamic acid preoptic area slices: effects of estradiol. *Journal of Neurochemistry*, **49**, 1732–9.

Everitt, B.J. (1990). Sexual motivation: a neural and behavioural analysis of the mechanisms underlying appetite and copulatory responses of male rats. *Neuroscience and Biobehavioral Reviews*, **14**, 217–32.

Everitt, B.J. and Fuxe, K. (1977). Dopamine and sexual behaviour in female rats. Effects of dopamine receptor agonists and sulpiride. *Neuroscience Letters*, **4**, 209–13.

Everitt, B.J. and Stacey, P. (1987). Studies of instrumental behavior with sexual reinforcement in male rats (*Rattus norvegicus*): II. Effects of preoptic area lesions, castration and testosterone. *Journal of Comparative Psychology*, **101**, 407–19.

Everitt, B.J., Fuxe, K., and Hokfelt, T. (1975a). Serotonin, catecholamines and sexual receptivity of female rats. Pharmacological findings. *Journal of Pharmacology*, **6**, 269–76.

Everitt, B.J., Fuxe, K., and Jonsson, G. (1975b). The effects of 5,7-dihydroxy-tryptamine lesions of ascending 5-hydroxytryptamine pathways on the sexual and aggressive behaviour of female rats. *Journal of Pharmacology*, **6**, 25–32.

Everitt, B.J., Cador, M., and Robbins, T.W. (1989). Interactions between the amygdala and ventral striatum in stimulus–reward associations: studies using a second-order schedule of sexual reinforcement. *Neuroscience*, **30**, 63–75.

Fernandez-Guasti, A., Larsson, K., and Beyer, C. (1985a). Potentiative action of α- and β-adrenergic receptor stimulation in inducing lordosis behavior. *Pharmacology, Biochemistry and Behavior*, **22**, 613–17.

Fernandez-Guasti, A., Larsson, K., and Beyer, C. (1985b). Prevention of proges-terone-induced lordosis behavior by alpha or beta adrenergic antagonists in ovariectomized estrogen-primed rats. *Pharmacology, Biochemistry and Behavior*, **22**, 279–82.

Fernandez-Guasti, A., Larsson, K., and Beyer, C. (1985c). Effect of bicuculline on sexual activity in castrated male rats. *Physiology and Behavior*, **36**, 235–7.

Fernandez-Guasti, A., Larsson, K., and Beyer, C. (1986a). GABAergic control of masculine sexual behavior. *Pharmacology, Biochemistry and Behavior*, **24**, 1065–70.

Fernandez-Guasti, A., Larsson, K., and Beyer, C. (1986b). Effect of bicuculline on sexual activity in castrated male rats. *Physiology and Behavior*, **36**, 235–7.

Fernandez-Guasti, A., Larsson, K., and Vega-Sanabria, J. (1986c). Depression of postejaculatory ultrasonic vocalization by (+)-bicuculline. *Behavioural Brain Research*, **19**, 35–9.

Fernandez-Guasti, A., Larsson, K., and Beyer, C. (1986d). Lordosis behavior and GABAergic neurotransmission. *Pharmacology, Biochemistry and Behavior*, **24**, 673–6.

Fernandez-Guasti, A., Ahlenius, S., Hjorth, S., and Larsson, K. (1987). Separation of dopaminergic and serotonergic inhibitory mechanisms in the mediation of estrogen-induced lordosis behaviour in the rat. *Pharmacology, Biochemistry and Behavior*, **27**, 93–8.

Fernandez-Guasti, A., Escalante, A., and Agmo, A. (1989). Inhibitory action of various $5HT_{1B}$ receptor agonists on rat masculine sexual behaviour. *Pharmacology, Biochemistry and Behavior*, **34**, 811–16.

Fernandez-Guasti, A., Escalante, A., Hong, E., and Agmo, A. (1990a). Behavioral actions of the serotonergic anxiolytic indorenate. *Pharmacology, Biochemistry and Behavior*, **37**, 83–8.

Fernandez-Guasti, A., Roldan-Roldan, G., and Saldivar, A. (1990b). Pharmacological manipulation of anxiety and male rat sexual behavior. *Pharmacology, Biochemistry and Behavior*, **35**, 263–7.

Ferrari, F. and Baggio, G. (1982). Reinforcement with naloxone of N-N-propylnorapomorphine (NPA) capability for stimulating male rat copulatory behavior. *Experientia*, **38**, 951–3.

Ferrari, F., Baggio, G., and Mangiafico, V. (1985). The dopamine autoreceptor agonist B-HT 920 markedly stimulates sexual behavior in male rats. *Experientia*, **41**, 636–8.

Finberg, J.P.M. and Vardi, Y. (1990). Inhibitory effect of 5-hydroxytryptamine on penile erectile function in the rat. *British Journal of Pharmacology*, **101**, 698–702.

Finkey and Vardi 1990

Foreman, M.M. and Hall, J.L. (1987). Effects of D_2-dopaminergic receptor stimulation on the lordotic response of female rats. *Psychopharmacology*, **91**, 96–100.

Foreman, M.M. and Moss, R.L. (1978a). Role of hypothalamic alpha and beta adrenergic receptors in the control of lordotic behavior in the ovariectomized-estrogen primed rat. *Pharmacology, Biochemistry and Behavior*, **9**, 235–41.

Foreman, M.M. and Moss, R.L. (1978b). Role of hypothalamic serotonergic receptors in the control of lordosis behavior in the female rat. *Hormone Research*, **10**, 97–106.

Foreman, M.M. and Moss, R.L. (1979). Role of hypothalamic dopaminergic receptors in the control of lordosis behavior in the female rat. *Physiology and Behavior*, **22**, 283–9.

Foreman, M.M. and Wernicke, J.F. (1990). Approaches for the development of oral drug therapies for erectile dysfunction. *Seminars in Urology*, **8**, 107–12.

Foreman, M.M., Hall, J.L., and Love, R.L. (1989). The role of the $5\text{-}HT_2$ receptor in the regulation of sexual performance of male rats. *Life Sciences*, **45**, 1263–70.

Forsberg, G., Bednar, I., Eneroth, P., and Södersten, P. (1987a). Naloxone reverses post-ejaculatory inhibition of sexual behaviour in female rats. *Journal of Endocrinology*, **113**, 429–34.

Forsberg, G., Bednar, I., and Södersten, P. (1987b). Naloxone stimulates sexual behaviour in lactating rats. *Journal of Endocrinology*, **113**, 423–7.

Forsberg, G., Bednar, I., Everoth, P., and Södersten, P. (1990). Beta-endorphin acts on the reproductive tract of female rats to suppress sexual receptivity. *Neuroscience Letters*, **115**, 92–6.

Frankfurt, M. and Azmitia, E. (1984). Regeneration of serotonergic fibers in the rat hypothalamus following unilateral 5,7-dihydroxytryptamine injection. *Brain Research*, **298**, 273–82.

Frankfurt, M., Renner, K., Azmitia, E., and Luine, V. (1985). Intrahypothalamic 5,7-dihydroxytryptamine: temporal analysis of effects on 5-hydroxytryptamine content in brain nuclei and on facilitated lordosis behavior. *Brain Research*, **340**, 127–33.

Gessa, G.L., Paglietti, E., and Quarantotti, B.P. (1979). Induction of copulatory behavior in sexually inactive rats by naloxone. *Science*, **204**, 203–5.

Gonzalez, M.J. Celis, M.E., Hole, D.R., and Wilson, C.A. (1993). The interaction of oestradiol, α-melanotrophin (αMSH) and noradrenaline within the ventromedial nucleus in the control of female sexual behaviour. *Neuroendocrinology*. In press.

Gonzalez-Mariscal, G. and Beyer, C. (1989). Blockade of LHRH-induced lordosis by α- and β-adrenergic antagonists in ovariectomized, estrogen primed rats. *Pharmacology, Biochemistry and Behavior*, **31**, 573–7.

Gorzalka, B.B. and Whalen, R.E. (1975). Inhibition not facilitation of sexual behavior by PCPA. *Pharmacology, Biochemistry and Behavior*, **3**, 511–13.

Gorzalka, B.B., Luck, K.A., and Tanco, S.A. (1991). Effects of the oxytocin fragment prolyl–leucyl–glycinamide on sexual behavior in the rat. *Pharmacology, Biochemistry and Behavior*, **38**, 273–9.

Gower, A.J., Berendsen, H.H.G., and Broekkamp, C.L. (1986). Antagonism of drug-induced yawning and penile erections in rats. *European Journal of Pharmacology*, **122**, 239–44.

Gray, G.D., Davis, H.N., and Dewsbury, D.A. (1974). Effects of L-dopa on the heterosexual copulatory behaviour of male rats. Short communication. *European Journal of Pharmacology*, **27**, 367–70.

Grierson, J.P., James, M.D., Pearson, J.R., and Wilson, C.A. (1988). The effect of selective D_1 and D_2 dopaminergic agents on sexual receptivity in the female rat. *Neuropharmacology*, **27**, 181–9.

Gunnet, J.W., Lookingland, K.L., and Moore, K.E. (1986). Comparison of the effects of castration and steroid replacement on incerto-hypothalamic dopaminergic neurones in male and female rats. *Neuroendocrinology*, **44**, 269–75.

Hamberger-Bar, R. and Rigter, H. (1975). Apomorphine: facilitation of sexual behaviour in female rats. *European Journal of Pharmacology*, **32**, 357–60.

Hamberger-Bar, R., Rigter, H., and Dekker, I. (1978). Inhibition of serotonin reuptake differentially affects heterosexual behavior of male and female rats. *Life Sciences*, **22**, 1827–36.

Hansen, S. and Ross, S.B. (1983). Role of descending monoaminergic neurons in the control of sexual behavior: effects of intrathecal infusions of 6-hydroxydopamine and 5,7-dihydroxytryptamine. *Brain Research*, **268**, 285–90.

Hansen, S., Stanfield, E.J., and Everitt, B.J. (1980). The role of ventral bundle noradrenergic neurones in sensory components of sexual behaviour and coitus-induced pseudopregnancy. *Nature*, **286**, 152–4.

Harlan, R., Shivers, B., and Pfaff, D.W. (1983). Midbrain microinfusions of prolactin increase the oestrogen-dependent behavior, lordosis. *Science*, **219**, 1451–3.

Herbert, J. (1989). Specific roles for β-endorphin in reproduction and sexual behaviour. In *Brain opioid systems in reproduction* (ed. R. Dyer and J. Bicknell), pp. 167–86. Oxford University Press.

Herbert, J. and McGregor, A. (1990). Interactions between steroids and opioids in the control of reproductive behaviour. *Journal of Reproduction and Fertility*. Abstract Series No 6, p. 3, Abstract S2.

Herndon, J.G. Jr., Caggiula, A.R., Sharp, D., Ellis, D., and Redgate, E. (1978). Selective enhancement of the lordotic component of female sexual behavior in rats following destruction of central catecholamine-containing systems. *Brain Research*, **141**, 137–51.

Hillegaart, V., Ahlenius, S., and Larsson, K. (1989). Effects of local application of 5-HT into the median and dorsal raphe nuclei on male rat sexual and motor behavior. *Behavioural Brain Research*, **33**, 279–86.

Hillegaart, V., Ahlenius, S., and Larsson, K. (1991). Region-selective inhibition of male rat sexual behavior and motor performance by localized forebrain 5HT injections: a comparison with effects produced by 8-OH-DPAT. *Behavioral Brain Research*, **42**, 169–80.

Hlinak, Z., Madlafousek, J., and Krejci, I. (1983). Effects of lisuride on pre-copulatory and copulatory behaviour of adult male rats. *Psychopharmacology*, **79**, 231–5.

Hoffman, N.W., Gerall, A.A., and Kalivas, P.W. (1987). Sexual refractoriness and locomotion effects on brain monoamines in the male rat. *Physiology and Behavior*, **41**, 563–9.

Holmgren, B., Urba-Holmgren, R., Trucios, N., Zermeno, M., and Eguibar, J.R. (1985). Association of spontaneous and dopaminergic-induced yawning and penile erections in the rat. *Pharmacology, Biochemistry and Behavior*, **22**, 31–5.

Hughes, A.M., Everitt, B.J., and Herbert, J. (1987a). Selective effects of beta-endorphin infused into the hypothalamus, pre-optic area and bed nucleus of the stria terminalis on the sexual and ingestive behaviour of male rats. *Neuroscience*, **23**, 1063–73.

Hughes, A.M., Everitt, B.J., Lightman, S.L., and Todd, K. (1987b). Oxytocin in the central nervous system and sexual behaviour in male rats. *Brain Research*, **414**, 133–7.

Hughes, A.M., Everitt, B.J., and Herbert, J. (1988). The effects of simultaneous or separate infusions of some pro-opiomelanocortin-derived peptides (beta-endorphin, melanocyte stimulating hormone, and corticotrophin-like intermediate polypeptide) and their acetylated derivatives upon sexual and ingestive behavior of male rats. *Neuroscience*, **27**, 689–98.

Hughes, A.M., Everitt, B.J., and Herbert, J. (1990). Comparative effects of preoptic area infusions of opioid peptides, lesions and castration on sexual behaviour in male rats: studies of instrumental behaviour, conditioned place preference and partner preference. *Psychopharmacology*, **102**, 243–56.

Hull, E.M., Bitran, D., Pehek, E.A., Warner, R.K., Band, L.C., and Holmes, G.M. (1986). Dopaminergic control of male sex behavior in rats: Effects of an intracerebrally-infused agonist. *Brain Research*, **370**, 73–81.

Hull, E.M., Bitran, D., Pehek, E.A., Holmes, G.M., Warner, R.K., Band, L.C., and Clemens, L.G. (1988a). Brain localization of cholinergic influence on male sex behavior in rats: agonists. *Pharmacology, Biochemistry and Behavior*, **31**, 169–74.

Hull, E.M., Pehek, E.A., Bitran, D., Holmes, G.M., Warner, R.K., Band, L.C., Bazzett, T., and Clemens, L.G. (1988b). Brain localization of cholinergic influence on male sex behavior in rats: antagonists. *Pharmacology, Biochemistry and Behavior*, **31**, 175–8.

Hull, E.M., Warner, R.K., Bazzett, T.J., Eaton, R.C., Thompson, J.T., and Scaletta, L.L. (1989). D2/D1 ratio in the medial preoptic area affects copulation of male rats. *Journal of Pharmacology and Experimental Therapeutics*, **251**, 422–7.

Hull, E.M., Bazzett, T.J., Warner, R.K., Eaton, R.C., and Thomson, J.T. (1990). Dopamine receptors in the ventral tegmental area modulate male sexual behavior in rats. *Brain Research*, **512**, 1–6.

Hunter, A.J., Hole, D.R., and Wilson, C.A. (1985). Studies into the dual effects of serotonergic pharmacological agents on female sexual behaviour in the rat: preliminary evidence that endogenous 5HT is stimulatory. *Pharmacology, Biochemistry and Behavior*, **22**, 5–13.

Irving, S.M., Goy, R.W., Haning, R.V., and Davis, G.A. (1981). Prostaglandins, clonidine and sexual receptivity in the guinea pig. *Brain Research*, **204**, 65–77.

James, M.D., Lane, S.M., Hole, D.R., and Wilson, C.A. (1989*a*). Hypothalamic sites of action of the dual effect of 5HT on female sexual behavior in the rat. In *Behavioral pharmacology of 5HT* (ed. P. Bevan, A.R. Cools, and T. Archer), pp. 73–8. Erlbaum, New York.

James, M.D., Hole, D.R., and Wilson, C.A. (1989*b*). Differential involvement of 5-hydroxytryptamine (5HT) in specific hypothalamic areas in the mediation of steroid-induced changes in gonadotrophin release and sexual behaviour in female rats. *Neuroendocrinology*, **49**, 561–9.

Johnson, M. and Everitt, B. (1988). *Essential reproduction* (3rd edn). Blackwell, Oxford.

Kalra, P.S., Simkins, J.W., Luttge, W.G., and Kalra, S.P. (1983). Effects on male sex behavior and preoptic dopamine neurons of hyperprolactinemia induced by MtTW15 pituitary tumors. *Endocrinology*, **113**, 2065–71.

Kalra, S.P., Clark, J.T., Sahu, A., Dube, M.G., and Kalra, P.S. (1988). Control of feeding and sexual behaviors by neuropeptide Y: physiological implications. *Synapse*, **2**, 254–7.

Kastin, A.J., Coy, D.H., Schally, A.V., and Zadina, J.E. (1980). Dissociation of effects of LH–RH analogs on pituitary regulation and reproductive behavior. *Pharmacology, Biochemistry and Behavior*, **13**, 913–14.

Kaufman, L.S., McEwen, B.S., and Pfaff, D.W. (1988). Cholinergic mechanisms of lordotic behavior in rats. *Physiology and Behavior*, **43**, 507–14.

Kerdelhue, B., Bethea, C.L., Ling, N., Chretien, M., and Weiner, R.I. (1982). β-endorphin concentrations in serum, hypothalamus and central gray of hypophysectomised and mediobasal hypothalamus lesioned rats. *Brain Research*, **231**, 85–91.

Kihlstrom, J.E. and Agmo, A. (1974). Some effects of vasopressin on sexual behaviour and seminal characteristics in intact and castrated rabbits. *Journal of Endocrinology*, **60**, 445–53.

Lauber, A.H. (1988). Bethanechol-induced increase in hypothalamic estrogen receptor binding in female rats is related to capacity for estrogen-dependent reproductive behavior. *Brain Research*, **456**, 177–82.

Lauber, A.H., Romano, G.J., Mobbs, C.V., Howells, R.D., and Pfaff, D.W. (1990). Estradiol induction of proenkephalin messenger RNA in hypothalamus: dose-response and relation to reproductive behavior in the female rat. *Molecular Brain Research*, **8**, 47–54.

Lee, R.L., Smith, E.R., Mas, M., and Davidson, J.M. (1990). Effects of intrathecal administration of 8OH-DPAT on genital reflexes and mating behavior in male rats. *Physiology and Behavior*, **47**, 665–9.

Leipheimer, R.E. and Sachs, B.D. (1988). GABAergic regulation of penile reflexes and copulation in rats. *Physiology and Behavior*, **42**, 351–7.

Lookingland, K.J. and Moore, K.E. (1984). Dopamine receptor-mediated regulation of incerto-hypothalamic dopaminergic neurones in the male rat. *Brain Research*, **304**, 329–38.

Luine, V.N. and McEwen, B.S. (1983). Sex differences in cholinergic enzymes of diagonal band nuclei in the rat preoptic area. *Neuroendocrinology*, **36**, 475–82.

Luine, V., Frankfurt, M., Rainbow, T.C., Biegon, A., and Azmitia, E. (1983). Intrahypothalamic 5,7-dihydroxytryptamine facilitates feminine sexual behavior and decreases [³H]imipramine binding and 5-HT uptake. *Brain Research*, **264**, 344–8.

Luine, V.N., Thornton, J.E., Frankfurt, M., and MacLusky, N.J. (1987). Effects of hypothalamic serotonin depletion on lordosis behavior and gonadal hormone receptors. *Brain Research*, **426**, 47–52.

Malmnas, W. (1973). Monoaminergic influence on testosterone-activating copulatory behaviour in the castrated male rat. *Act Physiologica Scandanavia* (Suppl.), **395**, 1–128.

Malmnas, W. (1976). The significance of dopamine, versus other catecholamines, for L-dopa induced facilitation of sexual behavior in the castrated male rat. *Pharmacology, Biochemistry and Behavior*, **4**, 521–6.

Marson, L. and McKenna, K.E. (1990). The identification of a brain stem site controlling spinal sexual reflexes in male rats. *Brain Research*, **515**, 303–8.

Mas, M., Gonzales-Mora, J.L., Louilot, A., Sole, C., and Gandalupe, T. (1990). Increased dopamine release in the nucleus accumbens of copulating male rats as evidenced by *in vivo* voltammetry. *Neuroscience Letters*, **110**, 303–8.

Masco, D., Weigel, R., and Carrer, H.F. (1986). Gamma aminobutyric acid mediates ventromedial hypothalamic mechanisms controlling the execution of lordotic responses in the female rat. *Behavioural Brain Research*, **19**, 153–62.

Mathes, C.W., Smith, E.R., Popa, B.R., and Davidson, J.M. (1990). Effects of intrathecal and systemic administration of buspirone on genital reflexes and mating behavior in male rats. *Pharmacology, Biochemistry and Behavior*, **36**, 63–8.

Mathews, D., Greene, S.B., and Hollingsworth, E.M. (1983). VMN lesion deficits in lordosis: partial reversal with pergolide mesylate. *Physiology and Behavior*, **31**, 745–8.

McCarthy, M.M., Malik, K.F., and Feder, H.H. (1990). Increased GABAergic transmission in medial hypothalamus facilitates lordosis but has the opposite effect in preoptic area. *Brain Research*, **507**, 40–4.

McIntosh, T.K. and Barfield, R.J. (1984*a*). Brain monoaminergic control of male reproductive behavior. I. Serotonin and the post-ejaculatory refractory period. *Behavioral Brain Research*, **12**, 255–65.

McIntosh, T.K. and Barfield, R.J. (1984*b*). Brain monoaminergic control of male reproductive behavior. II. Dopamine and the post-ejaculatory refractory period. *Behavioral Brain Research*, **12**, 267–73.

McIntosh, T.K. and Barfield, R.J. (1984*c*). Brain monoaminergic control of male reproductive behavior. III. Norepinephrine and the post-ejaculatory refractory period. *Behavioural Brain Research*, **12**, 275–81.

McIntosh, T.K., Vallano, M.L., and Barfield, R.J. (1980). Effects of morphine, beta-endorphin and naloxone on catecholamine levels and sexual behaviour in the male rat. *Pharmacology, Biochemistry and Behavior*, **13**, 435–41.

Mehrara, B.J. and Baum, M.J. (1990). Naloxone disrupts the expression but not the acquisition by male rats of a conditioned place preference response for an oestrous female. *Psychopharmacology*, **101**, 118–25.

Melis, M.R., Argiolas, A., and Gessa, G.L. (1987). Apomorphine-induced penile-erection and yawning: site of action in the brain. *Brain Research*, **415**, 98–107.

Menard, C.S. and Dohanich, G.P. (1989). Scopolamine inhibition of lordosis in naturally cycling female rats. *Physiology and Behavior*, **45**, 819–23.

Menard, C.S. and Dohanich, G.P. (1990). Physostigmine facilitation of lordosis in naturally cycling female rats. *Pharmacology, Biochemistry and Behavior*, **36**, 853–8.

Mendelson, S.D. and Gorzalka, B.B. (1984*a*). Serotonin antagonist pirenperone inhibits sexual behavior in the male rat: attenuation by quipazine. *Pharmacology, Biochemistry and Behavior*, **22**, 565–71.

Mendelson, S.D. and Gorzalka, B.B. (1984*b*). Cholecystokinin-octapeptide produces inhibition of lordosis in the female rat. *Pharmacology, Biochemistry and Behavior*, **21**, 755–9.

Mendelson, S.D. and Gorzalka, B.B. (1985*a*). Serotonin type 2 antagonists inhibit lordosis behavior in the female rat: reversal with quipazine. *Life Sciences*, **38**, 33–9.

Mendelson, S.D. and Gorzalka, B.B. (1985*b*). A facilitatory role for serotonin in the sexual behavior of the female rat. *Pharmacology, Biochemistry and Behavior*, **22**, 1025–33.

Mendelson, S.D. and Gorzalka, B.B. (1986*a*). Harmine reverses the inhibition of lordosis by the 5-HT$_2$ antagonists pirenperone and ketanserin in the female rat. *Pharmacology, Biochemistry and Behavior*, **25**, 111–15.

Mendelson, S.D. and Gorzalka, B.B. (1986*b*). 5HT$_{1A}$ receptors: differential involvement in female and male sexual behavior in the rat. *Physiology and Behavior*, **37**, 345–51.

Mendelson, S.D. and Gorzalka, B.B. (1986*c*). Effects of 5-HT$_{1A}$ selective anxiolytics on lordosis behavior: interactions with progesterone. *European Journal of Pharmacology*, **132**, 323–6.

Mendelson, S.D. and Gorzalka, B.B. (1988). Stimulation of beta-adrenoreceptors inhibits lordosis behavior in the female rat. *Pharmacology, Biochemistry and Behavior*, **29**, 717–23.

Mendenez-Abraham, E.M., Viesca, P.M., Plaza, A.V., and Marin, B. (1988). Modifications of the sexual activity in male rats following administration of antiserotoninergic drugs. *Behavioral Brain Research*, **30**, 251–8.

Meyerson, B.J. (1981). Comparison of the effects of β-endorphin and morphine on exploratory and socio-sexual behavior in the male rat. *European Journal of Pharmacology*, **69**, 453–63.

Michanek, A. and Meyerson, B.J. (1982). Influence of estrogen and progesterone on behavioral effects of apomorphine and amphetamine. *Pharmacology, Biochemistry and Behavior*, **16**, 875–9.

Miller, R.L. and Baum, M.J. (1987). Naloxone inhibits mating and conditioned place preference for an estrous female in male rats soon after castration. *Pharmacology, Biochemistry and Behavior*, **26**, 781–9.

Mitchell, J.B. and Stewart, J. (1989). Effects of castration, steroid replacement and sexual experience on mesolimbic dopamine and sexual behaviors in the male rat. *Brain Research*, **491**, 116–27.

Mitchell, J.B. and Stewart, J. (1990). Facilitation of sexual behaviors in the male rat associated with intra-VTA injection of opiates. *Pharmacology, Biochemistry and Behavior*, **35**, 643–50.

Mobbs, C.V., Romano, G.J., Schwartz-Giblin, S., and Pfaff, D.W. (1989). Biochemistry of a steroid-regulated mammalian mating behavior; heat-shock proteins and secretion, enkephalin and GABA. In *Neural control of reproductive function*, pp. 95–116. Alan R. Liss, New York.

Montemayor, M.E., Clark, A.S., Lynn, D.M., and Roy, E.J. (1990). Modulation by norepinephrine of neural responses to estradiol. *Neuroendocrinology*, **52**, 473–80.

Mora, S. and Diaz-Veliz, G. (1986). Pharmacological evidence of catecholaminergic involvement in the behavioral effects of luteinizing hormone releasing hormone in rats. *Pharmacology, Biochemistry and Behavior*, **24**, 433–8.

Moreines, J., Kelton, M., Luine, V.N., Pfaff, D.W., and McEwen, B.S. (1988). Hypothalamic serotonin lesions unmask hormone responsiveness of lordosis behavior in adult male rats. *Neuroendocrinology*, **47**, 453–8.

Moss, R.L. and Dudley, C.A. (1990). Differential effects of a luteinizing-hormone-releasing hormone (LHRH) antagonist analogue on lordosis behavior induced by LHRH and the LHRH fragment Ac-LHRH 5-10. *Neuroendocrinology*, **52**, 138–42.

Moss, R.L. and Foreman, M.M. (1976). Potentiation of lordosis behavior by interhypothalamic infusion of synthetic luteinizing hormone-releasing hormone. *Neuroendocrinology*, **20**, 176–81.

Moss, R.L. and McCann, S.M. (1973). Induction of mating behavior in rats by luteinizing hormone-releasing factor. *Science*, **181**, 177–9.

Moss, R.L., McCann, S.M., and Dudley, C.A. (1975). Releasing hormones and sexual behavior. *Progress in Brain Research*, **42**, 37–46.

Myers, B.M. and Baum, M.J. (1978). Facilitation by opiate antagonists of sexual performance in the male rat. *Pharmacology, Biochemistry and Behavior*, **10**, 615–18.

Myers, B.M. and Baum, M.J. (1980). Facilitation of copulatory performance in male rats by naloxone: effects of hypophysectomy, 17α-estradiol, and luteinizing hormone releasing hormone. *Pharmacology, Biochemistry and Behavior*, **12**, 365–70.

Nakajima, S. and McKenzie, G.M. (1986). Reduction of the rewarding effect of brain stimulation by a blockade of dopamine D_1 receptor with SCH 23390. *Pharmacology, Biochemistry and Behavior*, **24**, 919–23.

Nock, B. and Feder, H.H. (1979). Noradrenergic transmission and female sexual behavior of guinea pigs. *Brain Research*, **166**, 369–80.

Nock, B. and Feder, H.H. (1981). Neurotransmitter modulation of steroid action in target cells that mediate reproduction and reproductive behavior. *Neuroscience and Biobehavioral Reviews*, **5**, 437–47.

Nock, B. and Feder, H.H. (1984). α_1-Noradrenergic regulation of hypothalamic progestin receptors and guinea pigs lordosis behavior. *Brain Research*, **310**, 77–85.

O'Connor, L.H. and Feder, H.H. (1985). Estradiol and progesterone influence 5-hydroxytryptophan-induced myoclonus in male guinea pigs: sex differences in serotonin-steroid interactions. *Brain Research*, **330**, 121–5.

O'Connor, L., Nock, B., and McEwen, B.S. (1985). Quantitative autoradiography of $GABA_A$ receptors in rat forebrain: receptors distribution and effects. *Society of Neuroscience Abstract*, **11**, 223–5.

Pehek, E.A., Thompson, J.T., Eaton, R.C., Bazzett, T.J., and Hull, E.M. (1988). Apomorphine and haloperidol, but not domperidone, affect penile reflexes in rats. *Pharmacology, Biochemistry and Behavior*, **31**, 201–8.

Pfaff, D.W. (1973). Luteinizing hormone-releasing factor potentiates lordosis behavior in hypophysectomized ovariectomized female rats. *Science*, **182**, 1148–9.

Pfaff, D.W. (1980). In *Estrogens and brain function: a neuronal analysis of a hormone-controlled mammalian reproductive behavior*. Springer, New York.

Pfaff, D.W. and Schwartz-Giblin, S. (1988). Cellular mechanisms of female reproductive behaviors. In *The physiology of reproduction* (ed. E. Knobil, J. Neill and D.W. Pfaff), pp. 1487–567. Raven, New York.

Pfaus, J.G. and Gorzalka, B.B. (1987). Opioids and sexual behavior. *Neuroscience and Behavioral Reviews*, **11**, 1–34.

Pfaus, J.G. and Phillips, A.G. (1989). Differential effects of dopamine receptor antagonists on the sexual behavior of male rats. *Psychopharmacology*, **98**, 363–8.

Pfaus, J.G., Pendleton, N., and Gorzalka, B.B. (1986). Dual effect of morphiceptin on lordosis behavior: possible mediation by different opioid receptor subtypes. *Pharmacology, Biochemistry and Behavior*, **24**, 1461–4.

Pfaus, J.G., Damsma, G., Nomikos, G.G., Wenkstern, D.G., Blaha, C.D., Phillips, A.G., and Fibiger, H.C. (1990). Sexual behavior enhances central dopamine transmission in the male rat. *Brain Research*, **530**, 345–8.

Pleim, E.T., Matochik, J.A., Barfield, R.J., and Auerbach, S.B. (1990). Correlation of dopamine release in the nucleus accumbens with masculine sexual behavior in rats. *Brain Research*, **524**, 160–3.

Poggioli, R., Vergoni, A.V., Marrama, D., Giuliani, D., and Bertolini, A. (1990). NPY-induced inhibition of male copulatory activity is a direct behavioural effect. *Neuropeptides*, **16**, 169–72.

Quintin, L., Buda, M., Hilavic, G., Bardelay, C., Ghignone, M., and Piejol, J.F. (1986). Catecholamine metabolism in the rat locus coeruleus as studied by *in vivo* differential pulse voltammetry III. Evidence for the existence of an alpha-2-adrenergic tonic inhibition in behaving rats. *Brain Research*, **375**, 235–45.

Qureshi, G.A. and Södersten, P. (1986). Sexual activity alters the concentration of amino-acids in the cerebrospinal fluid of male rats. *Neuroscience Letters*, **70**, 374–8.

Qureshi, G.A., Bednar, I., Forsberg, B.G., and Södersten, P. (1988). GABA inhibits sexual behavior in female rats. *Neuroscience*, **27**, 169–74.

Qureshi, G.A., Forsberg, G., Bednar, I., and Södersten, P. (1989). Tryptophan, 5-HTP, 5-HT and 5-HIAA in the cerebrospinal fluid and sexual behavior in male rats. *Neuroscience Letters*, **97**, 227–31.

Raible, L.H. (1988). Inhibitory action of alpha-melanocyte stimulating hormone on lordosis in rats: possible involvement of serotonin. *Pharmacology, Biochemistry and Behavior*, **30**, 37–43.

Raible, L.H. and Gorzalka, B.B. (1986). Short and long term inhibitory actions of alpha-melanocyte stimulating hormone on lordosis in rats. *Peptides*, **7**, 581–6.

Rainbow, T.C., Snyder, L., Berck, D.J., and McEwen, B.S. (1984). Correlation of muscarinic receptor induction in the ventro-medial hypothalamic nucleus with the activation of feminine sexual behavior by oestradiol. *Neuroendocrinology*, **39**, 476–80.

Richmond, G. and Clemens, L.G. (1986a). Cholinergic mediation of feminine sexual receptivity: demonstration of progesterone independence using a progestin receptor antagonist. *Brain Research*, **373**, 159–63.

Richmond, G. and Clemens, L.G. (1986b). Evidence for involvement of midbrain central gray in cholinergic mediation of female sexual receptivity in rats. *Behavioral Neuroscience*, **100**, 376–80.

Richmond, G. and Clemens, L. (1988). Ventromedial hypothalamic lesions and cholinergic control of female sexual behavior. *Physiology and Behavior*, **42**, 179–82.

Rodriguez, M., Castro, R., Hernandez, G., and Mas, M. (1984). Different roles of catecholaminergic and serotoninergic neurons of the medial forebrain bundle on male rat sexual behavior. *Physiology and Behavior*, **33**, 5–11.

Rodriguez-Sierra, J.F. and Komisaruk, B.R. (1977). Effects of prostaglandin E₂ and indomethacin on sexual behavior in the female rat. *Hormones and Behavior*, **9**, 281–9.

Rodriguez-Sierra, J.F. and Komisaruk, B.R. (1982). Common hypothalamic sites for activation of sexual receptivity in female rats by LHRH, PGE₂ and progesterone. *Neuroendocrinology*, **35**, 363–9.

Sachs, B.D. and Meisel, R.L. (1988). The physiology of male sexual behaviour. In *The physiology of reproduction* (ed. E. Knobil, J. Neill and D.W. Pfaff), pp. 1393–485. Raven, New York.

Sakuma, Y. and Pfaff, D.W. (1983). Modulation of the lordosis reflex of female rats by LHRH; its antiserum and analogs in the mesencephalic central gray. *Neuroendocrinology*, **36**, 218–24.

Sala, M., Braida, D., Leone, M.P., Calcaterra, P., Monti, S., and Gori, E. (1990). Central effect of yohimbine on sexual behavior in the rat. *Physiology and Behavior*, **47**, 165–73.

Sawyer, C.H., Baldwin, D.M., and Haun, C.K. (1975). Effects of intraventricular injections of corticotrophins on hypothalamopituitary ovarian function and behavior in the female rabbit. In *Sexual behavior, pharmacology and biochemistry* (ed. M. Sandler and G.L. Gessa), pp. 259–68. Raven, New York.

Scaletta, L.L. and Hull, E.M. (1990). Systemic or intracranial apomorphine increases copulation in long-term castrated male rats. *Pharmacology, Biochemistry and Behavior*, **37**, 471–5.

Schmidt, A.W. and Peroutka, S.J. (1989). 5-hydroxytryptamine receptor 'families'. *FASEB Journal*, **3**, 2242–9.

Schultze, H.G. and Gorzalka, B.B. (1991). Oxytocin effects on lordosis frequency and lordosis duration following infusion into the medial pre-optic area and ventromedial hypothalamus of female rats. *Neuropeptides*, **18**, 99–106.

Schumacher, M., Coirini, H., Pfaff, D.W., and McEwen, B.S. (1990). Behavioral effects of progesterone associated with rapid modulation of oxytocin receptors. *Science*, **250**, 691–4.

Segal, D.S. and Whalen, R.E. (1970). Effect of chronic administration of *p*-chlorophenylalanine on sexual receptivity of the female rat. *Psychopharmacologia*, **16**, 434–8.

Segal, M., Shahami, E., and Jacobowitz, D.M. (1983). Phenylethylamine, norepinephrine and mounting behavior in the male rat. *Pharmacology, Biochemistry and Behavior*, **20**, 133–5.

Shivers, B.D., Harlan, R.E., and Pfaff, D.W. (1989). A subset of neurons containing immunoreactive prolactin is a target for estrogen regulation of gene expression in rat hypothalamus. *Neuroendocrinology*, **49**, 23–7.

Shrenker, P. and Bartke, A. (1985). Adrenalectomy does not prevent the hyperprolactinemic induced sexual behavior deficits in CDF male rats. *Life Sciences*, **36**, 1881–8.

Sietnieks, A. and Meyerson, B.J. (1982). Enhancement by progesterone of 5-hydroxytryptophan inhibition of the copulatory response in the female rat. *Neuroendocrinology*, **35**, 321–6.

Singer, J.J. (1972). Effects of *p*-chlorophenylalanine on the male and female sexual behavior of female rats. *Psychology Reports*, **30**, 891–3.

Sirinathsinghji, D.J.S. (1983*a*). Modulation of lordosis behavior of female rats by naloxone, β-endorphin and its antiserum in the mesencephalic central gray: possible mediation via GnRH. *Neuroendocrinology*, **39**, 222–30.

Sirinathsinghji, D.J.S. (1983*b*). GnRH in the spinal subarachnoid space potentiates lordosis behavior in the female rat. *Physiology and Behavior*, **31**, 717–23.

Sirinathsinghji, D.J.S. (1985). Modulation of lordosis behaviour in the female rat by corticotrophin releasing factor, β-endorphin and gonadotropin releasing hormone in the mesencephalic central gray. *Brain Research*, **336**, 45–55.

Sirinathsinghji, D.J.S. and Herbert, J. (1981). The effects of intracerebroventricular infusions of naloxone on sexual behaviour of male rats. *Proceedings of the 163rd Meeting of the Endocrine Society, London*, p. 6, Abstract No 12.

Sirinathsinghji, D.J.S., Rees, L.H., Rivier, J., and Vale, W. (1982). Corticotropin-releasing factor is a potent inhibitor of sexual receptivity in the female rat. *Nature*, **300**, 232–5.

Siranathsinghji, D.J.S., Whittington, P.E., Audsley, A., and Fraser, H.M. (1983). β-endorphin regulates lordosis in female rats by modulating LH-RH release. *Nature*, **301**, 62–3.

Sirinathsinghji, D.J.S., Whittington, P.E., and Audsley, A.R. (1986). Regulation of mating behaviour in the female rat by gonadotrophin-releasing hormone in the ventral tegmental area: effects of selective destruction of the A10 dopamine neurones. *Brain Research*, **374**, 167–73.

Smith, E.R. and Davidson, J.M. (1990). Yohimbine attenuates aging-induced sexual deficiencies in male rats. *Physiology and Behavior*, **47**, 631–4.

Smith, E.R., Maurice, J., Richardson, R., Walter, T., and Davidson, J.M. (1990). Effects of four beta-adrenergic receptor antagonists on male rat sexual behaviour. *Pharmacology, Biochemistry and Behavior*, **36**, 713–17.

Södersten, P., Larsson, K., Ahlenius, S., and Engel, J. (1976). Stimulation of mounting behavior but not lordosis behavior in ovariectomized female rats by *p*-chlorophenylalanine. *Pharmacology, Biochemistry and Behavior*, **5**, 329–33.

Södersten, P., Henning, M., Melin, P., and Ludin, S. (1983). Vasopressin alters female sexual behaviour by acting on the brain independently of alterations in blood pressure. *Nature*, **301**, 608–10.

Södersten, P., de Vries, G.J., Buijs, R.M., and Melin, P. (1985). A daily rhythm in behavioral vasopressin sensitivity and brain vasopressin concentrations. *Neuroscience Letters*, **58**, 37–41.

Södersten, P., Forsberg, G., Bednar, I., Eneroth, P., and Wiesenfeld-Hallin, Z. (1989). Opioid peptide inhibition of sexual behaviour in female rats. In *Brain opioid systems in reproduction* (ed. R. Dyer and J. Bicknell), pp. 203–15, Oxford University Press.

Stavy, M. and Herbert, J. (1989). Differential effects of beta-endorphin infused into the hypothalamic pre-optic area at various phases of the male rats' sexual behaviour. *Neuroscience*, **30**, 433–42.

Stefanick, M.L., Smith, E.R., Clark, J.T., and Davidson, J.M. (1982). Effects of a potent dopamine receptor agonist, RDS-127, on penile reflexes and seminal emission in intact and spinally transected rats. *Physiology and Behavior*, **29**, 973–8.

Stefanick, M.L., Smith, E.R., Szumowski, D.A., and Davidson, J.M. (1983). Reproductive physiology and behavior in the male rat following acute and chronic peripheral adrenergic depletion by guanethidine. *Pharmacology, Biochemistry and Behavior*, **23**, 55–63.

Stern, J.M. (1990). Multisensory regulation of maternal behavior and masculine sexual behavior: a revised view. *Neuroscience and Biobehavioral Reviews*, **14**, 183–200.

Tagliamonte, A., Fratta, W., Del Fiacco, F., and Gessa, G.L. (1974). Possible stimulatory role of brain dopamine in the copulatory behavior of male rats. *Pharmacology, Biochemistry and Behavior*, **2**, 257–60.

Thody, A.J. and Wilson, C.A. (1983). Melanocyte stimulating hormone and the inhibition of sexual behaviour in the female rat. *Physiology and Behavior*, **31**, 67–72.

Thody, A.J., Wilson, C.A., and Everard, D. (1979). Facilitation and inhibition of sexual receptivity in the female rat by α-MSH. *Physiology and Behavior*, **22**, 447–50.

Thody, A.J., Wilson, C.A., and Everard, D. (1981). α-Melanocyte stimulating hormone stimulates sexual behaviour in the female rat. *Psychopharmacology*, **74**, 153–6.

Uphouse, L., Montanez, M., Richards-Hill, R., Caldarola-Pastuszka, M., and Droge, M. (1991). Effects of 8OH-DPAT on sexual behaviours of the proestrus rat. *Pharmacology, Biochemistry and Behavior*, **39**, 635–40.

Varthy, I. and Etgen, A.M. (1989). Hormonal activation of female sexual behavior is accompanied by hypothalamic norepinephrine release. *Journal of Neuroendocrinology*, **1**, 383–8.

Verma, S., Chhina, G.S., Mohan Kumar, V., and Singh, B. (1989). Inhibition of male sexual behavior by serotonin application in the medial preoptic area. *Physiology and Behavior*, **46**, 327–30.

Vincent, P.A., Thornton, J., and Feder, H.H. (1987). Possible role of alpha-2-noradrenergic receptors in modulation of sexual behavior in female guinea pigs. *Neuroendocrinology*, **46**, 10–13.

Vincent, P.A. and Feder, H.H. (1988). Alpha-1- and alpha-2-noradrenergic receptors modulate lordosis behavior in female guinea pigs. *Neuroendocrinology*, **48**, 477–81.

Vitale, M.L., Parisi, M.N., Chiochio, S.R., and Tramezzani, J.H. (1984). Median eminence serotonin involved in the proestrus gonadotrophin release. *Neuroendocrinology*, **39**, 136–41.

Wallen, K. (1990). Desire and ability: hormones and the regulation of female sexual behaviour. *Neuroscience and Biobehavioral Reviews*, **14**, 233–41.

Ward, I.L., Crowley, W.R., Zemplan, F.P., and Margules, D.L. (1975). Monoaminergic mediation of female sexual behavior. *Journal of Comparative Physiology and Psychology*, **88**, 53–61.

Warner, R.K., Thompson, J.T., Markowski, V.P., Loucks, J.A., Bazzett, T.J., Eaton, R.J. *et al.* (1991). Microinjection of the dopamine antagonist CIS-Dupenthixol into the MPOA impairs copulation, penile reflexes, and sexual motivation in male rats. *Brain Research*, **540**, 177–82.

Watson, N.V. and Gorzalka, B.B. (1990). Relation of spontaneous wet dog shakes and copulatory behavior in male rats. *Pharmacology, Biochemistry and Behavior*, **37**, 825–9.

Wiesenfeld-Hallin, Z. and Södersten, P. (1984). Spinal opiates affect sexual behaviour in rats. *Nature*, **309**, 257–8.

Wiesner, J.B. and Moss, R.L. (1984). Beta-endorphin suppression of lordosis behavior in female rats: Lack of effect of peripherally-administered naloxone. *Life Sciences*, **34**, 1455–62.

Wiesner, J.B. and Moss, R.L. (1986*a*). Suppression of receptive and proceptive behavior in ovariectomized, estrogen-progesterone-primed rats by intraventricular beta-endorphin: studies of behavioral specificity. *Neuroendocrinology*, **43**, 57–62.

Wiesner, J.B. and Moss, R.L. (1986b). Behavioral specificity of β-endorphin suppression of sexual behavior: differential receptor antagonism. *Pharmacology, Biochemistry and Behavior*, **24**, 1235–9.

Wilson, C.A. and Hunter, A.J. (1985a). Effects and mechanisms of action of *p*-chlorophenylalanine (PCPA) on sexual behaviour in the female rat. In *Psychopharmacology of sexual disorders*. No. 4 in series Biological Psychiatry–New Prospects (ed. M. Segal), pp. 33–49. Libbey, London.

Wilson, C.A. and Hunter, A.J. (1985b). Progesterone stimulates sexual behaviour in female rats by increasing 5HT activity on $5HT_2$ receptors. *Brain Research*, **333**, 223–9.

Wilson, C.A., Thody, A.J., and Everard, D. (1979). Effect of various ACTH analogs on lordosis behavior in the female rat. *Hormones and Behavior*, **13**, 293–300.

Wilson, C.A., Bonney, R.C., Everard, D.M., and Wise, J. (1982). Mechanisms of action of *p*-chlorophenylalanine in stimulating sexual receptivity in the female rat. *Pharmacology, Biochemistry and Behavior*, **16**, 777–84.

Wilson, C.A., James, M.D., Grierson, J.P., and Hole, D.R. (1991a). Involvement of catecholaminergic systems in the zona incerta in the steroidal control of gonadotrophin release and female sexual behaviour. *Neuroendocrinology*, **53**, 113–23.

Wilson, C.A., Thody, A., Hole, D.R., Grierson, J.P., and Celis, M.E. (1991b). Interaction of estradiol, αMSH and dopamine in the regulation of sexual receptivity in the female rat. *Neuroendocrinology*, **54**, 14–22.

Winn, P. (1991). Cholinergic stimulation of substantia nigra effects on feeding, drinking and sexual behaviour in the male rat. *Psychopharmacology*, **104**, 208–14.

Witcher, J.A. and Freeman, M.E. (1985). The proestrous surge of prolactin enhances sexual receptivity in the rat. *Biology of Reproduction*, **32**, 834–9.

Witt, D.M. and Insel, T.R. (1991). A selective oxytocin antagonist attenuates progesterone facilitation of female sexual behavior. *Endocrinology*, **128**, 3269–76.

Zadina, J.E., Kastin, A.J., Fabre, L.A., and Coy, D.H. (1981). Facilitation of sexual receptivity in the rat by an ovulation-inhibiting analog of LHRH. *Pharmacology, Biochemistry and Behavior*, **15**, 961–4.

Zemplan, F.P., Trulson, M.E., Howell, R., and Hoebel, B.G. (1977). Influence of *p*-chloramphetamine on female sexual reflexes and brain monoamine levels. *Brain Research*, **123**, 347–56.

2

The effect of dopaminergic and serotonergic agents on the lordosis response in female rats

Sven Ahlenius

INTRODUCTION

The dorsiflexion of the back of the female rat in response to male mounting, the lordosis reflex, is the most clear expression of sexual behaviour in the female. In addition to this, the female solicits male sexual activity by distinct presenting postures, 'darting' and 'hopping', accompanied by wiggling of the ears. The receptive female is also characterized by olfactory, and possibly also auditory, cues (see, for example, Bermant 1967; Pfaff *et al.* 1973). Under laboratory conditions, however, appetitive aspects of the behaviour are not allowed to play normally. The mating test is a well directed performance on a small stage with prepared actors given several rehearsals. Thus, the copulatory performance is in focus not necessarily because of a higher *a priori* interest, or validity of the observations for sexual functions generally, but because of its greater accessibility and reliability—to the extent that it has often been used as a model for studies on mammalian brain–behaviour relationships (see Pfaff 1989).

The regulation of female rat lordosis behaviour by ovarian hormones is well documented (Boling and Blandau 1939; see Beach 1948; Young 1961). Thus, the behaviour is suppressed by ovariectomy and can be restored by sequential treatment with oestrogen and progesterone, or by treatment with high oestrogen doses. In the early sixties, Meyerson (1964*b*) made the interesting observation that lordosis could be induced by reserpine treatment in oestrogen-primed female rats. Reserpine produces a depletion of monoamine stores in the nervous system (see Carlsson 1965), and the results suggested a monoaminergic link, directly or indirectly via effects on regulatory mechanisms of hormone release, in the mediation of lordosis behaviour. Results from these studies, and additional experiments with drugs affecting monoaminergic neurotransmission, led to the suggestion of an inhibitory serotonergic tone in the mediation of lordosis behaviour in the female rat (Meyerson 1964*c*). These initial observations of a monoaminergic link in hormone-dependent behaviour opened a new area of investigation, as evidenced by reports from a number of different laboratories (see Ahlenius *et al.* 1975; Carter and Davis 1977; Meyerson and Malmnäs 1978).

This chapter will focus on experiments in this field performed at the Departments of Psychology and Pharmacology at the University of Göteborg. Two topics have been of primary interest.

1. Possible involvement of brain catecholamines. Although the initial experiments on hormone–monoamine interactions, as cited above, indicated a role for brain serotonin, they did not exclude a possible role also for brain catecholamines. The first series of experiments to be described below addressed this question.

2. Functional differentiation of 5-hydroxytryptamine (5-HT) receptor sub-types. Following the initial characterization of 5-HT$_1$ and 5-HT$_2$ receptors (Peroutka and Snyder 1979), evidence for further sub-types and subdivisions within the major categories have been put forward at an accelerated rate (see, for example, Peroutka 1988). The second part of this chapter will present evidence for specific and different roles for 5-HT$_1$ and 5-HT$_2$ receptors.

BRAIN DOPAMINE IN THE MEDIATION OF LORDOSIS BEHAVIOUR IN THE FEMALE RAT

The evidence for an inhibitory role of brain serotonin in the mediation of lordosis behaviour in the female rat was based on different lines of investigation. Firstly, there was an induction of lordosis behaviour by reserpine or tetrabenazine treatment in ovariectomized, oestrogen-primed animals (Meyerson 1964*b*), and lordosis could also be induced by treatment with the tryptophan hydroxylase inhibitor *p*-chlorophenylalanine (PCPA) in the same preparation (Meyerson and Lewander 1970). Secondly, lordosis behaviour induced by sequential oestrogen–progesterone pretreatment in ovariectomized female rats was inhibited by subsequent treatment with the 5-HT precursor 5-hydroxytryptophan (5-HTP), but less so after treatment with the catecholamine precursor dihydroxyphenylalanine (DOPA) (Meyerson 1964*a,c*). In the precursor experiments, the animals were pretreated with an inhibitor of monoamine oxidase (MAO). Finally, it was not possible to induce lordosis by chlorpromazine treatment in ovariectomized, oestrogen-primed females (Meyerson 1966).

Needless to say, the conclusions regarding the serotonergic involvement in female rat lordosis behaviour were highly dependent on proposed mechanisms of action for the respective drug treatment. By themselves, none of these treatments selectively affects brain serotonergic or catecholaminergic neurotransmission, and the weight of convergent evidence from the different approaches is very much limited by multiple and unpredictable actions of the drugs or the drug combinations on brain monoaminergic neurotransmission. Thus, both reserpine and tetrabenazine, in the high doses used, deplete brain catecholamine and serotonin stores (see Carlsson 1965). PCPA not only inhibits tryptophan hydroxylase irreversibly, but also produces a reversible inhibition of brain tyrosine hydroxylase (Koe and Weissman 1966). Furthermore, the monoamine precursors 5-HTP and DOPA were administered to animals treated with an unselective MAO inhibitor, and the aromatic L-amino acid decarboxylase is widely distributed in brain tissues. Both these factors may account for the formation of 5-HT or catecholamines at inappropriate sites resulting in unspecific effects, directly or indirectly (see, for example, Butcher *et al.* 1970).

On the background sketched above, we decided to examine further the effects of tetrabenazine and PCPA, with particular attention to the effects of these treatments on brain catecholamine neurotransmission. In a first series of experiments, we followed the time course of action of tetrabenazine on lordosis behaviour and on whole-brain monoamine levels in ovariectomized, oestrogen-primed female rats. We used two doses of tetrabenazine, 2 and 10 mg kg^{-1}, in these studies. Both doses induced lordosis behaviour to the same degree and with the same duration. The effects on brain monoamine levels differed, however. The high dose treatment produced a depletion of brain dopamine (DA), noradrenaline (NA), as well as 5-HT, whereas the low dose only depleted brain DA stores, suggesting an inhibitory role also for brain dopaminergic neurotransmission (Ahlenius *et al.* 1972*b*) (Fig. 2.1). In subsequent experiments, we examined in a similar fashion the effects of PCPA in a dose of 150 mg kg^{-1}. The results demonstrated that administration of this acute dose of PCPA produced an increased lordosis response and, as assessed in parallel experiments, a depletion of DA, NA, and 5-HT (Fig. 2.2).

In order to investigate the effects of tyrosine hydroxylase inhibition separately, we used the tyrosine hydroxylase inhibitor α-methyl-*p*-tyrosine (AMPT) (Udenfriend *et al.* 1965). Results from this experiment made it clear that the lordosis response was facilitated concomitantly with a depletion of brain catecholamines (Ahlenius *et al.* 1972*a*), again suggesting that depletion of brain catecholamines was a sufficient condition for the facilitation of lordosis behaviour in ovariectomized, oestrogen-treated female rats. A causal connection was demonstrated in a subsequent experiment where it was shown that the facilitation of lordosis produced by AMPT could be antagonized by treatment with L-DOPA (Ahlenius *et al.* 1975). Although these latter experiments did not differentiate between the catecholamines DA and NA, our initial study with tetrabenazine suggested that DA may be the responsible agent (cf. Fig. 2.1).

Continued studies in other laboratories indeed support the notion that brain DA has an inhibitory role in the mediation of female rat lordosis

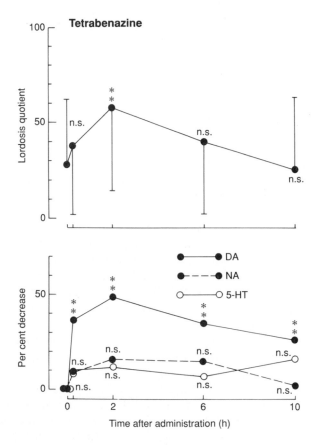

Fig. 2.1 Time course of action of tetrabenazine (2 mg kg^{-1}) on lordosis behaviour and on whole-brain monoamine levels in the oestrogen-primed, ovariectomized female rat. Statistical comparisons with controls, as indicated in the figure. For further details see Ahlenius *et al.* (1972*b*). Levels of statistical significance are indicated by n.s. ($p > 0.05$) and ** ($p < 0.01$).

behaviour. Thus, it was found that the selective DA receptor blocking agent pimozide facilitated lordosis behaviour in oestrogen-primed, ovariectomized females (Everitt *et al.* 1974, 1975). These observations were confirmed and extended in a recent report assigning a specific role for the DA D$_2$ receptor sub-type. By use of DA agonists and antagonists with selective affinity for the DA D$_1$ or the D$_2$ receptor site, it was concluded that there is an inhibitory DA D$_2$ receptor mediated mechanism in the control of female rat lordosis behaviour (Grierson *et al.* 1988).

   The basic model in the studies described so far has been the ovariectomized (sometimes also adrenalectomized, as discussed further below), oestrogen-primed female rat. It should be noted, however, that the same

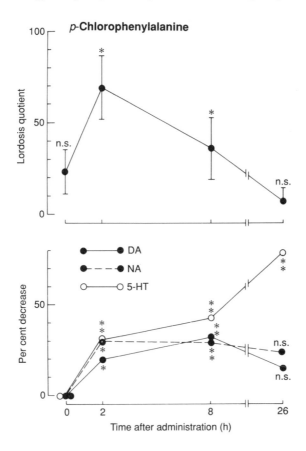

Fig. 2.2 Time course of action of *p*-chlorophenylalanine (150 mg kg^{-1}) on lordosis behaviour and whole-brain monoamine levels in the oestrogen-primed, ovariectomized female rat. Statistical comparisons with controls, as indicated in the figure. For further details see Ahlenius *et al.* (1972*a*). Levels of statistical significance are indicated by n.s. ($p > 0.05$) and ** ($p < 0.01$).

treatments which facilitate the display of lordosis might inhibit the response in fully receptive females. Furthermore, some dopaminergic agonists have been reported to have a biphasic pattern of effects: stimulation followed by inhibition (Sietnieks and Meyerson 1985; Foreman and Hall 1987; Grierson *et al.* 1988). The phasic effects may be due to preferential stimulation of inhibitory dopaminergic autoreceptors initially, followed by stimulation of postsynaptic receptors at higher doses. The anatomical site of the receptor population involved is not known, however, and this is a limiting factor in the interpretation of these findings. Thus, the intrinsic activity of a dopaminergic compound can be expected to interact with the receptor sensitivity pre- and postsynaptically, and this is of particular concern when discussing phasic effects induced by the treatment (see Carlsson 1983). The experiments using inhibitors of monoamine storage, or the experiments with inhibitors of monoamine synthesis, as described above (Ahlenius *et al.* 1972*a*,*b*; 1975), support the interpretation of autoreceptor-mediated effects by low agonist doses.

It is well known that the secretion of adrenocorticotrophic hormone (ACTH) release from the pituitary is under tonic noradrenergic inhibitory control in several species, including the rat (see Ganong 1974). It has been suggested that ACTH, as for example released by reserpine treatment, may release adrenal steroids, and that this mechanism could explain the facilitation of lordosis by drug treatments in ovariectomized, oestrogen-primed female rats (Feder and Ruf 1969; Paris *et al.* 1971; De Catanzaro and Gorzalka 1980). Such a mechanism may in fact explain a weak facilitation of lordosis by treatment with the DA-β-hydroxylase inhibitor FLA-63 in ovariectomized animals (Ahlenius *et al.* 1975). However, the pituitary–adrenal axis is probably not involved in the effects of dopaminergic drugs on the lordosis behaviour for two major reasons:

(1) in many of the studies cited above the experiments were performed on animals which were also adrenalectomized (e.g. Everitt *et al.* 1974, 1975; Grierson *et al.* 1988);

(2) the effects on ACTH by adrenergic drugs is primarily mediated via noradrenergic, rather than dopaminergic, mechanisms (see Meites and Sonntag 1981).

Taken together, the available evidence strongly suggests the existence of an inhibitory dopaminergic mechanism in the mediation of lordosis in the female rat. The specific receptor involved appears to be of the DA D_2 type. The pharmacological manipulations indicate a central site of action, although the precise location remains to be determined. Thus, in addition to the suggested inhibitory role for brain serotonin in the mediation of lordosis behaviour in the female rat, there is evidence that brain DA D_2 receptors also have a similar function.

5-HT$_1$ AND 5-HT$_2$ RECEPTOR MECHANISMS IN THE MEDIATION OF LORDOSIS BEHAVIOUR IN THE FEMALE RAT

Up to the recent introduction of new selective 5-HT agonists and antagonists, it was generally assumed that brain serotonin had an inhibitory function on sexual behaviour generally, in male as well as in female rats (see Meyerson and Malmnäs 1978; Larsson and Ahlenius 1985). It was thus of considerable interest when the serotonergic agonist 8-hydroxy-2-(di-*n*-

propylamino) tetralin (8-OHDPAT) (Arvidsson *et al.* 1981; Hjorth *et al.* 1982) was found to produce a marked facilitation of the male rat's sexual behaviour (Ahlenius *et al.* 1981). Following this initial observation of 8-OHDPAT as an anomalous serotonergic agent, a specific binding site, 5-HT$_{1A}$, has been described for this compound in brain tissue (Middlemiss and Fozard 1983; see Hamon *et al.* 1987). For further details on the effects of this and related serotonergic compounds on male rat sexual behaviour see Ahlenius and Larsson (1991). When administered to the female rat, however, 8-OHDPAT produced the suppression of lordosis expected by a serotonergic agonist (Ahlenius *et al.* 1986; Mendelson and Gorzalka 1986*b*; Fernandez-Guasti *et al.* 1987). Although this observation was in accord with the general view on the role of serotonin in the mediation of lordosis behaviour, other evidence as indicated above prompted further studies on the behavioural effects of this compound. It thus appeared that serotonergic inhibitory mechanisms of lordosis behaviour could be mediated via 5-HT$_{1A}$ receptors. The inhibition of lordosis by 8-OHDPAT was obtained with the same efficacy in ovariectomized animals where the behaviour was induced by oestrogen plus progesterone treatment as in animals given oestrogen alone. Furthermore, there was no facilitation of lordosis in animals maintained on a threshold dose of oestrogen (Ahlenius *et al.* 1986).

In a subsequent series of experiments we used a different model to further examine the role of 5-HT$_1$ and 5-HT$_2$ receptors in the mediation of female rat lordosis behaviour. Thus, we tested the ability of selective 5-HT$_1$ or 5-HT$_2$ antagonists to antagonize 5-HTP-induced suppression of lordosis behaviour (Ahlenius *et al.* 1989*b*). The lordosis response was induced by treating ovariectomized female rats with oestrogen alone (1.25 μg per animal for 3–4 days) or with oestrogen (1.25 μg per animal) plus progesterone (0.5 mg per animal). In order to enhance the selectivity of the 5-HTP treatment for serotonergic neurotransmission the animals were also given an inhibitor of peripheral 5-HTP decarboxylase (benserazide) as well as an inhibitor of neuronal 5-HT reuptake (zimeldine). As a typical 5-HT$_1$ antagonist we used (−)pindolol. This β-receptor blocking compound has also been demonstrated to possess antiserotonergic activity (Middlemiss *et al.* 1977; Costain and Green 1978), and has high affinity for the 5-HT$_{1A}$ receptor site (see Palacios *et al.* 1987). As a control for β-receptor mediated effects, we used the selective β-receptor blocking agent betaxolol (Cavero *et al.* 1983; Hoyer 1989). Pirenperone was selected as a 5-HT$_2$ antagonist (Colpaert *et al.* 1982; Hoyer *et al.* 1985).

The 5-HTP-induced suppression of lordosis was completely antagonized by the administration of (−)pindolol. Betaxolol had no effect, indicating that the effects of (−)pindolol were due to blockade of 5-HT receptors, rather than of β-adrenoceptors. (−)Pindolol was effective in both preparations of hormone treatment, oestrogen alone or oestrogen plus progesterone. Interestingly, pirenperone not only failed to antagonize the 5-HTP-induced

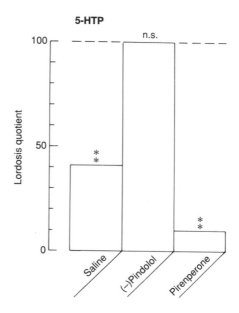

Fig. 2.3 Antagonism by (−)pindolol of 5-HTP-induced suppression of lordosis behaviour in the oestrogen-primed, ovariectomized female rat. All animals were treated with 5-HTP (25 mg kg^{-1}) before the administration of saline, (−)pindolol (2 mg kg^{-1}) or pirenperone (0.25 mg kg^{-1}). Statistical comparisons with oestrogen-treated controls (broken line), as shown in the figure. For further details see text and Ahlenius *et al.* (1989*b*). Levels of statistical significance are indicated by n.s. ($p > 0.05$) and ** ($p < 0.01$).

effects but also produced a further suppression of lordosis compared with 5-HTP-treated animals (Fig. 2.3).

Together these observations not only provide further support for an inhibitory 5-HT$_1$-receptor mediated link in the neural control of lordosis behaviour, but also suggest the possibility of an opposite, stimulatory role for the 5-HT$_2$ receptor. This is in agreement with conclusions reached by other investigators (Wilson and Hunter 1985; Mendelson and Gorzalka 1986*a*) based on results from other experimental models (see also Gorzalka *et al.* 1990).

As discussed in the previous section, it appears that central DA D$_2$ receptors have an inhibitory role similar to that proposed for 5-HT$_{1A}$ receptors. In agreement with this contention it has been found that the DA agonists apomorphine, quinpirole, and lisuride all suppress the display of lordosis behaviour (Sietnieks 1985; Fernandez-Guasti *et al.* 1987; Hlinak 1987).

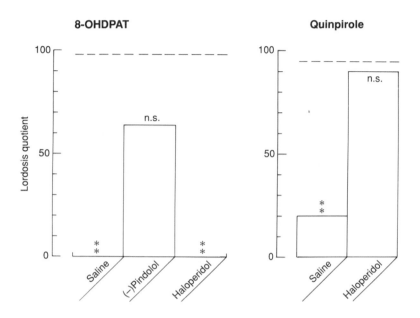

Fig. 2.4 Effects of (−)pindolol and haloperidol on 8-OHDPAT- or quinpirole-induced suppression of lordosis behaviour in oestrogen-primed, ovariectomized female rats. The animals were treated with 8-OHDPAT (0.25 mg kg^{-1}) or quinpirole (1.25 mg kg^{-1}) and treated with saline, (−)pindolol (2 mg kg^{-1}), or haloperidol (0.2 mg kg^{-1}). Statistical comparisons with oestrogen-treated controls (broken line), as shown in the figure. For further details see text and Fernandez-Guasti *et al.* (1987). Levels of statistical significance are indicated by n.s. ($p > 0.05$) and ** ($p < 0.01$).

Lisuride, however, has the interesting property of having agonist actions at both DA and 5-HT receptors (Kehr 1977). This, to some extent, also applies to 8-OHDPAT (Ahlenius *et al.* 1989*a*). Thus, in a separate series of experiments we investigated the effects of the 5-HT$_1$ receptor blocker (−)pindolol and the DA receptor blocking agent haloperidol on lisuride or 8-OHDPAT-induced suppression of lordosis. In both cases, the suppression of lordosis was antagonized by the administration of (−)pindolol, whereas haloperidol was ineffective. The suppression of lordosis produced by apomorphine or quinpirole was fully antagonized by the same dose of haloperidol (Fernandez-Guasti *et al.* 1987). These results provide further support for the operation of two separate mechanisms, one dopaminergic and one serotonergic, in the mediation of lordosis in the female rat (Fig. 2.4).

CONCLUDING REMARKS

As mentioned in the introduction, we have focused on one particular aspect of the female rat's sexual behaviour, the lordosis response. There is evidence to propose an inhibitory role for central dopaminergic (D_2) and serotonergic (5-HT_{1A}) inhibitory mechanisms in the physiological regulation of this behaviour. The interpretation of these findings for understanding the physiology of female rat reproductive behaviour is difficult, let alone generalizations across species to man. Nevertheless, attempts in this direction would be impossible without information of the kind presented here, even though there are pieces missing from the jigsaw puzzle. Inasmuch as the general scheme of supraspinal, spinal, and peripheral neural connections in urogenital and sexual functions in mammals are similar, it is possible that the exact neurotransmitter mechanisms discussed above could have retained a strategic position, although the means of expression might have changed in evolution. In the clinical context this means that we should look for possible side-effects on urogenital or sexual functions of selective DA D_2 receptor antagonists or agonists, as presently developed for treatment of schizophrenia and Parkinson's disease, respectively. Of particular interest is the new generation of anxiolytics, and possibly antidepressants, spearheaded by buspirone (see New 1990), which act as agonists at the 5-HT_{1A} receptor. New and selective compounds of this kind are now being developed in many laboratories in the pharmaceutical industry. Needless to say, it is important to identify possible side-effects. At the same time, however, the side-effects are clues to possible new therapies. It was also mentioned in the introduction that the clear and distinct response of lordosis behaviour has been a model system for studying the physiology of behaviour. The definition of neurotransmitter mechanisms participating in the mediation of this behavioural response can also be used to define and characterize the effects of new pharmacological agents. Our discoveries of the specific effects of 8-OHDPAT on central serotonergic neurotransmission exemplifies this latter approach, where we took advantage of the proposed role for serotonin in the mediation of male rat sexual behaviour (see Ahlenius and Larsson 1991).

REFERENCES

Ahlenius, S. and Larsson, K. (1991). Physiological and pharmacological implications of specific effects of 5-HT_{1A} agonists on rat sexual behavior. In *5-HT_{1A} agonists, 5-HT_3 antagonists and benzodiazepines: their comparative behavioural pharmacology* (ed. R.J. Rodgers and S.J. Cooper), pp. 281–315. John Wiley, Chichester, U.K.

Ahlenius, S., Engel, J., Eriksson, H., Modigh, K., and Södersten, P. (1972*a*). Importance of central catecholamines in the mediation of lordosis behaviour in ovariectomized rats treated with estrogen and inhibitors of monoamines synthesis. *Journal of Neural Transmission*, **33**, 247–55.

Ahlenius, S., Engel, J., Eriksson, H., and Södersten, P. (1972b). Effects of tetra-benazine on lordosis behaviour and on brain monoamines in the female rat. *Journal of Neural Transmission*, **3**, 155–62.

Ahlenius, S., Engel, J., Eriksson, H., Modigh, K., and Södersten, P. (1975). On the involvement of monoamines in the mediation of lordosis behavior. In *Sexual behavior: pharmacology and biochemistry* (ed. M. Sandler and G.L. Gessa), pp. 137–45. Raven, New York.

Ahlenius, S., Larsson, K., Svensson, L., Hjorth, S., Carlsson, A., Lindberg, P., Wikström, H., and Sanchez, D. (1981). Effects of a new type of 5-HT receptor agonist on male rat sexual behavior. *Pharmacology, Biochemistry and Behavior*, **15**, 785–92.

Ahlenius, S., Fernandez-Guasti, A., Hjorth, S., and Larsson, K. (1986). Suppression of lordosis behaviour by the putative 5-HT receptor agonist 8-OH-DPAT in the rat. *European Journal of Pharmacology*, **124**, 361–3.

Ahlenius, S., Hillegaart, V., and Wijkström, A. (1989a). Evidence for selective inhibition of limbic forebrain dopamine synthesis by 8-OH-DPAT in the rat. *Naunyn-Schmiedeberg's Archives of Pharmacology*, **339**, 551–6.

Ahlenius, S., Larsson, K., and Fernandez-Guasti, A. (1989b). Evidence for the involvement of central 5-HT$_{1A}$ receptors in the mediation of lordosis behavior in the female rat. *Psychopharmacology*, **98**, 440–4.

Arvidsson, L.E., Hacksell, U., Nilsson, J.L.G., Hjorth, S., Carlsson, A., Lindberg, P., Sanchez, D., and Wikström, H. (1981). 8-Hydroxy-2-(di-n-propylamino) tetralin, a new centrally acting 5-hydroxytryptamine receptor agonist. *Journal of Medicinal Chemistry*, **24**, 921–3.

Beach, F.A. (1948). *Hormones and behavior*. Cooper Square, New York.

Bermant, G. (1967). Copulation in rats. *Psychology Today*, **1**, 53–60.

Boling, J.L. and Blandau, R.J. (1939). The estrogen–progesterone induction of mating responses in the spayed female rat. *Endocrinology*, **25**, 359–64.

Butcher, L., Engel, J., and Fuxe, K. (1970). L-Dopa induced changes in central monoamine neurons after peripheral decarboxylase inhibition. *Journal of Pharmacy and Pharmacology*, **22**, 313–16.

Carlsson, A. (1965). Drugs which block the storage of 5-hydroxytryptamine and related amines. In *Handbook of experimental pharmacology* (ed. O. Eichler and A. Farah), pp. 529–92. Springer, Berlin.

Carlsson, A. (1983). Dopamine receptor agonists: intrinsic activity vs state of the receptor. *Journal of Neural Transmission*, **57**, 309–15.

Carter, C.S. and Davis, J.M. (1977). Biogenic amines, reproductive hormones and female sexual behavior: a review. *Biobehavioral Reviews*, **1**, 213–24.

Cavero, I., Lefevre-Borg, F., Manoury, P., and Roach, A.G. (1983). *In vitro* and *in vivo* pharmacological evaluation of betaxolol, a new potent and selective β_1-adrenoceptor antagonist. In *Betaxolol and other β_1-adrenoceptor antagonists* (ed. P.L. Morselli, J.R. Kilborn, I. Cavero, D.C. Harrison, and S.Z. Langer), pp. 31–42. Raven, New York.

Colpaert, F.C., Niemegeers, C.J.E., and Janssen, P.A.J. (1982). A drug discrimination analysis of lysergic acid diethylamide (LSD): *in vivo* agonist and antagonist effects of purported 5-hydroxytryptamine antagonists and of pirenperone, a LSD-antagonist. *Journal of Pharmacology and Experimental Therapeutics*, **221**, 206–14.

Costain, D.W. and Green, A.R. (1978). β-Adrenoceptor antagonists inhibit the behavioural responses of rats to increased brain 5-hydroxytryptamine. *British Journal of Pharmacology*, **64**, 193–200.

De Catanzaro, D. and Gorzalka, B.B. (1980). Effects of dexamethasone, cortico-sterone, and ACTH on lordosis in ovariectomized and adrenalectomized-ovariectomized rats. *Pharmacology, Biochemistry and Behavior*, **12**, 201–6.

Everitt, B.J., Fuxe, K., and Hökfelt, T. (1974). Inhibitory role of dopamine and 5-hydroxytryptamine in the sexual behavior of female rats. *European Journal of Pharmacology*, **29**, 184–91.

Everitt, B.J., Fuxe, K., Hökfelt, T., and Jonsson, G. (1975). Role of monoamines in the control by hormones of sexual receptivity in the female rat. *Journal of Comparative Physiology and Psychology*, **89**, 556–72.

Feder, H.H. and Ruf, K.B. (1969). Stimulation of progesterone release and estrous behavior by ACTH in ovariectomized rodents. *Endocrinology*, **84**, 171–4.

Fernandez-Guasti, A., Ahlenius, S., Hjorth, S., and Larsson, K. (1987). Separation of dopaminergic and serotonergic inhibitory mechanisms in the mediation of estrogen-induced lordosis behaviour in the rat. *Pharmacology, Biochemistry and Behavior*, **27**, 93–8.

Foreman, M.M. and Hall, J.L. (1987). Effects of D_2-dopaminergic receptor stimula-tion on the lordotic response of female rats. *Psychopharmacology*, **91**, 96–100.

Ganong, W.F. (1974). Brain mechanisms regulating the secretion of the pituitary gland. In *The neurosciences: third study program* (ed. F.O. Schmitt and F.G. Worden), pp. 549–63. MIT Press, Cambridge, MA, U.S.A.

Gorzalka, B.B., Mendelson, S.D., and Watson, N.V. (1990). Serotonin receptor subtypes and sexual behavior. *Annals of the New York Academy of Sciences*, **600**, 435–44.

Grierson, J.P., James, M.D., Pearson, J.R., and Wilson, C.A. (1988). The effect of selective D_1 and D_2 dopaminergic agents on sexual receptivity in the female rat. *Neuropharmacology*, **27**, 181–9.

Hamon, M., Emerit, M.B., El Mestikawy, S., Verge, D., Daval, G., Marquet, A., and Gozlan, H. (1987). Pharmacological, biochemical and functional properties of 5-HT_{1A} receptor binding sites labelled by [^{3}H]8-hydroxy-2-(di-*n*-propylamino) tetralin in the rat brain. In *Brain 5-HT_{1A} receptors* (ed. C.T. Dourish, S. Ahlenius, and P. Hutson), pp. 34–51. Ellis Horwood, Chichester, NJ, USA.

Hjorth, S., Carlsson, A., Lindberg, P., Sanchez, D., Wikström, H., Arvidsson, L.-E., Hacksell, U., and Nilsson, J.L.G. (1982). 8-Hydroxy-2-(di-*n*-propylamino) tetralin, 8-OH-DPAT, a potent and selective simplified ergot congener with central 5-HT-receptor stimulating activity. *Journal of Neural Transmission*, **55**, 169–88.

Hlinak, Z. (1987). Lisuride inhibits temporarily sexual behavior in female rats. *Pharmacology, Biochemistry and Behavior*, **27**, 211–15.

Hoyer, D. (1989) 5-Hydroxytryptamine receptors and effector coupling mechanism in peripheral tissues. In *The peripheral actions of 5-hydroxytryptamine* (ed. J.R. Fozard), pp. 72–99. Oxford University Press.

Hoyer, D., Engel, G., and Kalkman, H.O. (1985). Molecular pharmacology of 5-HT_1 and 5-HT_2 recognition sites in rat and pig brain membranes: radioligand binding studies with [^{3}H]5-HT, [^{3}H]8-OH-DPAT, ($-$)[^{125}I] iodocyanopindolol, [^{3}H]mesulergine and [^{3}H]ketanserin. *European Journal of Pharmacology*, **118**, 13–23.

Kehr, W. (1977). Effect of lisuride and other ergot derivatives on monoaminergic mechanisms in rat brain. *European Journal of Pharmacology*, **41**, 261–73.

Koe, B.K. and Weissman, A. (1966). *p*-Chlorophenylalanine: a specific depletor of brain serotonin. *Journal of Pharmacology and Experimental Therapeutics*, **154**, 499–516.

Larsson, K. and Ahlenius, S. (1985). Masculine sexual behavior and brain mono-amines. In *Psychopharmacology of sexual disorders* (ed. M. Segal), pp. 15–32. John Libbey, London.

Meites, J. and Sonntag, W.E. (1981). Hypothalamic hypophysiotropic hormones and neurotransmitter regulation: current views. *Annual Review of Pharmacology and Toxicology*, **21**, 295–322.

Mendelson, S.D. and Gorzalka, B.B. (1986*a*). Serotonin type 2 antagonists inhibit lordosis behavior in the female rat: reversal with quipazine. *Life Sciences*, **38**, 33–9.

Mendelson, S.D. and Gorzalka, B.B. (1986*b*). 5-HT$_{1A}$ receptors: differential in-volvement in female and male sexual behavior in the rat. *Physiology and Behavior*, **37**, 345–51.

Meyerson, B.J. (1964*a*). The effect of neuropharmacological agents on hormone-activated estrus behaviour in ovariectomised rats. *Archives of International Pharmacodynamics*, **150**, 4–33.

Meyerson, B.J. (1964*b*). Estrus behavior in spayed rats after estrogen or progester-one treatment in combination with reserpine or tetrabenazine. *Psychopharma-cologia* (Berlin), **6**, 210–18.

Meyerson, B.J. (1964*c*). Central nervous monoamines and hormone induced estrus behaviour in the spayed rat. *Acta Physiologica Scandinavia*, **63** (Suppl. 241), 1–32.

Meyerson, B.J. (1966). Oestrous behaviour in oestrogen treated ovariectomized rats after chlorpromazine alone or in combination with progesterone, tetrabenazine or reserpine. *Acta Pharmacologica et Toxicologica*, **24**, 363–76.

Meyerson, B.J. and Lewander, T. (1970). Serotonin synthesis inhibition and estrous behavior in female rats. *Life Sciences*, **9**, 661–71.

Meyerson, B.J. and Malmnäs, C.-O. (1978). Brain monoamines and sexual behavior. In *Biological determinants of sexual behavior* (ed. J.B. Hutchinson), pp. 521–54. Wiley, London.

Middlemiss, D.N. and Fozard, J.R. (1983). 8-Hydroxy-2-(di-*n*-propylamino)tetralin discriminates between subtypes of the 5-HT$_1$ recognition site. *European Journal of Pharmacology*, **90**, 151–3.

Middlemiss, D.N., Blakeborough, L., and Leather, S.R. (1977). Direct evidence for an interaction of β-adrenergic blockers with the 5-HT receptor. *Nature*, **267**, 289–90.

New, J.S. (1990). The discovery and development of buspirone, a new approach to the treatment of anxiety. *Medicinal Research Reviews*, **10**, 283–326.

Palacios, J.M., Pazos, A., and Hoyer, D. (1987). Characterization and mapping of 5-HT$_{1A}$ sites in the brain of animals and man. In *Brain 5-HT$_{1A}$ receptors* (ed. C.T. Dourish, S. Ahlenius, and P.H. Hutson), pp. 67–81. Ellis Horwood, Chichester, NJ, USA.

Paris, C.A., Resko, J.A., and Goy, R.W. (1971). A possible mechanism for the induction of lordosis by reserpine in spayed rats. *Biology of Reproduction*, **4**, 23–30.

Peroutka, S.J. (1988). 5-Hydroxytryptamine receptor subtypes: molecular, bio-chemical and physiological characterization. *TIPS*, **11**, 496–500.

Peroutka, S.J. and Snyder, S.H. (1979). Multiple serotonin receptors: differential binding of [^{3}H] 5-hydroxytryptamine, [^{3}H] lysergic acid diethylamide and [^{3}H] spiroperidol. *Molecular Pharmacology*, **16**, 687–99.

Pfaff, D.W. (1989). Features of a hormone-driven defined neural circuit for a mammalian behavior. Principles illustrated, neuroendocrine syllogisms, and multiplicative steroid effects. *Annals of the New York Academy of Sciences*, **563**, 131–47.

Pfaff, D.W., Lewis, C., Diakow, C., and Keiner, M. (1973). Neurophysiological analysis of mating behavior responses as hormone-sensitive reflexes. *Progress in Physiology and Psychology*, **5**, 253–97.

Sietnieks, A. (1985). Involvement of 5-HT_2 receptors in the LSD- and L-5-HTP induced suppression of lordotic behavior in the female rat. *Journal of Neural Transmission*, **61**, 65–80.

Sietnieks, A. and Meyerson, B.J. (1985). Effect of domperidone on apomorphine inhibition of the copulatory response and exploratory behaviour in the female rat. *Acta Pharmacologica et Toxicologica*, **57**, 160–5.

Udenfriend, S., Zaltzman-Nirenberg, P., and Nagatsu, T. (1965). Inhibitors of purified beef adrenal tyrosine hydroxylase. *Biochemical Pharmacology*, **14**, 837–45.

Wilson, C.A. and Hunter, A.J. (1985). Progesterone stimulates sexual behaviour in female rats by increasing 5-HT activity on 5-HT_2 receptors. *Brain Research*, **333**, 223–9.

Young, W.C. (ed.) (1961). The hormones and mating behavior. In *Sex and internal secretions* (ed. W.C. Young), pp. 1173–239. Williams and Wilkins, Baltimore, NJ, USA.

3

Animal models of human sexual behaviour

Ronald J. Barfield

INTRODUCTION

Human sexual behaviour is properly studied in humans; however, animal models provide insights and information not easily obtained from studies on people. Basic research with animal model systems can lead to the discovery of basic principles and mechanisms. For example, the use of the neurotoxin, N-methyl-4-phenyl-1,2,5,6-tetrahydropyridine HCL (MPTP), in rodents and primates has proved a useful model system for elucidating possible pathophysiologic mechanisms underlying Parkinson's disease (Langston *et al.* 1984). The discovery of such principles and mechanisms can lead to rational therapies for disorders traced to common mechanisms in humans. Basic research on healthy humans is at best difficult if at all possible.

The use of animal model systems can be viewed as an application of the comparative method. As such, it has inherent strengths and weaknesses. The strength of the comparative method is that the study of how different animals carry out related functions can lead to an understanding of basic mechanisms common among the species in question. For example, castration of male livestock leads to a decline in aggression resulting in ease of handling. Castration of men results in a reduction of sexual aggressive pathologies (Bradford 1988). The mechanism is not understood in detail, but it is reasonable to believe that common androgen-sensitive neural targets which mediate sex-related aggressive behaviour must be involved.

An animal model also has potential weaknesses. A behavioural or physiological end-point may appear alike in humans and animals, but in fact may be only analogous rather than homologous. For example, different kinds of aggressive expression may reflect different underlying motivational states, for example, sexual motivation, feeding, and so on and may be under the control of different underlying mechanisms and stimulus variables.

Thus for the comparative approach to be maximally effective, it is essential that there is a comprehensive understanding of the behaviour of the animal model as well as of the human, at least as far as possible. As Beach stated the problem, 'The validity of interspecific generalization can never exceed the reliability of intraspecific analysis; and the latter is an indispensable antecedent of the former' (Beach 1979). Development of a suitable animal model system is not always based on a comparative analysis. At times it is profitable to use an 'experimental model' in which one measures drug effects on a functional output apparently unrelated to the condition for which the drug is considered in humans. In such cases (for example, rotorod screening tests for sedatives) the results have good predictive value with respect to the effects on the human condition, but there should be no assumption of a common underlying mechanism. Whether a comparative animal model system or an experimental model system is chosen depends upon the behaviour to be studied and the strategies available. Either system may be useful or misleading so it is important to keep in mind the strength and weaknesses of the approach selected.

THE RAT AS AN ANIMAL MODEL FOR SEXUAL BEHAVIOUR

Although any number of species at various phylogenetic levels may serve as useful model systems, the rat is the most commonly used. For this reason I will describe rat sexual behaviour in some detail and illustrate the use of this model with examples based on studies in this species. The rat, however, is not suitable for questions related to all aspects of sexual behaviour so at times, reference will be made to studies employing other animal models.

The popularity of the rat as a model system is in part due to its practicality and in part to its suitability. Rats are relatively easy to handle, breed well in captivity, and are very hardy and adaptable. Their moderate size makes them good subjects for surgical procedures, and many can be housed in relatively small spaces. Rats possess a complex social organization and their behaviour is easy to observe in the laboratory.

Rats are an ideal subject for many kinds of behavioural studies ranging from developmental learning experiments to those concerned with sociosexual behaviour. They perform well with observers present and they possess a rich behavioural repertoire. Rats are territorial and highly social. Their social organization is probably polygynous with a dominant male defending a territory in which several females reside. These animals communicate with olfactory cues as well as ultrasonic vocalizations.

Although rats exhibit complex patterns of sociosexual behavioural interaction, their behaviour is highly predictable and is therefore easily replicated in laboratories around the world. For example, if a particular drug were tested for its effect on some aspect of rat sexual behaviour, it would be expected that results would be the same from laboratory to laboratory as long as the same methodology was used. These factors undoubtedly account for the fact that rats are employed in the majority of studies on all phases of reproductive behaviour.

Rat sociosexual behaviour

If we are to have a viable model for sexual behaviour we must, as Beach has advised, strive toward a complete understanding of the behaviour of the species in question (Beach 1979). With the rat, we probably come as close or closer than with any other species used as animal models. In describing rat sociosexual behaviour, the sexes will at times be discussed separately. But it must be kept in mind that the animals are in continuous interaction and that the behaviour of one subject is a critical variable that can influence the behaviour of the other subject under study.

Behaviour of the mating pair

The normal intact female comes into heat or behavioural oestrus on the third day of a four-day oestrous cycle, or some hours after parturition (post-partum oestrus). In fact, in nature, the female probably rarely exhibits oestrus cycles at all, except at the start of the breeding season. The rest of the time she is probably pregnant, lactating, or both.

As the female enters the third day of her cycle, oestradiol levels are high and progesterone begins to rise leading to proestrus. At this time, the female shows interest in the male, and increases scent marking; ultrasonic mating calls reach a peak (Matochik *et al.* 1992). As the time of oestrus and ovulation approaches, the female begins to exhibit proceptive behaviour (Beach 1976). This behaviour is sometimes referred to as solicitation activity and consists of a number of component responses. First, the female orients her body at right angles to the male and then turns and runs from him. At the end of her run she may exhibit some darting activity and sometimes a rapid rotation of the head on its long axis which results in 'ear wiggling' (McClintock 1984). During her orienting or running behaviour she may also emit ultrasonic mating calls. These calls have a complex structure and occur at frequencies well beyond the range of human hearing, around 50 kHz (Thomas and Barfield 1985).

If the female is with a sexually active male, he follows as she runs away. During this time he may emit ultrasonic mating calls similar to those of the female (Sales 1972). These calls increase the rate of female solicitation behaviour. After a brief bout of running, depending on the space available, the female stops in a crouched posture. The male might sniff or nudge the female leading to her assumption of the 'lordosis posture', an exaggerated dorsiflexion of the spine which exposes her perineal region. At times, the female assumes the lordosis posture only after the male mounts, with pelvic thrusting and palpation of her torso with his forepaws. As the male makes several shallow thrusts, the penis moves closer to the vagina. If the female is receptive she orients her vaginal orifice toward the probing penis.

A brief insertion (intromission) usually, but not always, occurs following such a mount with thrusting. This intromission lasts only a fraction of a second (0.25–0.5 s). The male and female generally separate after an intromission and both groom their genitals. The next episode of mounting will occur 30 s to 5 min after the previous intromission. The time depends on the size of the cage and individual variation in mating speed. The average interval between intromission is about 5 min in a large enclosure compared with 30–60 s in the small test cages most commonly used.

Either the male or the female may initiate the next bout of mounting and intromission and both sexes possess a similar copulatory rhythm. After about 10 to 12 regularly spaced intromissions, the male ejaculates. Following ejaculation, the male enters a post-ejaculatory refractory period. The female, for her part, displays a longer latency before attempting to reinitiate copulation following an intromission.

Approximately 30 s after ejaculation, the male begins to emit a 22 kHz ultrasonic post-ejaculatory call (Barfield and Geyer 1972). These monotonic whistles continue for about 4 min. After cessation of 22 kHz calling, the male becomes alert and within 1–2 min reinitiates mounting.

During the time the male emits the 22 kHz vocalization, he exhibits a sleep-like electroencephalographic (EEG) pattern. In contrast, when moving or sniffing about the cage, an alert, awake EEG pattern is evident (Barfield and Geyer 1975).

The male and female continue to interact as before, but the male ejaculates after only three to five intromissions. Another series of intromissions follows a somewhat longer second post-ejaculatory refractory period and the pattern repeats for four to eight ejaculations. When the male does not reinitiate a bout of mounting and intromission for 30 min after the previous ejaculation, he is considered to be sexually exhausted (Sachs and Barfield 1976).

Sexual reflexes

The genital reflexes of male rats can be observed in both intact as well as spinalectomized animals. A male is placed on its back and gentle pressure is applied at the base of the penis, leading to erections, 'flips' (rapid dorsal flips of the phallus), 'cups' (a flaring response of the glans) and, at times ejaculation. These responses represent penile actions which occur during actual copulation, but can be isolated in this manner to study mechanisms of control independently of behavioural interaction with other animals (Sachs 1983).

Females, too, exhibit lordosis reflexes in response to manual stimulation of the flanks or to vaginal–cervical stimulation. Again this form of analysis allows controlling mechanisms to be studied independently of behavioural interaction with a potential mate.

Measures of sexual behaviour

From the complex interactions described above, numerous objective measures can be obtained. Experiments are usually designed not to observe the entire complex sequence of sexual behaviour, but rather to assess specific measures. As will be illustrated later, this can lead to misleading or erroneous conclusions.

Female measures

There are five proceptive responses that can be objectively scored:

(1) marking behaviour—the female drags her perineum over an object depositing some sebaceous substance or urine;

(2) ultrasonic mating calls—50 kHz vocalizations can be counted using an ultrasonic detector commonly known as a bat detector;

(3) darting or hopping behaviour—a stiff-legged rapid movement distinct from walking or running;

(4) ear wiggling—rapid rotation of the head which results in an apparent vibration of the ears;

(5) orientation—the female orients at right angles to the male before running away.

Each of these responses is measured in terms of frequency per unit time. In addition, the latency to the first display of each pattern can also serve as a useful measure.

These proceptive responses are generally considered to be indicative of the female's sexual motivation, as they require her initiative.

The display of the lordosis response is generally considered to be an indication of receptivity, in contrast to proceptivity. Lordosis is a reflexive response to mounting by the male. This is not to say, however, that the ease of elicitation of the lordosis response does not vary with the sexual motivation of the female. Lordosis is generally measured in terms of the lordosis quotient (LQ). This measure is derived by dividing the number of lordosis responses observed by the number of mounts received from a sexually experienced male. Usually the LQ is based on a test consisting of ten mounts by the male. In addition, the intensity of the lordosis response is sometimes assessed according to a numerical score of one to three (Hardy and DeBold 1971). This so-called lordosis score (LS) may be a reliable indicator of overall female sexual responsiveness.

Measures of male sexual behaviour

The male displays a number of responses which serve to attract and orient the female to his presence. He, like the female, emits ultrasonic mating calls, exhibits scent markings, and may also nuzzle, nudge, or sniff the female when he encounters her. All of these responses can be counted and expressed as a frequency measure or in terms of the latency to the first response in a test.

Male copulatory activity, on the other hand, presents a rich array of basic measures that can then be used to derive more complex indices of male sexual activity. Mounts, intromissions, and ejaculations can all be counted and expressed in terms of frequency and they can be expressed in terms of latency to the first appearance of a particular response. In addition, the actual temporal patterning of these responses can be expressed so that one can reveal a picture of not only how many instances of a response occurred but how these responses were distributed in time (Sachs and Barfield 1976).

The post-ejaculatory refractory period and its associated post-ejaculatory 22 kHz vocalization can also be described in terms of the duration for which these phases of the sexual response persist.

Derived measures

The rate of copulation can be expressed by dividing the latency until ejaculation by the number of intromissions that occur before ejaculation. This ratio yields the average interval between intromissions. This rate measure may reflect sexual motivation or merely fluctuations in the oscillator that drives the temporal patterning of male sexual behaviour.

Another useful measure is that of the ratio of mount to intromissions in a copulatory sequence. This measure of copulatory efficiency (sometimes called 'hit rate') is a much more useful measure of sexual activity than mount frequency would be. Mount frequency by itself may only reflect the inability of a male to gain insertion a high proportion of the time.

Measures of genital reflexes

The frequency and temporal patterning of phallic responses provides a valuable model for the assessment of the effects of drugs and hormones on reflexive components of these male sexual responses. As these responses are elicited in both intact and spinalectomized animals the relative contribution of cerebral and spinal mechanisms can be evaluated. In addition it is possible to evaluate psychogenic or behavioural influences on these basic processes.

To which aspects of human sexual response can the foregoing measures be related? This is the crux of the problem. An attempt at such an assignment must be cautious. Just because a behaviour pattern in a model system seems to reflect the human condition, this does not necessarily make it a true reflection. For example, to use mount frequency as a measure of male sexual motivation could be very misleading—observations of mating pairs of rats reveal that large numbers of mounts reflect an inefficient copulatory reaction on the part of the male, an uncooperative female, or poor communication between the mating pair. Similarly, rapid mating (including the rapid attainment of ejaculation) could on one hand be considered as a reflection of increased sexual desire, but on the other hand it might prove a good animal model for premature ejaculation.

COORDINATION OF REPRODUCTIVE BEHAVIOUR

From a biological point of view, the functional significance of sexual behaviour is reproduction. This is an obvious, but often overlooked, point. The patterns of behaviour and their underlying mechanisms have evolved in a manner consistent with the maximization of reproductive success. Therefore, to understand the mechanisms that govern sexual behaviour, it is essential to understand their role in the reproductive process of the species. No one would consider a study of feeding disorders without a basic appreciation of nutritional processes, yet often we study sexual behaviour without an appreciation of the reproductive processes that they serve.

The biological foundation of reproductive processes is phylogenetically old and very conservative for reasons that are obvious. What has changed over time are the details of patterns of behaviour and the expression of the underlying mechanisms. On the other hand the fundamental mechanisms remain under the control of the same hypothalamic, brainstem, and spinal mechanisms.

Insights into how mechanisms function in one species may lead to an understanding of functions in another provided that there is an understanding of where the particular behavioural elements fit in the reproductive process. For example, would a large number of intromissions in the male rat be indicative of a high level of mating activity, or would, rather, the more rapid attainment of ejaculation following fewer intromissions? Would then fewer intromissions be indicative of an optimal pattern of mating behaviour with respect to the reproductive process? As will be discussed below, attainment of ejaculation after a short time and relatively fewer intromissions may in fact be reproductively maladaptive.

Coordination of reproductive activity in the rat

The multiple intromission–multiple ejaculation pattern in rats is explicable in terms of the attainment of pregnancy by the female. In some strains of laboratory rat and probably in the wild, females becomes pregnant only after receiving a large number of intromissions (10 to 20) and more than one ejaculation from the male (Austin and Dewsbury 1986; Barfield, unpublished results). The neuroendocrine apparatus of the female counts the number of intromissions and measures the intervals between them. Only when there is sufficient vaginal–cervical stimulation is the neuroendocrine reflex triggered resulting in a release of luteotrophic hormone (LTH) which maintains the corpus luteum in a manner analogous to the action of chorionic gonadotrophin in humans. Thus the female does not become pregnant merely as a result of sperm being present in her reproductive tract. The female must have stimulation sufficient to trigger LTH release and sperm transport (Adler and Toner 1986). Therefore, the sexual behaviour of the species directly affects reproductive physiology. Parenthetically, in some so-called reflexly ovulating species such as cats and rabbits, copulatory stimulation is required to trigger the ovulatory surge of LH (Everett 1961). In all probability, copulatory stimulation may, at times, lead to an advancement of ovulation in so-called spontaneously ovulating species, which may explain why there is a higher than expected number of pregnancies resulting from rape (Zarrow and Clark 1968; Clark and Zarrow 1971).

The multiple intromission pattern serves two functions. First, it leads to ejaculation by the male and, secondly, it triggers the luteotrophic response of the female which is necessary for pregnancy. Both the male and female count and time the intervals between intromissions. For each sex, there is an optimal number of intromissions and an optimal interval between them. The optimal interval for the female is upwards of five minutes with the effectiveness of each intromission dropping off as intervals become shorter or longer (Edmonds *et al.* 1972). Similarly, in the male, too long an interval between intromissions results in a delay in ejaculation or failure to ejaculate at all (Sachs and Barfield 1976).

Following ejaculation, the male refractory period serves not only to curb the sex drive and ultimately to quell it, but it is also necessary to allow the newly impregnated female to transport sperm effectively through her reproductive tract on the way to fertilization of the ova. Should another male mate with the female before about six minutes has elapsed, the pregnancy is blocked due to the disruption of the sperm plug and interruption of sperm transport. During the refractory period the male is hyperaggressive to other males (Thor and Flannelly 1979) but may show an interest in the female and actively prevent others from mating with her (Barfield and Thomas 1986). After about three ejaculations, the male will allow another to mate with the female that he has already successfully impregnated. It appears, therefore, that the male protects his parental investment only so long as is necessary in order to ensure his paternity.

It has been suggested that the clutching reaction observed in female rhesus monkeys may signal that orgasm has occurred (Zumpe and Michael 1968). After exhibiting the clutching reaction the female often exhibits contractions of her lower abdomen. At times, the female rushes away from the male leaving him ejaculating into thin air. One might speculate that in such species, the function of the female's orgasm is to synchronize the orgasm of the male with hers so that her reproductive contractions could aid in the transport of semen at the time of its delivery. Were this true, it would suggest an alteration of our thoughts on simultaneous orgasm and demonstrate just how maladaptive a premature ejaculation would be in a reproductive as well as in a behavioural context.

This brief account of reproduction coordination in rats demonstrates that optimality for reproductive success is not equivalent to a greater quantity of events or to greater rapidity or intensity of responses. Rather we see that reproductively optimal intromission and ejaculatory behaviour proceeds at a moderate pace. This suggests that our behavioural end-points ought not appear on a monotonic scale, but rather should be modal for the species involved. Thus an agent that speeds the rate of copulation in our rat model may very well be disruptive sexually in a human application.

DOMESTICATION OF THE HUMAN SPECIES

Our animal models are domesticated species and the process of domestication results in an alteration of reproductive behaviour and physiology. Therefore we can only speculate on the natural conditions and biological significance of patterns of reproductive behaviour.

Humans, too, have been domesticated. As we have practised husbandry on our domesticated species such as hens (300 eggs per year) or dairy cattle (constant lactation), we regulate our own reproduction and as a result may have altered fundamental patterns of human sexual behaviour.

In our early human ancestors, reproductive maturity probably did not anticipate physical maturity as today it does so dramatically. Young adults mated, pregnancy ensued, and pregnancy and lactation occupied the next 20 to 30 months. There were probably no ovulatory cycles during intensive lactation and probably a general reduction in female sexual behaviour (Stern 1986). How males' sexual behaviour might have been affected by such a reproductive pattern remains an interesting question.

In modern society we speak of 'normal' menstrual cycles, but in our ancient ancestors menstrual cycles were probably very abnormal and indicative of reproductive inactivity due to social or physiological problems. Indeed, in ancient Greece mental illness in barren women ('hysteria') was attributed to the inability to conceive (Katchadourian and Lunde 1975).

Thus menstrual cycles are a product of our own domestication and in these terms many problems both sexual as well as clinical/pathological may be understood better. Women did not evolve to display perpetual cyclic sexual appetites, nor does an ovary that proceeds through 13 ovulatory cycles a year reflect a biological entity that is the human female. Finally, in the application of the comparative method, to profit from the use of an animal model, we must also maintain a cross-cultural perspective. Norms of human sexuality vary broadly from culture to culture and certainly within modern western societies (Ford and Beach 1951).

APPLICATION OF THE MODEL

Profitable application of an animal model requires both a thorough understanding of the behaviour of the model species as well as a thorough and objective understanding of the human behaviour in question. In order for the model to be useful therapeutically, it is necessary to have as thorough an understanding as possible of the relationship between behavioural elements and their underlying causal mechanisms. Clearly, there are deficiencies in both areas; but acknowledging this, we can still proceed, with reasonable caution.

A functional analysis of masculine copulatory behaviour in the rat reveals cohorts of related behavioural responses. Based on factor analysis, Sachs (1978) posed four such cohorts: an initiation factor, a hit-rate factor, an intromission count factor, and a copulatory rate factor. These functionally related groups of behaviour patterns could be the product of a fewer or of a greater number of neural mechanisms. There is no reason to expect a one-to-one relationship between neural structures and their neuromodulators and the behaviour that they affect. More likely, the behavioural output is the result of a complex integration among a variety of neural systems, some essentially sexual (e.g. spinal mechanisms governing sexual reflexes or hypothalamic neural targets of sex hormones involved in the mediation of sexual responses) and others multipurpose (e.g. sensory, locomotory, and perceptual).

Numerous brainstem, limbic, and spinal structures are involved in the control of both male (Sachs 1978) and female (Pfaff 1980) rats. These structures may or may not have common neurochemical neuromodulatory control. In addition, it is not generally possible to relate particular aspects of the total behaviour pattern with particular subsystems.

Sex hormones exert effects on sexual behaviour by integrating neural components resulting in a coordinated behavioural output. Neurotransmitters function in the mediation of transmission within and between neural elements as well as by acting as integrative modulators of coordinated neural outputs. Thus treatment with a drug that affects neuroendocrine or neurochemical systems may have numerous effects at different levels and these effects may or may not be coordinated, leading to results that are difficult to interpret. For example, Lee *et al.* (1990) report paradoxical effects of 8-OHDPAT on genital reflexes and mating behaviour in male rats. Similarly, Cagiano *et al.* (1989) showed that D_2 agonists such as quin-pirole and antagonists (raclopride) both bring about a significant reduction in intromission frequency. This would suggest that intromission frequency by itself may not be a reliable index of pharmacologic effects on sexual behaviour in the rat.

A final point, and one of critical significance, is the choice of subjects to be studied. Normal, healthy animals might be considered to be displaying optimal levels of behaviour. Therefore pharmacologic agents, whether agonists or antagonists, may only show deleterious effects in a true sense. Following this logic one should devise experiments such that behaviour is altered toward an optimum or away from the optimum response. For example, Smith and Davidson (1990) demonstrated that yohimbine stimulates sexual responses in older rats that normally were deficient in this behaviour.

Determining what is normal or optimal for a given species is also difficult. Rarely can we observe and measure the behaviour of a model species in the natural environment. The experimenter creates the environment in which the animal's behaviour will be observed. A variable as basic as cage size can have a profound effect on the rate of mating in rats (McClintock 1984; Barfield and Thomas 1986). In addition, the condition and behaviour of the stimulus subject can have marked effects on the behaviour of the experimental animal.

Given a particular sexual dysfunction in the human, the choice of an appropriate physiological or behaviour end-point in an animal model is by no means simple or obvious. Initially, a distinction should be made between motivational versus performance or functional deficits although it should be recognized that with complex behaviour a complete dichotomy is somewhat artificial.

Consideration of motivational deficits such as inhibited sexual desire (ISD) would suggest an end-point that would not be confounded by behavioural or stimulus variables from another animal. An operant approach provides the purest tests of motivational factors (Everitt *et al.* 1987) although there can still remain problems of interpretation of results. For example, a drug could affect learning or perception in addition to sexual behaviour.

Another measure that reflects motivational state would be proceptive behaviour of the female or courtship behaviour of the male. Vocalization and scent marking in the absence of a potential mate can reveal deficits in interest in mating without confounding stimuli from another animal. On the other hand, observation of patterns of initiation with another animal reveal effects on other facets of behavioural interaction. Assessment of how one sex responds to cues from the other could be important. For example, the rate of darting by the female in response to vocalizations from the male may reflect her sexual interest (Thomas *et al.* 1982).

Functional or performance end-points should be assessed according to the analogous behavioural deficit in humans. Effects of a drug on premature ejaculation might be assessed in an animal model by looking for retardation of the rate or the number of intromissions preceding ejaculation without an attendant impediment to normal copulation. Anxiolytic drugs reduce 'anxiety'-induced reductions in the number of intromissions in rats (Fernandez-Guasti *et al.* 1990). Whether this suggests a rational therapy for this dysfunction in humans is not known at this time.

The rat model system also provides an opportunity to assess drug effects on erectile dysfunction, both of an organic or psychogenic nature. Purely organic dysfunction can be assessed in a spinalized animal whereas behaviourally induced dysfunctions can be evaluated in the intact animal.

SUMMARY

Use of animal models for human sexual behaviour is an application of the comparative method and as such carries with it assets and liabilities. As Beach pointed out, to maximize the effect of this inherently insightful approach, one must understand the behaviour and underlying mechanisms of the model species as well as that of humans.

The rat is the most widely used animal model system for sexual behaviour. This is attributed to the practicality of this laboratory animal as well as its suitability for the investigation of basic questions concerning regulatory mechanisms underlying sociosexual behaviour. Rat sociosexual behaviour is complex, and different situational variables can lead to different behavioural outcomes. It is therefore important to devise experimental approaches that will be free of confounding variables. Measures of rat sexual behaviour are based on our perception of behavioural units and are often combined to yield derived measures. As derived measures are composed of multiple behavioural elements, there is a risk of obtaining confusing or paradoxical results.

The understanding of reproductive coordination is a key to gaining understanding of the behavioural and motivational significance of elements of reproductive behaviour in both humans and animal models. Furthermore, it is important to be aware that the reproductive behaviour and physiology of both humans and laboratory animals have been subject to domestication and that this has led to alterations in basic patterns of behaviour and their functional significance.

Animal models can be useful if, in their application, one takes into account the concept of optimality of behaviour in terms of its functional significance rather than just simple increases or decreases in behavioural output.

REFERENCES

Adler, N.T. and Toner, J.P. (1986). The effects of copulatory behavior on sperm transport and fertility in rats. *Annals of the New York Academy of Sciences*, **474**, 21–32.

Austin, D. and Dewsbury, D.A. (1986). Possible influence of strain differences on pregnancy initiation in laboratory rats. *Physiology and Behavior*, **37**, 621–6.

Barfield, R.J. and Geyer, L.A. (1972). Sexual behaviour: ultrasonic postejaculatory song of the male rat. *Science*, **176**, 1349–50.

Barfield, R.J. and Geyer, L.A. (1975). The ultrasonic postejaculatory vocalization and the postejaculatory refractory period of the male rat. *Journal of Comparative and Physiological Psychology*, **88**, 723–34.

Barfield, R.J. and Thomas, D.A. (1986). The role of ultrasonic vocalizations in the regulation of reproduction in rats. *Annals of the New York Academy of Sciences*, **474**, 33–43.

Beach, F.A. (1976). Sexual attractivity, proceptivity, and receptivity in female mammals. *Hormones and Behavior*, **7**, 105–33.

Beach, F.A. (1979). Animal models for human sexuality. In *Sex, hormones, and behavior* (ed. Ciba Foundation), pp. 113–43. Symposium 62, Excerpta Medica.

Bradford, J.M.W. (1988). Organic treatment for the male sexual offender. *Annals of the New York Academy of Sciences*, **528**, 193–202.

Cagiano, R., Barfield, R.J., White, N.R., Pleim, E.T., and Cuomo, V. (1989). Mediation of rat postejaculatory 22 kHz ultrasonic vocalization by dopamine D_2 receptors. *Pharmacology, Biochemistry and Behavior*, **34**, 53–8.

Clark, J.H. and Zarrow, M.X. (1971). Influence of copulation on time of ovulation in women. *American Journal of Obstetrics and Gynecology*, **109**, 1083–5.

Edmonds, S., Zoloth, S.R., and Adler, N.T. (1972). Storage of copulatory stimulation in the female rat. *Physiology and Behavior*, **8**, 161–4.

Everett, J.W. (1961). The mammalian female reproductive cycle and its controlling mechanisms. In *Sex and internal secretions* (ed. W.C. Young), Vol. 1, pp. 497–555. Williams and Wilkins, Baltimore.

Everitt, B.J., Fray, P., Kostarczyk, E., Taylor, S., and Stacey, P. (1987). Studies of instrumental behaviour with sexual reinforcement in male rats (*Rattus norvegicus*): I. Control by brief visual stimuli paired with a receptive female. *Journal of Comparative Psychology*, **101**, 395–406.

Fernandez-Guasti, A., Roldan-Roldan, G., and Saldivar, A. (1990). Pharmacological manipulation of anxiety and male rat sexual behaviour. *Pharmacology, Biochemistry and Behavior*, **35**, 263–8.

Ford, C.S. and Beach, F.A. (1951). *Patterns of sexual behaviour*. Harper, New York.

Hardy, D.F. and DeBold, J.F. (1971). Effects of mounts without intromission upon the behavior of female rats during the onset of estrogen-induced heat. *Physiology and Behavior*, **7**, 643–5.

Katchadourian, H.A. and Lunde, D.T. (1975). *Fundamentals of human sexuality* (2nd edn). Holt, Rinehart and Winston, New York.

Langston, J.W., Irwin, I., Langston, E.B., and Forno, L.S. (1984). Pargyline prevents MPTP-induced parkinsonism in primates. *Science*, **225**, 1480–2.

Lee, R.L., Smith, E.R., Mas, M., and Davidson, J.M. (1990). Effects of intrathecal administration of 8-OH-DPAT on genital reflexes and mating behavior in male rats. *Physiology and Behavior*, **47**, 665–70.

Matochik, J.A., White, N.R., and Barfield, R.J. (1992). Variations in scent marking and ultrasonic vocalizations by Long–Evans rats across the estrous cycle. *Physiology and Behavior*, **51**, 783–6.

McClintock, M.K. (1984). Group mating in the domestic rat as a context for sexual selection: consequences for the analysis of sexual behaviour and neuroendocrine responses. *Advances in the Study of Behavior*, **14**, 1–50.

Pfaff, D.W. (1980). *Estrogens and brain function*. Springer, New York.

Sachs, B.D. (1978). Conceptual and neural mechanisms of masculine copulatory behavior. In *Sex and behavior* (ed. T.E. McGill, D.A. Dewsbury, and B.D. Sachs), pp. 267–96. Plenum, New York.

Sachs, B.D. (1983). Potency and fertility: hormonal and mechanical causes and effects of penile actions in rats. In *Hormones and behavior in higher vertebrates* (ed. J. Balthazart, E. Prove, and R. Gilles), pp. 86–110. Springer, Berlin.

Sachs, B.D. and Barfield, R.J. (1976). Functional analysis of masculine copulatory behavior in the rat. In *Advances in the study of behavior* (ed. J.S. Rosenblatt, R.A. Hinde, E. Shaw, and C. Beer), Vol. 7, pp. 92–154. Academic Press, New York.

Sales, G.D. (1972). Ultrasound and mating behaviour in rodents with some observations on other behavior situations. *Journal of Zoology*, **168**, 149–64.

Smith, E.R. and Davidson, J.M. (1990). Yohimbine attenuates aging-induced sexual deficiencies in male rats. *Physiology and Behavior*, **47**, 631–4.

Stern, J.M. (1986). Licking, touching, and suckling: contact stimulation and maternal psychobiology in rats and women. *Annals of the New York Academy of Sciences*, **474**, 95–107.

Thomas, D.A. and Barfield, R.J. (1985). Ultrasonic vocalization of the female rat (*Rattus norvegicus*) during mating. *Animal Behaviour*, **33**, 720–5.

Thomas, D.A., Howard, S.B., and Barfield, R.J. (1982). Male-produced ultrasonic vocalizations and mating patterns in female rats. *Journal of Comparative and Physiological Psychology*, **96**, 807–15.

Thor, D.H. and Flannelly, K.J. (1979). Copulation and intermale aggression in rats. *Journal of Comparative and Physiological Psychology*, **93**, 223–8.

Zarrow, M.X. and Clark, J.H. (1968). Ovulation following vaginal stimulation in a spontaneous ovulator and its implications. *Journal of Endocrinology*, **40**, 343–52.

Zumpe, D. and Michael, R.P. (1968). The clutching reaction and orgasm in the female rhesus monkey (*Macaca mulatta*). *Journal of Endocrinology*, **40**, 117–23.

4

Experimental approaches for the development of pharmacological therapies for erectile dysfunction

Mark M. Foreman[†] and Paul C. Doherty

INTRODUCTION

During the past fifteen years, both academic and pharmaceutical laboratories have targeted major research efforts in the physiology, pathophysiology, and pharmacology of sexual response. The discoveries stemming from this research have in turn resulted in a variety of clinical trials using different therapeutic strategies for sexual disorders in both men and women. These sexual disorders include dysfunctions of the desire, arousal, and orgasmic phases of the sexual response cycle as described by Kaplan (1979). These phases cover the full range of sexual responses starting with the integration of sensory inputs with cognitive, emotional, and desire components for the initiation of sexual activity; progressing to the vasocongestion of the genitalia; and terminating with the physiological and perceptual changes associated with orgasm. The following review will focus on one of these disorders, erectile dysfunction in the male, and will outline some of the characteristics of the pathophysiology, the patient population, and the experimental approaches for the development of pharmacotherapies.

ERECTILE PHYSIOLOGY AND PATHOLOGY

Under normal conditions, the sequence of responses leading to erection represents a self-amplifying process within a network of interconnected regulatory sites in the brain, the brainstem, the spinal cord, and the neuro-vascular network of the genitalia (Sachs and Meisel 1988; Bancroft 1989). The initial phase of genital arousal involves both a reduction of the descending inhibition of efferent neuronal activity from the thoracolumbar (T12–L3) and sacral (S2–S4) segments of the spinal cord and an increased sensitivity to afferent sensory responses from the genitalia (Bancroft 1989).

[†] Author to whom correspondence should be addressed.

The augmented activity within this neural network initiates the subsequent processes involved in the induction of tumescence and rigidity of the erectile tissue within the penis. The enlargement of the sinusoidal spaces for maximum tumescence and the compression of these blood-engorged spaces for rigidity (Aboseif and Lue 1988) increase the afferent neuronal activity from the tactile sensory receptors within the erectile tissue (Johnson and Kitchell 1987; Johnson, personal communication). During coitus, the increased activity from these afferent sensory fibres acts as a positive feedback limb of the sexual response cascade facilitating the maintenance of erection and lowering the response threshold for the ejaculatory reflex (Johnson and Kitchell 1987).

Erectile dysfunction is defined as the inability to achieve or maintain erection sufficient for successful intercourse. Currently, the most common diagnostic classification of erectile dysfunction subdivides aetiologies as being either organic or psychogenic in origin. Organic erectile dysfunction includes any aetiology that can be defined by standard clinical evaluations, such as neurologic, endocrinologic, vascular, and drug-induced dysfunctions (Fig. 4.1). Psychogenic erectile dysfunction is generally considered to be a consequence of psychiatric, emotional, or interpersonal disorders which indirectly effect the responsiveness of the neural network regulating erectile response (Fig. 4.1). However, psychogenic classification in many cases also encompasses any idiopathic disorder since this category includes disorders that do not have an organic origin that can be detected by current tests.

With the advent of new diagnostic methods, the proportion of patients who are classified as having either organic or psychogenic aetiologies has changed from predominantly psychogenic to equal or predominantly organic distributions. Table 4.1 contains a summary of recent data on the proportions of patients with either organic, psychogenic, or mixed aetiologies from

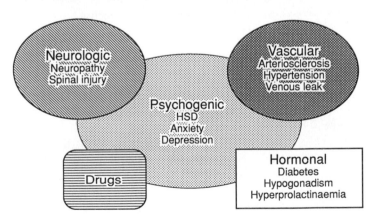

Fig. 4.1   Causes of erectile dysfunction.

Table 4.1 Incidence of psychogenic and organic erectile dysfunction

Reference	Number of patients	Mean age or age range	Diagnosis		
			Organic	Psychogenic	Mixed
Ellis *et al.* 1987	300	25–85	50.0	31.0	19.0
Melman *et al.* 1988	406	19–79	28.8	39.7	31.5
Gall *et al.* 1990	324	19–72	43.6	9.4	46.0
Nogueira *et al.* 1990	200	47.6	62.0	38.0	*
Cumming and Pryor 1991	86	19–79	42.0	58.0	*
Virag *et al.* 1991	615	48	25.2	27.5	47.3
		Average	41.9	33.9	36.0

* No estimate of mixed aetiology.

six urologic sexual dysfunction clinics. Thirty-four per cent of these patients were diagnosed as having psychogenic dysfunction compared with 42 per cent with organic causes and 36 per cent with a mixed organic and psychogenic dysfunction. The addition of the new category of mixed dysfunction is a recognition that emotional stress often accompanies the physical complaint of erectile failure, making the separation of a primary and secondary diagnosis difficult. The difficulty in treating these disorders may also increase as the patient reacts to his dysfunction. This may necessitate the use of combined pharmacotherapies to treat erectile dysfunction that is caused and exacerbated by coincidental and sequential physical and affective disorders.

The major psychiatric and emotional disorders that are thought to reduce erectile capacity include depression, anxiety, and hypoactive sexual desire (HSD). Although the impact of depression and anxiety on sexual interest and response has been recognized for decades (Howell et al. 1987; Kaplan 1988; Patterson and O'Gorman 1989; Bancroft 1989), the role of HSD in disorders of sexual response is a relatively recent conceptual discovery (Kaplan 1979, 1985; Leif 1985; Leiblum and Rosen 1988). HSD has been given the status of a separate affective disorder to account for the fact that many patients have suppressed sexual interest independent of interpersonal problems, emotional or other psychiatric disorders (American Psychiatric Association 1987). HSD has been cited as 'one of the most frequent complaints of couples seeking professional help' and it is 'the most resistant to therapeutic intervention and carries the poorest prognosis' (Schreiner-Engel and Schiavi 1986; Leiblum and Rosen 1988). Considering the incidence and prognosis of HSD, the success of treating erectile dysfunction may depend upon whether HSD is a primary or secondary cause. In a recent multi-centre study to evaluate the efficacy of a pharmacological agent, 30 per cent (113 patients) of the males recruited had a primary diagnosis of HSD and 47 per cent of these males (53 patients) also had a secondary diagnosis of erectile impairment (Segraves and Segraves 1991). Among the 258 male patients in this study who were classified as having a primary diagnosis of erectile dysfunction (69 per cent of total erectile dysfunction sample), 20 per cent of these patients also had secondary or tertiary diagnoses of low sexual drive (Segraves and Segraves 1990).

One major aetiological factor for erectile dysfunction that is associated with all of the major subgroups of psychogenic and organic causes of erectile dysfunction is the age of the patient (Verwoerdt et al. 1969; Schiavi 1985; Segraves 1988a; Bancroft 1989; Carroll et al. 1990). Kinsey and co-workers (1948) and others (Martin 1981; Hegeler and Mortensen 1978) documented an age-related decline in sexual activity in men. This decrease in sexual activity occurred progressively with ageing, but the rate of this decline appeared to be highest in the men beyond 65 years of age (Fig. 4.2). In contrast to the normal population, the age-related decline in sexual

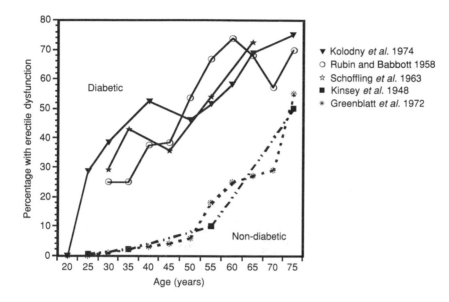

Fig. 4.2   Effect of diabetes and age on erectile dysfunction.

response is dramatically amplified in the diabetic population (Fig. 4.2). The acceleration of the decline in sexual response in diabetic patients can be attributed to an induction of central and peripheral neuropathies and vascular disease that are also observed in the elderly population (Rubin and Babbott 1958; Schiavi and Hogan 1979; Boura *et al.* 1986; Dyck *et al.* 1987; Lincoln *et al.* 1987; Lal 1988; Saenz de Tejada and Goldstein 1988; Bancroft 1989; Saenz de Tejada *et al.* 1989*a,b*; Whitehead *et al.* 1990; Blanco *et al.* 1990).

However, it is incorrect to assume from these studies that erectile disorders do not affect significant numbers of men younger than 65. Frank and co-workers (1978) at the University of Pittsburgh surveyed 100 'happily married' couples. Although the men in this study were among the least likely to have sexual disorders because of their age (mean of 37.4 years) and contented marital status, nine per cent of the males reported problems with erectile failures (Fig. 4.3). In a survey of 212 general outpatients (mean age of 35 years) by Schein and co-workers (1988) from Case Western Reserve University, erectile response problems were reported by 27 per cent of this sample, which presumably included all ranges of marital contentment (Fig. 4.3).

It is also incorrect to assume that patients seeking medical help for erectile dysfunction are primarily elderly. Although the frequency of erectile dysfunction is highest in the oldest population, the impact of impotence on the lives of men may be greater in younger age groups when sexual drive is

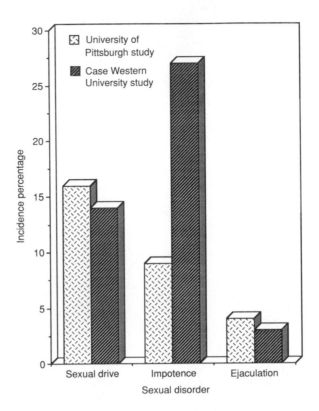

Fig. 4.3   Incidence of sexual dysfunction in men. (From Frank *et al.* 1978; Schein *et al.* 1988.)

higher. This assumption is supported by the summary of percentages of patients seeking medical help for erectile dysfunction (Fig. 4.4). The number of patients seeking help for erectile dysfunction is greatest between the ages of 40 and 60, which may represent the composite of the incidence and the impact of dysfunction. In another study (Slag *et al.* 1983) of 1180 male outpatients who were screened for erectile disorders, the average age of impotent patients who did not wish further diagnostic evaluation was 66.9 compared with 59.4 for patients who were willing to undergo evaluation. In a recent pharmaceutical study, the average age of men willing to undergo evaluation and participate was 54.2 years (Segraves and Segraves 1990). Since different aetiological factors may be responsible for erectile dysfunction within various age groups, the age of the men selected for a clinical trial could affect the apparent efficacy of a pharmacological agent targeted for a particular type of sexual disorder.

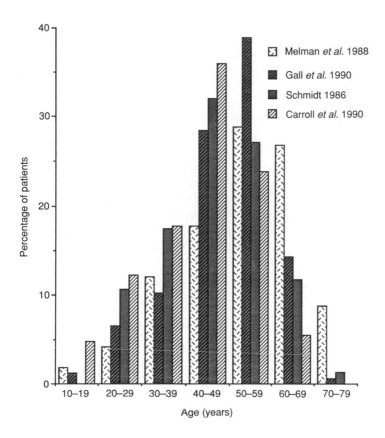

Fig. 4.4 Distribution of patients seeking treatment for erectile dysfunction within age groups.

APPROACHES FOR PHARMACOTHERAPIES

Currently, the most common pharmacological therapies used for erectile dysfunction include hormonal therapies to reverse endocrinopathies such as hypogonadism and hyperprolactinaemia, neuropharmacological therapies such as yohimbine, trazodone, and buspirone for psychogenic dysfunctions (Othmer and Othmer 1987; Morales *et al.* 1987*a,b*; Riley *et al.* 1989; Susset *et al.* 1989; Lal *et al.* 1990), and intrapenile injections of vasodilators (Lee *et al.* 1989; Lue 1989; Virag *et al.* 1991) for any form of erectile failure except arteriogenic or venogenic incompetence of the penile vascular tree. Since the only approved pharmacotherapies are those for endocrinopathies and the others are either marginally effective or involve intrapenile injection, a large clinical need exists for improved therapies for erectile dysfunction.

The three main therapeutic strategies that are being pursued have been previously classified as the psycho-, neuro-, and vascular pharmacologic approaches (Foreman and Wernicke 1990). Each of these approaches represents a different site of drug actions within the neurovascular pathways controlling erectile response. The *psychopharmacologic* approaches encompass drug therapies that primarily affect the behavioural components of sexual response, that is sexual drive or libido, through the alteration of neuronal activity within the brain centre responsible for the initiation of sexual response. Other components of sexual response are enhanced through the interconnections within this neural pathway. The *neuropharmacologic* approaches encompass drug-induced changes in neuronal activity associated with the brainstem and spinal neuropathways controlling erection. Neuropharmacologic therapies lower the erectile reflex threshold by directly amplifying the neuronal firing rate within the efferent limb of the erectile response reflex. The *vascular pharmacologic* approaches encompass any drug-induced alteration of smooth muscle responses within the penile vasculature. The current intrapenile vascular pharmacologic therapies bypass the neurovascular control and directly elicit an erection. However, some of the newer approaches under investigation are designed to correct defects in the control of vascular smooth muscle induced by diabetes or ageing processes. The different pharmacologic approaches represent not only different sites and mechanisms of action of pharmacologic agents but also the different disciplines and philosophies of the investigators who have developed these strategies. It should be noted that pharmacological agents can have effects at several sites in the response pathway, so this classification is restricted to responses and not agents.

Psychopharmacological approaches

The psychopharmacologic approaches have been developed by behavioural pharmacologists with the purpose of reactivating sexual response in dysfunctional patients by augmenting the activity of the neurones in the brain component of the sexual response pathway. These strategies are based upon a recognition that the level of sexual drive is an important factor for both the expression of sexual behaviour and the alteration of response thresholds of the erectile reflexes. The research strategies for development of psychopharmacological therapies have stemmed from three types of studies. First, the studies that have identified the area of the brain which regulates sexual drive and the types of transmitters within this area have provided the foundation for the neural control of sexual drive and its relationship to peripheral sexual reflexes. Second, the studies that have evaluated the effects of pharmacologic agents on the sexual behaviour of laboratory animals have provided a characterization of the types of receptors involved with this response. Finally, the clinical observations in which alterations in libido and subsequently peripheral sexual responses were seen to be side-effects of existing pharmacological agents have provided the clinical relevance of the laboratory studies as well as alternative pharmacological approaches for the control of the erectile response in man.

Identification and characterization of a sexual drive centre

The medial preoptic area (MPOA) of the ventral diencephalon has been identified as a brain area which has characteristics of a sexual drive centre in a variety of mammalian species (Sachs and Meisel 1988). In the initial neuroanatomical studies which attempted to localize the sexual drive centre, electrical stimulation and lesions of this area were found to amplify and suppress, respectively, the expression of sexual behaviour (Sachs and Meisel 1988). This region of the ventral diencephalon has extensive neural interconnections with other diencephalic areas, the limbic system, and the cerebral cortex. These neural pathways may represent anatomical substrates for biological, emotional, and cognitive components of the control of sexual behaviour (Levine 1984; Simerly and Swanson 1986, 1988; Sachs and Meisel 1988; Foreman and Wernicke 1990). This neural area also has interconnections with more caudal areas of the sexual response pathway which may form the anatomical bridge between the behavioural and physiological components of the sexual response (Skagerberg et al. 1982; Simerly and Swanson 1988; Wagner and Clemens 1991). Further correlations between anatomical interconnections and function were provided by neurophysiological and neurochemical studies. These studies demonstrated that the electrical activity and neurotransmitter changes in the MPOA paralleled changes in sexual behaviour (Mas et al. 1987; Oomura et al. 1988; Pfaus et al. 1990; Eaton et al. 1991). The neuronal activity within the preoptic area also appeared to be coordinated with the activity of other ventral diencephalic areas (such as the dorsomedial hypothalamic nucleus and ventromedial hypothalamic nucleus) as the sexual response developed (Oomura et al. 1988).

The endocrinologic studies established that the activity of neurones in these diencephalic areas is influenced by gonadal steroids and polypeptide hormones, through interactions with intracellular or membrane receptors for these hormones (Grant and Stumpf 1975; Sachs and Meisel 1988). All of the effects of systemic administration of steroid and polypeptide hormones on sexual behaviour were duplicated by the direct application of these hormones into these sites (Grant and Stumpf 1975; Foreman and Moss 1977, 1979; Sachs and Meisel 1988). Gonadal hormones not only affect the responsiveness of neurones in the MPOA but also affect the types of synaptic contacts and neuronal clustering such that sexual dimorphism can be demonstrated in histological studies of this area (Simerly et al. 1985; Allen et al. 1989). The sexual dimorphism induced by these hormones has been assumed to be important for the development of behavioural patterns and peripheral responses.

The neurochemical studies of the preoptic region have identified a variety of transmitters of which dopamine, noradrenalin, and serotonin have been studied the most extensively in sexual pharmacology. The preoptic region of the diencephalon receives synaptic inputs from serotonin and noradrenergic neurones, which are located in the nucleus raphe dorsalis and nucleus locus coeruleus, respectively, of the brainstem. This preoptic region contains a cluster of neurones which comprise the rostral component of the incerto-hypothalamic dopamine system (Grant and Stumpf 1975). The pharmacological evaluations of monoaminergic receptor subtypes have provided correlations to clinical responses as well as the foundations for many of the therapeutic approaches.

Psychopharmacological alteration of sexual drive

The observations of increased libido in parkinsonian, psychiatric, and impotent patients receiving the catecholamine precursor, L-dopa, stimulated research on the pharmacological control of sexual behaviour (Barbeau 1969; Yaryura-Tobias *et al.* 1970; Benkert *et al.* 1972; Brown *et al.* 1978; Buffum 1982; Segraves 1989). In laboratory animals, increased sexual behaviour can be induced by altering catecholamine metabolism through increasing synthesis with L-dopa (Malmnas 1976) or decreasing degradation with a monoamine oxidase B inhibitor, deprenyl (Dallo *et al.* 1986; Knoll *et al.* 1989). Amphetamine, a catecholamine-releasing agent, also increases sexual behaviour in rats and libido in men (Angrist and Gershon 1976; Dallo *et al.* 1986). These results are suggestive of an involvement of dopaminergic and/or adrenergic receptors in the control of sexual drive.

The theory of dopaminergic receptor involvement is further supported by the observations of increased libido in patients treated with dopamine agonists such as apomorphine (Benkert 1980) and pergolide (Jeanty *et al.* 1984) and dopamine reuptake inhibitors such as nomifensine (Freed 1983) and bupropion (Crenshaw *et al.* 1987). In animal studies, selective activation of D_2-dopaminergic receptors by the systemic administration of agonists such as apomorphine or quinelorane increases sexual behaviour in rats at doses which do not elicit other responses (Bitran and Hull 1987; Foreman and Hall 1987). These effects, in laboratory animals, were antagonized by dopamine antagonists that can penetrate the blood–brain barrier, but not by a peripherally active antagonist, suggesting that the receptors mediating these effects were located behind the blood–brain barrier (Foreman and Hall 1987). The effects observed with systemic administration of apomorphine or quinelorane can be replicated by direct infusion of these substances into the MPOA suggesting that the dopaminergic receptors within this area may contribute to this effect (Hull *et al.* 1989; Scaletta and Hull 1990).

Since L-dopa, amphetamine, and deprenyl affect the activity of all catecholaminergic neurones, it is possible that adrenergic receptors may also be involved in the regulation of sexual drive. In male rats, systemic administration of either prazosin, an α_1-adrenergic antagonist, or clonidine, an α_2-adrenergic agonist, suppresses mating behaviour, whereas yohimbine, an α_2-adrenergic antagonist, increases sexual behaviour (Clark *et al.* 1985; Bitran and Hull 1987). The blockade of postsynaptic (α_1) receptors or the stimulation of presynaptic (α_2) autoreceptors would result in a decrease in central noradrenergic activity, which could explain the similar reductions in sexual drive (Clark *et al.* 1985). The only beneficial effects of systemically or intracranially administered (Clark *et al.* 1985; Sala *et al.* 1990) yohimbine on sexual response which have been consistently documented in laboratory studies are the behavioural-drive-enhancing effects. Therefore, the psychopharmacologic effects of yohimbine may be responsible for its reported efficacy in the treatment of subgroups of patients with erectile dysfunction (Morales *et al.* 1987*a,b*; Riley *et al.* 1989; Susset *et al.* 1989). Other α_2-adrenergic antagonists with different properties such as idazoxan, imiloxan (Smith *et al.* 1987), and atizepamezole (Linnankoski *et al.* 1991) are currently being evaluated in preclinical and clinical studies.

Serotonin has been proposed to be an inhibitory transmitter in the control of sexual drive (Bitran and Hull 1987; Foreman *et al.* 1989; Gorzalka *et al.* 1990). This proposal is based on three types of experimental evidence. First, direct or indirect augmentation of 5-HT activity by the administration of the precursor, 5-hydroxytryptophan; 5-HT reuptake inhibitors; 5-HT releasers; or a variety of postsynaptic agonists results in a suppression of sexual behaviour in male rats (Bitran and Hull 1987; Foreman *et al.* 1989, 1990). These effects correlate with the clinical reports of suppressed libido and sexual response in patients treated with the 5-HT releasing agent, fenfluramine (Pinder *et al.* 1975) or the 5-HT reuptake inhibitors, seratraline and fluoxetine (Doogan and Caillard 1988; Zajecka *et al.* 1991). Second, reduction of the activity of 5-HT neurones by the administration of 5-HT autoreceptor agonists (5-HT$_{1A}$ agonists) such as 8-OHDPAT and buspirone increases sexual behaviour in male rats and rhesus monkeys (Ahlenius and Larsson 1987; Glaser *et al.* 1987; Pomerantz 1991*b*). In clinical studies, buspirone elevated libido in male and female patients with generalized anxiety (Othmer and Othmer 1987). Third, the suppression of serotonergic activity through the destruction of 5-HT neurones, inhibition of 5-HT synthesis, or blockade of 5-HT receptors results in an increase in sexual behaviour in laboratory studies (Bitran and Hull 1987; Foreman *et al.* 1988; Menendez *et al.* 1988; Sachs and Meisel 1988). Clinical studies focusing on the suppression of serotonergic activity have been attempted with *para*-chlorophenylalanine, a 5-HT synthesis inhibitor, and methysergide, a 5-HT antagonist, but the positive results were questionable and difficult to reproduce due to the neurotoxicity (e.g. PCPA) and nonselectivity (e.g. methysergide) of the agents, the small patient samples, and the ambiguous diagnostic and efficacy criteria (Benkert 1980; Buffum 1982). A new, highly selective $5\text{-HT}_{1C/2}$ antagonist, amesergide (LY237733), has been shown to induce and amplify sexual behaviour in male rats in doses as low as 100 ng kg^{-1}, which is 10 000 times below any other detectable response to this agent (Foreman *et al.* 1988). This agent has the potency and selectivity to become a useful tool in evaluating the clinical efficacy of this approach.

Since a variety of transmitters are known to influence sexual behaviour, the monoaminergic receptors represent only a few of the possible approaches for the psychopharmacologic treatment of erectile dysfunction (Bitran and Hull 1987; Murphy 1988; Sachs and Meisel 1988; Dornan and Malsbury 1989). However, since the non-monoaminergic effects have not been evaluated with the same detail in either laboratory or clinical studies, the clinical utility of these approaches remains unknown.

Neuropharmacological approaches

The neuropharmacological approaches are employed by pharmacologists to elicit spontaneous erections or to increase efferent cavernosal nerve activity and subsequently increase penile blood pressure. These approaches encompass any drug therapy that can improve or induce peripheral sexual responses through alteration of neuronal activity in the brain–spinal–genitalia pathway.

The neural network controlling sexual reflex responses

In addition to the behavioural organization functions of the neurones within the preoptic region of the ventral diencephalon, this area has also been thought to influence the response thresholds for sexual reflexes through connections with other integrative areas further downstream in the response pathway. Some of these areas include the dorsomedial, ventromedial, and paraventricular nuclei of the hypothalamus, the ventral tegmental area of the midbrain (Sachs and Meisel 1988), the paragigantocellular (PGC) region of the brainstem reticular formation (Marson and McKenna 1990), and the spinal cord (Skagerberg *et al.* 1982; Wagner and Clemens 1991). The PGC is of particular interest because it has recently been proposed to be a sexual reflex control centre which has the capacity to generate a tonic suppression of sexual reflexes (Marson and McKenna 1990). Connections between the PGC and the spinal cord segments containing the pudendal nerve motorneurones and preganglionic neurones of the parasympathetic pelvic nerve have been demonstrated and alterations in neuronal activity within the PGC have been recorded following genital stimulation. The PGC also is known to be involved in the control of blood pressure, heart rate, respiration, and analgesia, which are homeostatic responses that are altered during sexual function (Andrezik *et al.* 1981). The firing rate of neurones in the PGC can be altered by the application of pharmacologic agents such as GABA, 5-HT, morphine, enkephalin, nicotine, and noradrenalin (Glazer *et al.* 1981; Lovick 1985, 1987; Rasmussen and Aghajanian 1989) and thus a variety of neuropharmacologic approaches can be proposed for therapies that affect neuronal responses within this area.

Descending from the brainstem, the next major regulatory sites for the neural control of sexual response are located in the lumbar and sacral regions of the spinal cord. Two reflex neuropathways appear to regulate these vascular responses (Krane and Siroky 1981; Bennett *et al.* 1988; de Groat and Booth 1990; Steers 1990). The first is the psychogenic pathway which evokes genitalia arousal from perceptual responses generated in the brain. The psychogenic erectile responses are elicited primarily through the thoracolumbar (T12–L3) efferent autonomic fibres. The second is the reflexogenic pathway which allows for genitalia arousal through the discharge of the efferent neural fibres from the sacral (S2–S4) parasympathetic nerves in response to afferent sensory stimulation carried by the pudendal nerve from the genitalia. These regions control parasympathetic and sympathetic output to the vascular beds of the corpora cavernosa and contain motorneurones that innervate the bulbocavernosus muscles of the penis. The responses of these reflex pathways are chronically suppressed by descending inhibitory fibres from the ventral diencephalon and the paragigantocellular region of the brainstem (Skagerberg *et al.* 1982; Marson and McKenna 1990; Wagner and Clemens 1991). As in the case of the brainstem regulatory loci, the transmitters that impinge on or are secreted by these spinal neurones have not been completely identified. However, descending serotonin, substance P, and oxytocin immunoreactive fibres and enkephalin immunoreactive connections from spinal interneurones have been identified in these areas (Skagerberg *et al.* 1982; Micevych *et al.* 1986; Mas *et al.* 1987; Wagner and Clemens 1991).

As in the case of the preoptic area, neuronal clusters within these spinal regions form sexually dimorphic groupings of neurones that contain androgen receptors which appear to be important for the establishment of neural connections and the control of programmed cell death (Fishman and Breedlove 1985; Forger and Breedlove 1986; Allen *et al.* 1989; Senglaub and Arnold 1989). The programmed cell death of neurones within the preoptic area and the spinal cord is observed at different ages and may be partly responsible for the development of patterns of sexual response as well as the deterioration of these responses with ageing. One potential area for pharmacological intervention in the neuropathology of sexual response is the prevention or reversal of peripheral autonomic neuropathies associated with diabetes or ageing. Recent information on this subject has been summarized in prior reviews and research publications (Dyck *et al.* 1987;

Lincoln *et al.* 1987; Saenz de Tejada and Goldstein 1988; Blanco *et al.* 1990).

Neuropharmacologic control of erection

In addition to the effects on libido, dopaminergic, adrenergic, and serotonergic agents also affect erectile response in men and laboratory animals without changing sexual behaviour. These effects were first noted as side-effects in patients treated with L-dopa (Barbeau 1969; Brown *et al.* 1978) or dopaminergic agonists (Benkert 1980; Jeanty *et al.* 1984). More recently, subcutaneously administered apomorphine has been shown to induce penile erections reproducibly in normal and impotent patients (Danjou *et al.* 1989; Lal *et al.* 1989; Segraves *et al.* 1991). The magnitude of the erectile response is dose related (Lal *et al.* 1989; Segraves *et al.* 1991) and appears to be mediated by D_2 dopaminergic receptors within the central nervous system, since only centrally acting antagonists block this response (Lal *et al.* 1989). This acute response to dopaminergic receptor stimulation is not accompanied by increases in libido and therefore appears to be a neuropharmacologic rather than psychopharmacologic effect (Danjou *et al.* 1989). Although erections have been noted as side-effects of oral dopaminergic agonist therapy, the incidence and reproducibility of this response appears to be greater with subcutaneous administration. Since this response is highly reproducible and dose related, it has been proposed as a diagnostic test for selection of patients who would benefit from dopaminergic agonist therapy (Lal *et al.* 1989; Segraves *et al.* 1991). This test could be an inexpensive and rapid method to evaluate the response of the spinal cord to genitalia components of the sexual pathway, but the co-administration of a peripherally acting antagonist may be required to prevent the nausea and orthostatic hypotension that is seen in some patients (Lal *et al.* 1989; Segraves *et al.* 1991). In parallel to these clinical studies, dopaminergic agonist-induced erections have also been observed in rats (Gower *et al.* 1984; Doherty *et al.* 1991) and rhesus monkeys (Pomerantz 1990, 1991*a*). The dopaminergic receptors that mediate these effects are also behind the blood–brain barrier (Doherty *et al.* 1991; Pomerantz 1991*a*) and may be within the spinal cord. This assumption is based upon the identification of dopaminergic pathways connecting the ventral diencephalon with the lumbar spinal cord (Skagerberg *et al.* 1982), the observed changes in dopamine and its metabolites in the lumbar spinal cord during mating activity (Mas *et al.* 1987), and the stimulatory effects of intraspinal infusions of the dopaminergic agonist, lisuride, on sexual responses (Hansen 1982).

Unlike dopamine, serotonin appears to have different effects on the central and peripheral components of the sexual response. Although the serotonergic innervation of the MPOA is thought to suppress the expression of sexual behaviour (as described above), pharmacological amplification of serotonergic activity through the administration of serotonin-releasing agents or agonists also induces spontaneous erections in rats and rhesus monkeys (Szele *et al*. 1988; Berendsen *et al*. 1990). The erectogenic effects of serotonin have been proposed to be mediated by the 5-HT_{1C} receptor sub-type (Berendsen *et al*. 1990). These effects may contribute to the induction of priapism in patients treated with the antidepressant, trazodone (Scher *et al*. 1983; Bardin and Krieger 1990; Saenz de Tejada *et al*. 1991*a*). The trazodone metabolite, *meta*-chlorophenylpiperazine (mCPP), is a serotonergic agonist that induces erections in rats and rhesus monkeys (Szele *et al*. 1988; Berendsen *et al*. 1990) and selectively increases the firing rate of the penile nerve in rats (Steers and de Groat 1989). There have also been recent clinical observations that trazodone can induce increases in nocturnal erections and is beneficial for some impotent patients (Lal *et al*. 1990; Adaikan *et al*. 1991). These studies are suggestive that a serotonergic agonist may be useful for erectile dysfunction particularly if the stimulatory effects on erection can be separated from the inhibitory effects on sexual drive by development of highly selective 5-HT_{1C} agonists.

In addition to the involvement of monoamines in the control of the erectile responses, major roles for peptidergic, cholinergic, opioid, and GABA receptors have been proposed based on preliminary laboratory and clinical studies (Charney and Heninger 1986; Bitran and Hull 1987; Pfaus and Gorzalka 1987; Sachs and Meisel 1988; Fabbri *et al*. 1989; Argiolas and Gessa 1991). For example, endorphin receptors have been theorized to mediate the inhibitory effects of morphine on sexual function. In a single-blind study in comparison with placebo, naltrexone (an opiate antagonist) produced significant increases in both sexual performance and the number of morning and spontaneous erections (Fabbri *et al*. 1989). Another opiate antagonist, naloxone, has also been found to exert a synergistic effect with yohimbine in inducing erections (Charney and Heninger 1986). This additive effect of a psychopharmacologic agent (yohimbine) and a neuropharmacologic agent (naloxone) may represent a more effective approach for the treatment of erectile dysfunction than singular therapies. A combined therapeutic strategy would involve simultaneously increasing the activity or response of different regions of the sexual response pathway.

Vascular pharmacological control of sexual responses

The vascular pharmacologic approaches have been used by urologists and vascular pharmacologists with the intention of either inducing erections or correcting defects in the vascular beds of the penis. The primary research focus in this area is the pharmacological control of relaxation of the corpora cavernosal smooth muscle for the induction of erection. The three vascular pharmacologic approaches for the treatment of erectile dysfunction which are currently being evaluated include direct smooth muscle relaxation (e.g.

by papaverine and nitroglycerine), neuroreceptor modulation of smooth muscle responses (e.g. by α_1-adrenergic receptor blockade), and modification of the endothelial control of penile smooth muscle relaxation (e.g. by PGE_1). All of these approaches have been attempted with direct intrapenile injection of a variety of pharmacologic agents (Morales *et al.* 1987*a*; Lee *et al.* 1989; Lue 1989; Virag *et al.* 1991) but oral or alternative delivery methods such as application of transdermal patches or topical creams to the genitalia using these same approaches (Cavallini 1991) have not been as successful, primarily due to lower efficacy or systemic side-effects.

The challenge in targeting the end-organ responses for pharmacologic therapy is to minimize or eliminate systemic side-effects. This could be accomplished by creating a drug that has selectivity for the penile tissue responses either through dose selection or the identification of a receptor type that predominates in penile tissue. Basic science studies on the pharmacologic control of neurotransmission and smooth muscle contractility within the corpora cavernosa have been initiated with the hope of identifying unique characteristics of penile neuromuscular response or disease-induced changes in this regulation that would be amenable to systemic pharmacologic therapies. These initial studies have focused on the localization of catecholaminergic, cholinergic, and peptidergic transmitters within the cavernosal tissue and the characterization of the smooth muscle responses to agonists and antagonists for these receptors (Adaikan *et al.* 1981, 1991; Gu *et al.* 1983; Hedlund *et al.* 1984; Hedlund and Andersson 1985*a*; Lincoln *et al.* 1987; Saenz de Tejada *et al.* 1988*a,b*; Truex and Foreman 1989; Blanco *et al.* 1990; Traish *et al.* 1990). Additional receptors for putative autocrine substances such as the purinergic transmitters, prostaglandins, thromboxane, nitric oxide, and endothelin secreted from either the nerve terminals or endothelial cells have also been demonstrated (Hedlund and Andersson 1985*b*; Saenz de Tejada *et al.* 1988*a*, 1991*b*; Holmquist *et al.* 1990; Kim *et al.* 1991). The large range of interactions possible among all of these neuromuscular modulators presents a fertile research area for potential pharmacotherapies for vascular erectile disorders.

One promising pharmacotherapeutic approach is to elicit changes in smooth muscle response through effects on the vascular endothelium. The vascular endothelium has a major role in controlling smooth muscle tone through the release of a variety of relaxation and contraction factors. Some of these factors secreted by the endothelium include relaxation factors such as nitric oxide and prostaglandins such as PGE_1, and contraction factors such as endothelin and thromboxane (Hedlund and Andersson 1985*b*; Holmquist *et al.* 1990; Kim *et al.* 1991). In the corpora cavernosa, the relaxation effects of acetylcholine on smooth muscle are thought to be mediated by endothelia-derived relaxation factor(s) and this endothelial response appears to be changed in both experimentally induced diabetes and in tissue from diabetic patients (Fortes *et al.* 1983; Boura *et al.* 1986;

Adaikan *et al.* 1991). Another endothelial-dependent process that is increased in diabetes is the synthesis of thromboxanes which induce smooth muscle contraction (Gerrand *et al.* 1980). Therefore, one approach for the treatment of the vascular complications associated with diabetes (such as erectile dysfunction) is the use of thromboxane synthesis inhibitors and receptor antagonists, which would theoretically shift arachidonic acid metabolism toward the production of prostaglandins, or block the actions of thromboxanes thereby augmenting relaxation responses of smooth muscle. The use of intrapenile injection of PGE_1 is an example of how a deficit in an endothelial-dependent regulatory process can be bypassed in pharmacological therapy.

PROJECTIONS FOR PHARMACOTHERAPIES FOR ERECTILE DYSFUNCTION

Recent discoveries from physiological, pathophysiological, and pharmacological research on sexual responses have provided several major contributions towards the development of therapies for erectile dysfunction. First, these studies have defined regulatory roles for different components of the sexual response pathway stretching from the ventral diencephalon to the genitalia. Second, a variety of strategies for pharmacotherapies have been developed through the identification of the transmitters, receptors, and biochemical processes involved with responses at each level of this pathway. Finally, a variety of clinical trials have been initiated based upon the responses of novel pharmacological agents in newly developed animal models. In the near future, it should be possible to treat impotent patients with drugs that have been tailored for their specific sexual disorder regardless of whether it is a form of psychogenic dysfunction, neurogenic dysfunction, vasculogenic dysfunction, or a sexual disorder resulting from combined aetiologies. These new pharmacological approaches can be expected to have varied efficacy depending upon the cause of the dysfunction. Thus, the development of more reliable diagnostic techniques will be critical for the success of these therapies. Many of the pharmacological agents, e.g. dopaminergic and serotonergic agonists, may be useful diagnostic tools as well as pharmacotherapies.

Although the oral therapies are the most preferred, alternative routes of administration may be required for different pharmacotherapies. Currently, there are potential oral therapies under development which represent each of these pharmacological strategies. Examples of therapies that may be useful for the treatment of psychogenic disorders resultant from anxiety, depression, and hypoactive sexual desire include the α_2-antagonists, D_2-dopaminergic agonists, the 5-HT_{1A} agonists, and 5-HT_2 antagonists. An example of a therapy that may restore erectile function through the reduction of the erectile reflex response threshold is the opiate antagonist, naltrexone. However, neuropharmacologic therapies which are targeted for an acute induction of an erection may require parenteral administration in order to override the descending inhibition of the erectile response. One example of this type of therapy is the subcutaneous administration of dopaminergic agonists. The use of 5-HT_{1C} agonists to induce erections may also fall into this category. A possible example of an oral vascular pharmacological therapy is thromboxane synthesis inhibitor or receptor antagonist. However, the intrapenile administration of pharmacological agents is still the most efficacious pharmacotherapy for erectile dysfunction. Although some patients with psychogenic disorders may not respond (Diederic *et al.* 1991), this therapeutic approach can be expected to continue to have a major role in treating erectile dysfunction.

ACKNOWLEDGEMENTS

The authors acknowledge the efforts of Mr J.L. Hall, Mr R.L. Love, Ms A.M. McNulty, and Ms P. Wisler, who are the current active members of the technical staff in the Sexual Dysfunction Research Program within the Lilly Research Laboratories and Dr J.F. Wernicke, Dr A. Ridolfo, Dr J. McNay, Dr C. Samson, Dr J. Bay, Dr W. Offen, Mr V. Line, Ms D. Hildebrand, Ms L. Houpt, and Mr J. Bailey, the members of the Clinical Investigations Division within the Lilly Research Laboratories who have been responsible for the development of clinical trial methods for the evaluation of the safety and efficacy of pharmacological agents used for the treatment of sexual disorders in men and women. These individuals have been responsible for some of the new discoveries in sexual pharmacology.

REFERENCES

Aboseif, S.R. and Lue, T.F. (1988). Hemodynamics of penile erection. *Urologic Clinics of North America*, **15**, 1–7.

Adaikan, P.G., Karim, S., Kottegoda, S., and Ratnam, S. (1981). Cholinoreceptors in the corpus cavernosum muscle of the human penis. *Journal of Autonomic Pharmacology*, **3**, 107–11.

Adaikan, P.G., Lan, L.C., Nag, S.C., and Ratnam, S.S. (1991). Physio-pharmacology of human penile erection—autonomic/nitrergic neurotransmission and receptors of the human corpus cavernosum. *Asia Pacific Journal of Pharmacology*, **6**, 213–27.

Ahlenius, S. and Larsson, K. (1987). Evidence for a unique pharmacological profile of 8-OH-DPAT by evaluation of its effects on male rat sexual behaviour. In *Brain 5-HT$_{1A}$ Receptors* (ed. C.T. Dourish, S. Ahlenius, and P.H. Hutson), pp. 185–98. Ellis Horwood, Chichester.

Allen, L.S., Hines, M., Shryne, J.E., and Gorski, R.A. (1989). Two sexually dimorphic cell groups in the human brain. *Journal of Neuroscience*, 9, 497–506.

American Psychiatric Association (1987). Diagnostic and statistical manual of mental disorders (DSM-III R). APA, Washington, DC.

Andrezik, J.A., Chan-Palay, V., and Palay, S.L. (1981). The nucleus paragiganto-cellularis lateralis in the rat. Demonstration of afferents by the retrograde transport of horseradish peroxidase. *Anatomical Embryology*, 161, 373–90.

Angrist, B. and Gershon, S. (1976). Clinical effects of amphetamine and L-dopa on sexuality and aggression. *Comprehensive Psychiatry*, 17, 715–22.

Argiolas, A. and Gessa, G.L. (1991). Central functions of oxytocin. *Neuroscience and Biobehavioral Reviews*, 15, 217–31.

Bancroft, J. (1989). *Human sexuality and its problems* (2nd edn). Churchill Livingstone, Edinburgh, UK.

Barbeau, A. (1969). L-Dopa therapy in Parkinson's disease: a critical review of nine years' experience. *Canadian Medical Association Journal*, 101, 59–69.

Bardin, E.D. and Krieger, J.N. (1990). Pharmacological priapism: comparison of trazodone- and papaverine-associated cases. *International Journal of Urology and Nephrology*, 22, 147–52.

Benkert, O. (1980). Pharmacotherapy for impotence. *Modern Problems in Pharmacopsychiatry*, 15, 158–73.

Benkert, O., Crombach, G., and Kockott, G. (1972). Effect of L-dopa on sexually impotent patients. *Psychopharmacologia*, 23, 91–5.

Bennett, C.J., Seager, S.W., Vasher, E.A., and McGuire, E.J. (1988). Sexual dysfunction and electroejaculation in men with spinal cord injury: review. *Journal of Urology*, 139, 453–7.

Berendsen, H.H.G., Jenck, F., and Broekkamp, C.L.E. (1990). Involvement of 5-HT$_{1C}$ receptors in drug induced penile erections in rats. *Psychopharmacology*, 101, 57–61.

Bitran, D. and Hull, E.M. (1987) Pharmacological analysis of male rat sexual behavior. *Neuroscience and Biobehavioral Reviews*, 11, 365–89.

Blanco, R., Saenz de Tejada, I., Goldstein, I., Krane, R.J., Wotiz, H.H., and Cohen, R.A. (1990). Dysfunctional penile cholinergic nerves in diabetic impotent men. *Journal of Urology*, 144, 278–80.

Boura, A.L.A., Hodgson, W.C., and King, R.G. (1986). Changes in cardiovascular sensitivity of alloxan-treated diabetic rats to arachidonic acid. *British Journal of Pharmacology*, 89, 613–18.

Brown, E., Brown, G.M., Kofman, O., and Quarrington, B. (1978). Sexual function and affect in Parkinsonian men treated with L-dopa. *American Journal of Psychiatry*, 135, 1552–5.

Buffum, J. (1982). Pharmacosexology: the effects of drugs on sexual function. *Journal of Psychoactive Drugs*, 14, 5–44.

Carroll, J.L., Ellis, D.J., and Bagley, D.H. (1990). Age-related changes in hormones in impotent men. *Urology*, 36, 42–6.

Cavallini, G. (1991). Minoxidil versus nitroglycerin: a prospective double-blind controlled trial in transcutaneous erection facilitation for organic impotence. *Journal of Urology*, 146, 50–3.

Charney, D.S. and Heninger, G.R. (1986). Alpha$_2$-adrenergic and opiate receptor blockade, synergistic effects on anxiety in healthy subjects. *Archives of General Psychiatry*, 43, 1037–41.

Clark, J.T., Smith, E.R., and Davidson, J.M. (1985). Evidence for modulation of sexual behavior by alpha adrenoceptors in male rats. *Neuroendocrinology*, **41**, 36–43.

Crenshaw, T., Goldberg, J., and Stern, W. (1987). Pharmacologic modification of psychosexual dysfunction. *Journal of Sex and Marital Therapy*, **13**, 239–50.

Cumming, J. and Pryor, J.P. (1991). Treatment of organic impotence. *British Journal of Urology*, **67**, 640–3.

Dallo, J., Lekka, N., and Knoll, J. (1986). The ejaculatory behavior of sexually sluggish male rats treated with (−)deprenyl, apomorphine, bromocriptine and amphetamine. *Polish Journal of Pharmacology and Pharmacy*, **38**, 251–5.

Danjou, P., Alexandre, L., Warot, D., Lacomblez, L., and Puech, A.J. (1989). Assessment of erectogenetic properties of apomorphine and yohimbine. *British Journal of Clinical Pharmacology*, **26**, 733–9.

de Groat, W.C. and Booth, A.M. (1980). Physiology of male sexual function. *Annals of Internal Medicine*, **92**, 329–31.

Diederic, W., Stief, C.G., Lue, T.F., and Tanagho, E.A. (1991). Sympathetic inhibition of papaverine induced erection. *Journal of Urology*, **146**, 195–8.

Doherty, P.C., Wisler, P.A., and Foreman, M.M. (1991). Effects of quinelorane on yawning, penile erection and sexual behavior in the male rat. *Society for Neuroscience Abstracts*, **17**, 328.

Doogan, D.P. and Caillard, V. (1988). Sertraline: a new antidepressant. *Journal of Clinical Psychiatry*, **49** (Suppl.), 46–51.

Dornan, W. and Malsbury, C.W. (1989). Neuropeptides and male sexual behavior. *Neuroscience and Biobehavioral Reviews*, **13**, 1–15.

Dyck, P.J., Thomas, P.K., Asbury, A.K., Winegrad, A.I., and Porte, D. (1987). *Diabetic neuropathy*. W.B. Saunders, Philadelphia, PA.

Eaton, R.C., Moses, J., and Hull, E.M. (1991). Copulation increases dopamine activity in the medial preoptic area. *Society for Neuroscience Abstracts*, **17**, 328.

Ellis, L.R., Nellans, R.E., Kramer-Levien, D.J., Stewart Knoepfler, G., and Knoepfler, P. (1987). Evaluation of the first 300 patients treated at an outpatient center for male sexual dysfunction. *Western Journal of Medicine*, **147**, 296–300.

Fabbri, A., Jannini, A., Gnessi, L., Moretti, C., Ulisse, S., Franzese, A., Lazzari, R., Fraioli, F., Frajese, G., and Isidori, A. (1989). Endorphins in male impotence: evidence for naltrexone stimulation of erectile activity in patient therapy. *Psychoneuroendocrinology*, **14**, 103–11.

Fishman, R.B. and Breedlove, S.M. (1985). The androgenic induction of spinal sexual dimorphism is independent of supraspinal afferents. *Brain Research*, **355**, 255–8.

Foreman, M.M. and Hall, J.L. (1987). Effects of D_2-dopaminergic receptor stimulation on male rat sexual behavior. *Journal of Neural Transmission*, **68**, 153–70.

Foreman, M.M. and Moss, R.L. (1977). Effects of subcutaneous injections and intrahypothalamic infusions of releasing hormones upon lordotic response to repetitive mating. *Hormones and Behavior*, **8**, 219–34.

Foreman, M.M. and Moss, R.L. (1979). Roles of gonadotropins and releasing hormones in the hypothalamic control of lordosis behavior in the female rat. *Journal of Comparative Physiology and Psychology*, **93**, 556–65.

Foreman, M.M. and Wernicke, J.F. (1990). Approaches for the development of oral drug therapies for erectile dysfunction. *Seminars in Urology*, **8**, 107–12.

Foreman, M.M., Hall, J.L., and Love, R.L. (1988). Effects of LY237733, a selective 5-HT_2 receptor antagonist, on copulatory behavior of male rats. *Society for Neuroscience Abstracts*, **14**, 344.

Foreman, M.M., Hall, J.L., and Love, R.L. (1989). The role of the 5-HT$_2$ receptor in the regulation of sexual performance of male rats. *Life Sciences*, **45**, 1263–70.

Foreman, M.M., Hall, J.L., and Love, R.L.(1990). Acute effects of fenfluramine and pCA on copulatory behavior of male rats. *Society for Neuroscience Abstracts*, **16**, 388.

Forger, N.G. and Breedlove, S.M. (1986). Sexual dimorphism in human and canine spinal cord: role of early androgen. *Proceedings of the National Academy of Science, USA*, **83**, 7527–31.

Fortes, Z.B., Leme, J.G., and Scivoletto, R. (1983). Vascular reactivity in diabetes: role of the endothelial cell. *British Journal of Pharmacology*, **79**, 771–81.

Frank, E., Andersson, C., and Rubenstein, D. (1978). Frequency of sexual dysfunction in normal couples. *New England Journal of Medicine*, **299**, 111–15.

Freed, E. (1983). Increased sexual function with nomifensine. *Medical Journal of Australia*, **1**, 551.

Gall, H., Bahren, W., Holzki, G., Scherb, W., Sparwasser, C., and Ziegler, U. (1990). Ergebnisse nach multidisziplinarer abklarung bei patienten mit erektiler dysfunktion. *Hautarzt*, **41**, 353–9.

Gerrand, J.M., Stuart, M.J., Rao, G.H.R., Steffes, M.W., Mauer, S.M., Brown, D.M., and White, J.G. (1980). Alterations in the balance of prostaglandin and thromboxane synthesis in diabetic rats. *Journal of Laboratory and Clinical Medicine*, **95**, 950–8.

Glaser, T., Dompert, W.U., Schuurman, T., Spencer, D.P., and Traber, J. (1987). Differential pharmacology of the novel 5-HT$_{1A}$ receptor ligands 8-OH-DPAT, BAY R 1531 and ipsapirone. In *Brain 5-HT$_{1A}$ receptors* (ed. C.T. Dourish, S. Ahlenius, and P.H. Hutson), pp. 106–19. Ellis Horwood, Chichester.

Glazer, E.J., Steinbusch, H., Verhofstad, A., and Basbaum, A.I. (1981). Serotonin neurons in the nucleus raphe dorsalis and paragigantocellularis of the cat contain enkephalin. *Journal of Physiology*, **77**, 241–5.

Gorzalka, B.B., Mendelsohn, S.D., and Watson, N.V. (1990). Serotonin receptor subtypes and sexual behavior. *Annals of the New York Academy of Sciences*, **600**, 435–46.

Gower, A.J., Berendsen, H.H.G., Princen, M.M., and Broekkamp, C.L.E. (1984). The yawning–penile erection syndrome as a model for putative dopamine autoreceptor activity. *European Journal of Pharmacology*, **103**, 81–9.

Grant, L.D. and Stumpf, W.E. (1975). Hormone uptake sites in relation to CNS biogenic amine systems. In *Anatomical Neuroendocrinology* (ed. W.E. Stumpf and L.D. Grant), pp. 445–63. Karger, Basel.

Greenblatt, R.B., Jungck, E.C., and Blum, H. (1972). Endocrinology of sexual behavior. *Medical Aspects of Human Sexuality*, **6**, 110–31.

Gu, J., Polak, J.M., Probert, L., Isalm, K.N., Marangos, P.J., Mina, S., Adrain, T.E., McGregor, G.P., O'Shaughessy, J., and Bloom, S.R. (1983). Peptidergic innervation of the human male genital tract. *Journal of Urology*, **130**, 386–91.

Hansen, S. (1982). Spinal control of sexual behavior: effects of intrathecal administration of lisuride. *Neuroscience Letters*, **33**, 329–32.

Hedlund, H. and Andersson, K.-E. (1985*a*). Effects of some peptides on isolated human penile erectile tissue and cavernous artery. *Acta Physiologica Scandinavia*, **124**, 413–19.

Hedlund, H. and Andersson, K.-E. (1985*b*). Contraction and relaxation induced by some prostanoids in isolated human penile erectile tissue and cavernous artery. *Journal of Urology*, **134**, 1245–50.

Hedlund, H., Andersson, K.-E., and Mattisson, A. (1984). Pre- and postjunctional adreno- and muscarinic receptor functions in isolated human corpus spongiosum urethrae. *Journal of Autonomic Pharmacology*, **4**, 241–9.

Hegeler, S. and Mortensen, M. (1978). Sexuality and ageing. *British Journal of Sexual Medicine*, **5**, 16–19.

Holmquist, F., Andersson, K.-E., and Hedlund, H. (1990). Actions of endothelin on isolated corpus cavernosum from rabbit and man. *Acta Physiologica Scandinavia*, **139**, 113–22.

Howell, J.R., Reynolds, C.F., Thase, M.E., Frank, E., Jennings, J.R., Houck, P.R., Berman, S., Jacobs, E., and Kupfer, D.J. (1987). Assessment of sexual function, interest and activity in depressed men. *Journal of Affective Disorders*, **13**, 61–6.

Hull, E.M., Warner, R.K., Bazzett, T.J., Eaton, R.C., Thompson, J.T., and Scalletta, L.L. (1989). D_2/D_1 ratio in the medial preoptic area affects copulation of male rats. *Journal of Pharmacology and Experimental Therapeutics*, **251**, 422–7.

Jeanty, P., Van den Kerchove, M., Lowenthal, A., and DeBruyne, H. (1984). Pergolide therapy in Parkinson's disease. *Journal of Neurology*, **231**, 148–52.

Johnson, R.D. and Kitchell, R.L. (1987). Mechanoreceptor response to mechanical and thermal stimuli in the glans penis of the dog. *Journal of Neurophysiology*, **57**, 1813–36.

Kaplan, H.S. (1979). *Disorders of Sexual Desire*. Brunner Mazel, New York.

Kaplan, H.S. (1985). Comprehensive evaluation of disorders of sexual desire: introduction and overview. In *Comprehensive Evaluation of Disorders of Sexual Desire* (ed. H.S. Kaplan), pp. 1–16. American Psychiatric Press, Washington DC.

Kaplan, H.S. (1988). Anxiety and sexual dysfunction. *Journal of Clinical Psychiatry*, **49** (Suppl. 10), 21–5.

Kim, N., Azadzoi, K.M., Goldstein, I., and Saenz de Tejada, I. (1991). A nitric oxide-like factor mediates nonadrenergic-noncholinergic neurogenic relaxation of penile corpus cavernosum smooth muscle. *Journal of Clinical Investigation*, **88**, 112–18.

Kinsey, A.C., Pomeroy, W.B., and Martine, C.E. (1948). *Sexual Behavior in the Human Male*. W.B. Saunders, Philadelphia.

Knoll, J., Dallo, J., and Yen, T. (1989). Striatal dopamine, sexual activity and lifespan longevity of rats treated with (−)deprenyl. *Life Sciences*, **45**, 525–31.

Kolodny, R.C., Kahn, C.B., Goldstein, H.H., and Barnett, D.M. (1974). Sexual dysfunction in diabetic men. *Diabetes*, **23**, 306–9.

Krane, R.J. and Siroky, M.B. (1981). Neurophysiology of erection. *Urologic Clinics of North America*, **8**, 91–102.

Krane, R.J., Goldstein, I., and Saenz de Tejada, I. (1989). Impotence. *New England Journal of Medicine*, **321**, 1648–59.

Lal, S. (1988). Apomorphine in the evaluation of dopaminergic function in man. *Progress in Neuro-psychopharmacology and Biological Psychiatry*, **12**, 117–64.

Lal, S., Tesfaye, Y., Thavundayil, J., Thompson, T.R., Kiely, M.E., Nair, N.P.V., Grassino, A., and Dubrovsky, B. (1989). Apomorphine: clinical studies on erectile impotence and yawning. *Progress in Neuro-psychopharmacology and Biological Psychiatry*, **13**, 329–39.

Lal, S., Rios, O., and Thavundayil, J.X. (1990). Treatment of impotence with trazodone; a case report. *Journal of Urology*, **143**, 819–20.

Lee, L.M., Stevenson, W.D., and Szasz, G. (1989). Prostaglandin E$_1$ versus phentol-amine-papaverine for the treatment of erectile impotence: a double blind comparison. *Journal of Urology*, **141**, 549–50.

Leiblum, S.R. and Rosen, R.C. (1988). Introduction: changing perspectives on sexual desire. In *Sexual desire disorders* (ed. S.R. Leiblum and R.C. Rosen), pp. 1–20. Guilford Press, New York.

Leif, H.I. (1985). Evaluation of inhibited sexual desire. Relationship aspects. In *Comprehensive evaluation of disorders of sexual desire* (ed. H.S. Kaplan), pp. 61–76. American Psychiatry Press, Washington DC.

Levine, S.B. (1984). An essay on the nature of sexual desire. *Journal of Sex and Marital Therapy*, **10**, 83–96.

Lincoln, J., Crowe, R., Blacklay, P., Pryor, J., Lumley, J., and Burnstock, G. (1987). Changes in the VIPergic, cholinergic and adrenergic innervation of the human penile tissue in diabetic and non-diabetic impotent males. *Journal of Urology*, **137**, 1053–9.

Linnankoski, I., Gronosoos, M., Carlson, S., and Pertovaara, A. (1991). Atizepam-ezole, and alpha-2-adrenoreceptor increases sexual behavior in male monkeys. *Society for Neuroscience Abstracts*, **17**, 282.

Lovick, T.A. (1985). Projections from the diencephalon and mesencephalon to nucleus paragigantocellularis lateralis in the cat. *Neuroscience*, **14**, 853–61.

Lovick, T.A. (1987). Tonic GABAergic and cholinergic influences on pain control and cardiovascular control neurons in the nucleus paragigantocellularis lateralis of the rat. *Pain*, **31**, 401–9.

Lue, T.F. (1989). Intracavernous drug administration: its role in diagnosis and treatment of impotence. *Seminars in Urology*, **8**, 100–6.

Malmnas, C.O. (1976). The significance of dopamine, versus other catecholamines, for the L-dopa induced facilitation of sexual behavior in the castrated male rat. *Pharmacology, Biochemistry and Behavior*, **4**, 521–6.

Marson, L. and McKenna, K. (1990). The identification of a brainstem site controlling spinal sexual reflexes. *Brain Research*, **515**, 303–8.

Martin, C.E. (1981). Factors affecting sexual functioning in 60–79 year old married males. *Archives of Sexual Behavior*, **10**, 399–420.

Mas, M., Rodriguez del Castillo, A., Guerra, M., Davidson, J.M., and Battner, E. (1987). Neurochemical correlates of male sexual behavior. *Physiology and Behavior*, **41**, 341–5.

Melman, A., Tiefer, L., and Pederson, R. (1988). Evaluation of first 406 patients in urology department based center for male sexual dysfunction. *Urology*, **32**, 6–10.

Menendez, A.E., Moran, V.P., Velasco, P.A., and Marin, B. (1988). Modifications of the sexual activity of male rats following administration of antiserotonergic drugs. *Behavioral Brain Research*, **30**, 251–8.

Micevych, P.E., Coquelin, A., and Arnold, A.P. (1986). Immunohistochemical distribution of substance P, serotonin and methionine enkephalin in sexually dimorphic nuclei of the rat lumbar spinal cord. *Journal of Comparative Neurology*, **248**, 235–44.

Mikhalidas, D.P., Jeremy, J.Y., Shoukry, K., and Virag, R. (1990). Eicosanoids, impotence and pharmacologically induced erections. *Prostaglandins, Leukotrienes and Essential Fatty Acids*, **40**, 239–42.

Morales, A., Condra, M., Owen, J., Fenemore, J., and Surridge, D.H. (1987*a*). Oral and transcutaneous pharmacologic agents in the treatment of impotence. *Urologic Clinics of North America*, **15**, 87–93.

Morales, A., Condra, M., Owen, J., Fenemore, J., and Harris, C. (1987*b*). Is yohimbine effective in the treatment of impotence? Results of a controlled trial. *Journal of Urology*, **137**, 1168–72.

Murphy, M.R. (1988). Endogenous opiates and the mechanisms of male sexual behavior. In *Psychopharmacology of Sexual Disorders* (ed. M. Segal), pp. 51–62. John Libbey, London.

Nogueira, M.C., Herbaut, A.G., and Wespes, E. (1990). Neurophysiological invest-igations of two hundred men with erectile dysfunction. *European Urology*, **18**, 37–41.

Oomura, Y., Aou, S., Koyama, Y., Fujita, I., and Yoshimatsu, H. (1988). Central control of sexual behavior. *Brain Research Bulletin*, **20**, 863–70.

Othmer, E. and Othmer, S. (1987). Effect of buspirone on sexual dysfunction in patients with generalized anxiety disorder. *Journal of Clinical Psychiatry*, **48**, 201–3.

Patterson, D.G. and O'Gorman, E.C. (1989). Sexual anxiety in sexual dysfunction. *British Journal of Psychiatry*, **155**, 374–8.

Pfaus, J.G. and Gorzalka, B. (1987). Opioids and sexual behavior. *Neuroscience and Biobehavioral Reviews*, **11**, 1–34.

Pfaus, J.G., Damsma, G., Nomikos, G.G., Wenkstern, D.G., Blaha, C.D., Phillips, A.G., and Fibiger, H.C. (1990). Sexual behavior enhances central dopaminergic transmission in the male rat. *Brain Research*, **530**, 345–8.

Pinder, R.M., Brogen, R.N., Sawyer, P.R., Speight, T.M., and Avery, G.S. (1975). Fenfluramine: a review of its pharmacological properties and efficacy in obesity. *Drugs*, **10**, 241–323.

Pomerantz, S.D. (1990). Apomorphine facilitates erection in the rhesus monkey. *Pharmacology, Biochemistry and Behavior*, **35**, 659–64.

Pomerantz, S.D. (1991*a*). Quinelorane (LY163502): a D_2 dopaminergic receptor agonist, acts centrally to facilitate sexual behavior of rhesus monkeys. *Pharmacology, Biochemistry and Behavior*, **39**, 123–8.

Pomerantz, S.D. (1991*b*). 5-HT$_{1A}$ agonists, 8-OH-DPAT and ipsapirone, lower the ejaculatory threshold of rhesus monkeys. *Society for Neuroscience Abstracts*, **17**, 149.

Rasmussen, K. and Aghajanian, G.K. (1989). Withdrawal-induced activation of the locus coerulus neurons in opiate-dependent rats: attenuation by lesions of the nucleus paragigantocellularis. *Brain Research*, **505**, 346–50.

Riley, A.J., Goodman, R.S., Kellett, J.M., and Orr, R. (1989). Double blind trial of yohimbine hydrochloride in the treatment of erection inadequacy. *Sexual and Marital Therapy*, **4**, 17–26.

Rubin, A. and Babbott, D. (1958). Impotence and diabetes mellitus. *Journal of the American Medical Association*, **168**, 498–500.

Sachs, B.D. and Meisel, R.L. (1988). The physiology of male sexual behavior. In *The Physiology of Reproduction* (ed. E. Knobil, J.D. Neill, and L.L. Ewing), Vol. 2, pp. 1393–423. Karger, New York.

Saenz de Tejada, I. and Goldstein, I. (1988). Diabetic penile neuropathy. *Urologic Clinics of North America*, **15**, 17–22.

Saenz de Tejada, I., Goldstein, I., and Krane, R. (1988*a*). Local control of penile erection: nerves, smooth muscle and endothelium. *Urologic Clinics of North America*, **15**, 9–15.

Saenz de Tejada, I., Blanco, R., Goldstein, I., Azadozoi, K., de las Morenas, A., Krane, R., and Cohen, R. (1988*b*). Cholinergic neurotransmission in human corpus cavernosum. I. Responses of isolated tissue. *American Journal of Physiology*, **254**, H459–67.

Saenz de Tejada, I., Kim, N., Lagan, I., Krane, R., and Goldstein, I. (1989*a*). Regulation of adrenergic activity in penile corpus cavernosum. *Journal of Urology*, **142**, 1117–21.

Saenz de Tejada, I., Goldstein, I., Azadzoi, K., Krane, R., and Cohen, R.A. (1989*b*). Impaired neurogenic and endothelium-mediated relaxation of smooth muscle from diabetic men with impotence. *New England Journal of Medicine*, **320**, 1025–30.

Saenz de Tejada, I., Ware, C.J., Blanco, R., Pittard, J.T., Nadig, P.W., Azadzoi, K., Krane, R., and Goldstein, I. (1991*a*). Pathophysiology of prolonged penile erection associated with trazadone use. *Journal of Urology*, **145**, 60–4.

Saenz de Tejada, I., Carson, M.P., de las Morenas, A., Goldstein, I., and Traish, A.M. (1991*b*). Endothelin: localization, synthesis, activity and receptor types in human penile corpus cavernosum. *American Journal of Physiology*, **261**, H1078–85.

Sala, M., Braida, D., Leone, M.P., Calcaterra, P., Monti, S., and Gori, E. (1990). Central effect of yohimbine on sexual behavior in the rat. *Physiology and Behavior*, **47**, 165–73.

Scaletta, L.L. and Hull, E.M. (1990). Systemic or intracranial apomorphine increases copulation in long-term castrated male rats. *Pharmacology, Biochemistry and Behavior*, **37**, 471–5.

Schein, M., Zyzanski, S.J., Levine, S., Medalie, J.H., Dickman, R.L., and Alemangno, S.A. (1988). The frequency of sexual problems among family practice patients. *Family Practice Research Journal*, **7**, 122–34.

Scher, M., Krieger, J., and Juergens, S. (1983). Trazodone and priapism. *American Journal of Psychiatry*, **140**, 1362–3.

Schiavi, R.C. (1985). Evaluation of impaired sexual desire: biological aspects. In *Comprehensive evaluation of disorders of sexual desire* (ed. H.S. Kaplan), pp. 35–46. American Psychiatric Press, Washington DC.

Schiavi, R.C. and Hogan, B. (1979). Sexual problems in diabetes mellitus: psychological aspects. *Diabetes Care*, **2**, 9–17.

Schmidt, C.W. (1986). Common male sexual disorders: impotence and ejaculation. In *Clinical management of sexual disorders* (2nd edn) (ed. J.K. Meyer, C.W. Schmidt, Jr, and T.N. Wise), pp. 173–87. American Psychiatric Press, Washington DC.

Schoffling, K., Federlin, K., Ditschuneit, H., and Pfeiffer, E.F. (1963). Disorders of sexual function in male diabetics. *Diabetes*, **12**, 519–27.

Schreiner-Engel, P. and Schiavi, R.C. (1986). Lifetime psychopathology in individuals with low sexual desire. *Journal of Nervous and Mental Disorders*, **174**, 646–51.

Segraves, K.B. and Segraves, R.T. (1991). Hypoactive sexual desire disorder: prevalence and comorbidity in 906 subjects. *Journal of Sex and Marital Therapy*, **17**, 55–9.

Segraves, R.T. (1988*a*). Hormones and libido. In *Sexual desire disorders* (ed. S.R. Leiblum and R.C. Rosen), pp. 271–313. Guilford Press, New York.

Segraves, R.T. (1988*b*). Drugs and desire. In *Sexual desire disorders* (ed. S.R. Leiblum and R.C. Rosen), pp. 313–47. Guilford Press, New York.

Segraves, R.T. (1989). Effects of psychotropic drugs on human erection and ejaculation. *Archives of General Psychiatry*, **46**, 275–84.

Segraves, R.T. and Segraves, K.B. (1990). Categorical and multiaxial diagnosis of male erectile disorder. *Journal of Sex and Marital Therapy*, 16, 208–14.

Segraves, R.T., Bari, M., Segraves, K., and Spirnak, P. (1991). Effect of apomorphine on penile tumescence in men with psychogenic impotence. *Journal of Urology*, 145, 1174–5.

Senglaub, D.R. and Arnold, A.P. (1989). Hormonal control of neuron number in sexually dimorphic spinal nuclei of the rat: I. Testosterone-regulated death in the dorsolateral nucleus. *Journal of Comparative Neurology*, 280, 622–9.

Simerly, R.B. and Swanson, L.W. (1986). The organization of neural inputs to the medial preoptic nucleus of the rat. *Journal of Comparative Neurology*, 246, 312–42.

Simerly, R.B. and Swanson, L.W. (1988). Projections of the medial preoptic nucleus: a phaseolus vulgaris leucoagglutinin anterograde tract-tracing study in the rat. *Journal of Comparative Neurology*, 270, 209–42.

Simerly, R.B., Swanson, L.W., and Gorski, R.A. (1985). Reversal of sexually dimorphic distribution of serotonin-immunoreactive fibers in the medial preoptic nucleus by treatment with perinatal androgen. *Brain Research*, 340, 91–8.

Skagerberg, G., Bjorklund, A., Lindvall, O., and Schmidt, R.H. (1982). Origin and termination of the diencephalo-spinal dopamine system in the rat. *Brain Research Bulletin*, 9, 237–44.

Slag, M.F., Morley, J.E., Elson, M.K., Trence, D.L., Nelson, C.J., Nelson, A.E., Kinlaw, W.B., Beyer, S., Nuttall, F.Q., and Shafer, R.B. (1983). Impotence in medical clinical outpatients. *Journal of the American Medical Association*, 249, 1736–40.

Smith, E.R., Lee, R.L., Schnur, S.L., and Davidson, J.M. (1987). Alpha$_2$-adrenoceptor agonists and male sexual behavior. *Physiology and Behavior*, 41, 7–14.

Steers, W.D. (1990). Neural control of penile erection. *Seminars in Urology*, 8, 66–79.

Steers, W.D. and de Groat, W.C. (1989). Effects of *m*-chlorophenylpiperazine on penile and bladder function in rats. *American Journal of Physiology*, 257, R1441–9.

Susset, J., Tessier, C., Wincze, J., Bansal, S., Malhotra, C., and Schwacha, M.G. (1989). Effect of yohimbine hydrochloride on erectile impotence: a double-blind study. *Journal of Urology*, 141, 1360–3.

Szele, F.G., Murphy, D.L., and Garrick, N.A. (1988). Fenfluramine, *m*-chlorophenylpiperazine and other serotonin re-uptake agonists and antagonists on penile erections in non-human primates. *Life Sciences*, 43, 1297–303.

Traish, A.M., Carson, M.P., Kim, N., Goldstein, I., and Saenz de Tejada, I. (1990). Characterization of muscarinic acetylcholine receptors in human penile corpus cavernosum studies on whole tissue and cultured endothelium. *Journal of Urology*, 144, 1036–40.

Truex, L.L. and Foreman, M.M. (1989). Pharmacological studies on K$^+$-evoked release of ^{3}H-norepinephrine from rat corpus cavernosum. *Proceedings of the Society for Neuroscience*, 15, 631.

Verwoerdt, A., Pfeiffer, E., and Wand, H.S. (1969). Sexual behavior in senescence. II. Patterns of sexual activity and interest. *Geriatrics*, 24, 137–54.

Virag, R., Shoukry, K., Floresco, J., Nollet, F., and Greco, E. (1991). Intracavernous self-injection of vasactive drugs in the treatment of impotence: 8-Year experience with 615 cases. *Journal of Urology*, 145, 287–93.

Wagner, C.K. and Clemens, L.G. (1991). Projections of the paraventricular nucleus of the hypothalamus to the sexually dimorphic region of the spinal cord. *Brain Research*, **539**, 254–62.

Whitehead, E.D., Klyde, B.J., Zussman, S., and Salkin, P. (1990). Diagnostic evaluation of impotence. *Postgraduate Medicine*, **88**, 123–38.

Yaryura-Tobias, J., Diamond, B., and Merlis, S. (1970). The action of L-dopa on schizophrenic patients (a preliminary report). *Current Therapeutic Research*, **12**, 528–31.

Zajecka, J., Fawcett, J., Schaff, M., Jeffriess, H., and Guy, C. (1991). The role of serotonin in sexual dysfunction: fluoxetine-associated orgasm dysfunction. *Journal of Clinical Psychiatry*, **52**, 66–8.

5

Evaluation of drug effects on
human sexual function

Alan J. Riley and Elizabeth J. Riley

INTRODUCTION

In spite of the upsurge in research activity in the area of sexual functioning which followed the work of Masters and Johnson (1966, 1970), there have been few attempts to investigate the effect of drugs on human sexual function. Renshaw (1978) concludes her review, *Sex and drugs*, with the request for scientific evaluation of drug effects on sexual function, viz. 'Sexual side effects of needed medications must not only be noted but carefully and scientifically studied by physicians, since these may offer important avenues of understanding of the many unresolved riddles of the neurophysiology of the human sexual response'. Investigation of the effect of drugs on human sexual function may also suggest possible new pharmacotherapeutic approaches to the management of sexual dysfunction.

Much of the literature on human sexual pharmacology is based on anecdotal reports volunteered by patients of changes in their sexual function occurring, or more accurately, reported, during treatment with a particular drug. Less commonly, a more systematic enquiry into patients' sexual behaviour by means of questionnaires grafted on to clinical trials undertaken for other purposes have been reported. There have been few well controlled studies undertaken specifically to investigate sexual effects of drugs.

Reported sexual side-effects of drugs

There are three ways by which side-effects may be elicited: by spontaneous reporting by the patient, by direct questioning, or by the use of symptom-finding questionnaires. The spontaneous reporting approach is open to many biases. Patients may well volunteer adverse sexual effects but they may not comment so readily on beneficial or sexually enhancing effects a drug may have. Hence there is a bias towards reporting only negative effects. Spontaneous reporting is dependent upon the relationship between the patient and the doctor. Some patients feel unable to discuss aspects of their sexual behaviour with a particular doctor so that drug-induced changes may be unreported. There is probably also a sex difference—men may feel able to discuss sexual problems with their doctors whereas women may be more reluctant to do so, which is one of the reasons that accounts for the fact that at least 90 per cent of published sexual effects of drugs relate to males. Fortunately, more women now than in the past are able to discuss aspects of their sexual behaviour with their physicians. Physicians may also be less inclined to ask elderly patients about their sexual function which will lead to under-reporting of drug-induced changes in sexual function. This is particularly significant in view of high use of chronic medication in elderly patients. Under-reporting of sexual side-effects of drugs in the literature also probably occurs from failure of doctors to report them even when the patient has brought them to his or her attention.

Spontaneous reporting is the least satisfactory approach to eliciting sexual side-effects of drugs. Direct questioning of the patient by the doctor is better but not ideal, as it is open to any of the biases mentioned above. It is, however, more effective at detecting sexual effects. In a study that evaluated three antihypertensive agents, the incidence of impotence was found to be 10 per cent by spontaneous reporting and 26 per cent by direct questioning (Pritchard *et al.* 1968). Detection of sexual symptoms during drug treatment is improved by the use of symptom-finding questionnaires. Obviously, their use depends on pre-planning and designing, knowing what questions to ask, and the design of an appropriate questionnaire. Observations from a study of patients on antihypertensive treatment serve to illustrate the improved efficiency of this method of eliciting sexual symptoms compared with direct questioning—while no patient complained of decreased libido on direct questioning, 37 per cent reported this symptom when completing a questionnaire (Costa *et al.* 1979).

The design of a questionnaire deserves careful consideration. We are talking here about questionnaires used in trials that are not set up specifically to investigate sexual issues. It is axiomatic that the questions must be easily understood by the patients but this sometimes causes problems in the sexual area. Not all patients are willing to answer questions relating to their sexual functioning. For example, in a symptom-finding study in hypertensive men and women in which a very simple questionnaire was used, almost seven per cent of respondents who answered questions about peripheral vascular symptoms omitted to respond to questions about their sexual function (Riley *et al.* 1987). Ideally the questionnaire should be capable of identifying drug effects on the different components of sexual behaviour and response (drive, arousal, orgasm, ejaculation, and satisfaction) but some patients lack the necessary knowledge to enable such differentiation to be made. Furthermore, the more sexually explicit a questionnaire is, the lower is the response rate. In the questionnaire study alluded to above where the questions relating to sexual function formed only a small part of the instrument a relatively high response rate (68.3 per cent) was achieved. In contrast, Butler (1976) distributed a much more detailed questionnaire relating to sexual function to groups of women and obtained a response rate of only 36 per cent.

The occurrence of a reported sexual effect during drug treatment must be critically assessed. A patient may use a newly prescribed drug as a scapegoat for a pre-existing sexual difficulty. It is therefore essential to obtain a comprehensive sexual history before accepting that the symptom is, in fact, drug-induced. Many conditions for which drugs are given are associated with increased risk of sexual difficulties. Indeed, this increased incidence of sexual difficulties may obscure drug-induced changes.

An important procedure in assessing alleged side-effects of drugs is to withdraw the drug ('de-challenge') and then re-introduce the drug ('re-challenge') and observe what happens to the symptom. If it disappears on de-challenge and then reappears on re-challenge the likelihood that the symptom is drug induced is greatly increased. Re-challenge should be undertaken with matched placebo control to reduce the psychological effect resulting from the patient taking a tablet already associated, in his or her mind, with causing the particular symptom. Ideally, placebo-controlled re-challenge should be conducted double-blindly, but unfortunately not all pharmaceutical companies are willing or able to supply matching placebo and active tablets for this purpose. Sometimes this problem can be overcome by encapsulating the tablets locally.

The procedure of de-challenge and re-challenge has two important pitfalls in the case of suspected drug-induced sexual effects. De-challenge may not be associated with improvement in sexual function because a secondary psychogenic dysfunction could be superimposed on the primary (drug-induced) dysfunction causing the sexual symptom to persist after the drug is withdrawn despite the drug being initially implicated. In addition, de-challenge may not be associated with a rapid alleviation of the sexual symptom where the causative drug induced sexual dysfunction through endocrine mechanisms where some time may be taken after drug withdrawal for the endocrine status to return to normal.

LABORATORY STUDIES

The effects of drugs on sexual function can be studied in the laboratory in much the same way as drug effects on other body systems are investigated. They can be studied in healthy volunteers or in patients presenting with a defined sexual dysfunction. The design of laboratory studies of sexual function must take into account the volunteers or patients who participate, the stimulus used to induce the sexual response, and the means by which the sexual response is assessed and recorded.

Volunteers

Not all people are willing to participate in studies of their sexual behaviour or response. A questionnaire concerning sexual experience and behaviour was distributed to 200 women who had not previously taken part in a laboratory study of their sexual response (Riley 1990). Only 72 (36 per cent) questionnaires were returned completed, and of these respondents only 16 (i.e. eight per cent of the total number of women who received the questionnaire) expressed willingness to participate in sexual response studies. It is not known how many of these women would actually take part when the details of the study were discussed with them. Wolchick *et al.* (1983) found that only 15 per cent of a sample of female psychology undergraduates, already self-selected by their willingness to take part in a sexual questionnaire study, indicated interest in participating in a study which assessed vaginal responses to sexually explicit stimuli, once the methods involved were described. Considering, perhaps artificially, the observations of these two studies, it appears that less than two per cent of women would be willing to take part in sexual response studies. Figures relating to willingness of men to participate in such studies are not available but are probably comparable or slightly higher. The question arises as to whether the small proportion of people who are willing to participate are representative of the general population with respect to sexual responding in laboratory studies.

There are increasing data suggesting that people who volunteer for studies differ in several ways from non-volunteers. A higher incidence of psychopathology has been found in volunteers (Lasagna and von Felsinger 1954; Pollin and Perlin 1958). However, no differences on personality characteristics such as social desirability, psychopathic deviance, social participation, or authoritarianism were found between volunteers and non-volunteers for sexual questionnaire or interview studies (Baker and Perlman 1975). In contrast, a study of young unmarried male and female psychology students showed that, compared with non-volunteers, students who volunteer for a sexual behaviour study appeared to be more sexually permissive, had more non-coital experiences, dated more frequently, and held more liberal attitudes (Kaats and Davis 1971). Wolchick *et al.* (1983) reported that potential volunteers for a sexual response study had a higher frequency of masturbation than non-volunteers; a difference also found by Riley (1990). Volunteers for a study involving vaginal measures of sexual arousal differed from non-volunteers in that they had more exposure to commercialized erotic material, were exposed to these materials at an earlier age, reported less sexual fear, and had experienced more sexual trauma (Wolchick *et al.* 1983).

Patients who volunteer to take part in studies may also differ in many important aspects from those who do not volunteer. For example, in-patient alcoholics who volunteered to participate in an intrusive study of sexual function differed from non-volunteers in that they showed a greater interest in sex, reported less satisfaction with sex, and were more concerned about sexual functioning (Nirenberg *et al.* 1991). In addition there was a greater incidence of premature ejaculation and of negative sexual experiences in the volunteers.

It has been suggested that sexual arousal patterns are influenced by previous sexual experience (Griffitt 1975). Hence, in the light of the differences between volunteers and non-volunteers mentioned above, people who participate in laboratory sex studies might show different arousal patterns to non-volunteers. However, Heiman (1977) failed to show that the amount of previous sexual experience affected the degree of sexual arousal induced by listening to erotic audiotapes in the laboratory.

There are two levels of selection of volunteers for sexual response studies. First there is the self-selection by the people themselves as to whether they are willing to participate or not. This may involve influences from their sexual partner, although the importance of this aspect has not been addressed in studies. Secondly, from the people who have volunteered, the investigator must select those subjects who are suitable for the particular study. Thus, if we are wanting to study the effect of a drug that may inhibit sexual arousal in women, there is little point in recruiting women who are unable to experience sexual arousal in response to the selected stimulus in the laboratory.

An important limitation of studies in healthy volunteers is that the volunteers may respond maximally to sexual stimulation thereby not providing a means for demonstrating a sexually enhancing property of a drug.

Stimulus

The human sexual response can be invoked by a variety of stimuli. These can be grouped broadly into those that are generated in the brain, either intrinsically (fantasy) or by processing external stimuli perceived by the special senses, and those that involve direct physical stimulation of the erogenous body zones (masturbation). When designing laboratory investigations for studying the effect of drugs on the sexual response it is important to select an appropriate stimulus.

Fantasy has been used to induce sexual arousal in laboratory studies and some studies have shown significant correlation between subjective assessment and physiological measurement of sexual arousal induced by this mode of stimulation (Heiman 1977; Schreiner-Engel *et al.* 1981*a*). However, not all subjects can become sexually aroused in response to fantasy (Stock and Geer 1982) and very few people are capable of attaining orgasm by fantasy alone. Fantasy has, however, been used as the stimulus in a study of drug effect on human sexual response. Gillman and Lichtigfeld (1983) reported their study of the effects of breathing nitrous oxide on orgasm in women. Seven women were studied but unfortunately only one of these women attained orgasm during the study. This occurred irrespective of whether she inhaled nitrous oxide or air. The remaining six volunteers experienced at least mild genital sensations during fantasy which were enhanced by nitrous oxide. If the object of this study had been to investigate the effect of nitrous oxide on sexual arousal, then fantasy may have been an appropriate stimulus. As it is, nitrous oxide was not an appropriate stimulus to study drug effects on orgasm.

Sexual arousal can be induced by exposing volunteers to erotic material. This may be achieved by the subject reading erotic stories, listening to erotic narration, or by viewing erotic visual images presented by slides, films, or video tapes. The way erotic material is presented and the instructions that accompany it may influence the sexual response induced. When using recorded stories, the sex of the narrator can affect the degree of sexual arousal induced. An interesting study in men showed that greater subjective arousal but not greater physiological responding occurred when the narrator was female than when the same story was narrated by a man (Hall *et al.* 1985). Dekker *et al.* (1985) have illustrated the influence prior instruction can have on sexual arousal induced by listening to erotic narration. They found that sexual arousal was lower when the volunteers were instructed to attend to the description of the situations and events in a story than when they were told to attend to the images of sexual feelings in such situations. These are important considerations that need to be borne in mind when designing studies on the effect of drugs on sexual response where multiple experimental sessions are usually required.

Erotic material presented by video is now, perhaps, the most convenient stimulus for studies on the effect of drugs on the sexual response, but it has limitations. Few men or women are able to experience orgasm in response to such a stimulus and therefore it is inappropriate for studying the effects of drugs on orgasm, unless it is expected that the drug will lower the threshold for orgasm. Furthermore, in men, penile erection in response to visual erotic stimuli appears to be androgen independent (Bancroft and Wu 1983; Kwan *et al.* 1983) and therefore this would not be an appropriate mode of stimulation for an investigation of an anti-androgen on male sexual response. The hormonal determinants of sexual arousal induced by visual erotic stimuli in women have yet to be elucidated.

If the objective of the study is to investigate the effect of a drug on ejaculation and/or orgasm, direct genital stimulation is probably the most appropriate stimulus since it is the most certain of the various modes of stimulation to induce orgasm and ejaculation. Wagner and Levin (1980) used direct clitoral self-stimulation in their study of the effect of muscarinic blockade on sexual arousal and climax. In an attempt to standardize clitoral stimulation, we use a vibrator in our studies of drug effects on female sexual response (Riley and Riley 1981, 1983, 1986). In men, a vibrating sheath has been used as the stimulus in a pharmacological study (Riley *et al.* 1982). Finally, heterosexual love play including sexual intercourse has been used in some studies on the effects of drugs on the sexual response (Fox 1970; Wagner and Levin 1980; Riley unpublished observations). The subject will be exposed to a variety of stimuli including visual, tactile, auditory, genital, and fantasy. Although intercourse is a very important model on which to study the effects of drugs it is the least satisfactory from a research methodological point of view because it is impossible to control for the various external and internal stimuli to which the subject is exposed.

Rather than inducing the sexual response by the use of external stimuli, some studies have examined the effect of drugs on nocturnal penile erections (Kowalski *et al.* 1985; Goldstein 1986). Nocturnal erections are androgen dependent and induced by central mechanisms linked to sexual drive (Bancroft and Wu 1983; O'Carroll *et al.* 1985). Thus studying the effect of a drug on nocturnal erections provides a means of investigating how the drug affects central arousablility.

Evaluation of response

Assessment of drug effects on the human sexual response may be based on either subjective or objective phenomena. Subjective assessment usually relies on the volunteer completing rating scales either during or following sexual stimulation. While scientifically it is valuable to have objective assessment, it is also important to know how the volunteer perceived their sexual arousal. Drugs may influence the interaction between cognitive and physiological events associated with sexual arousal. For example, Malatesta *et al.* (1982) in their study of the effects of alcohol on sexual response in women found that subjective sexual arousal and orgasmic pleasurability showed a positive linear relationship to the level of intoxication, although physiological and behavioural accompaniments showed significant depression at higher blood-alcohol levels.

Evaluation of sexual arousal

Numerous rating scales have been developed for the subjective assessment of sexual arousal. These range in complexity from a simple ordinal rating of sexual arousal from 'no sexual arousal' (score 1) to 'very strong sexual arousal' (score 7) (Abramson *et al.* 1981) to scales that rate individually separate physiological events associated with sexual arousal. For example, Wincze *et al.* (1976) for their studies of female sexual response developed an 'awareness of physiological changes' score (APC). The APC involves the volunteer rating each of the following events on a scale ranging from zero (no change) to 5 (imagined maximum response): vaginal lubrication, breast swelling, nipple erection, skin flushing, pelvic warmth, increased heart rate, increased breathing rate, increased muscle tone, and less awareness of the environment. When using such a scale in studies involving drug effects it is essential to consider that the drug may effect one or more of these physiological changes by a direct pharmacological effect without affecting the sexual response, which may complicate the assessment of the effect of the drug on sexual arousal when this type of scale is employed.

Early studies of the human sexual response assessed sexual arousal by monitoring heart rate, blood pressure, finger temperature, electrodermal responses, and pupillary response but none of these parameters are useful in this context because they fail to differentiate sexual arousal from other kinds of arousal (Zuckerman 1971). Monitoring the temperature of the breasts in women, or groin (Wincze *et al.* 1977), or forehead (Hoon *et al.* 1976) have been used and have been shown to correlate with sexual arousal in some subjects.

The physiological changes that are specific to sexual arousal are genital vasocongestion and erection. Various methods for monitoring sexual arousal based on detecting these genital changes have been developed.

Objective assessment of sexual arousal in men involves recording penile erection, generally by means of a strain gauge applied to the penis. The most widely used method is the mercury in silastic rubber strain gauge (Fisher *et al.* 1965). In recent years solid-state semiconductor strain gauges have been developed (Bancroft 1974) as well as photoelectric cells for recording pulse amplitude from the dorsal penile artery of the penis (Bancroft and Bell 1985). Strain gauges measure changes in circumference or diameter of the penis but an important characteristic of the erect penis is an increase in penile rigidity. It is now possible to measure and record penile rigidity by means of 'RigiScan', an ingenious apparatus developed by Bradley *et al.* (1985). The apparatus is portable and recording can be undertaken in the volunteer's home. RigiScan can be used for real-time monitoring of penile rigidity and tumescence (Silva *et al.* 1990). In addition to recording nocturnal erections, RigiScan provides a means of recording acute drug effects on penile erection, such as following intracorporeal injection of drugs and for monitoring penile responses during exposure to erotic stimuli.

Methods used for assessing sexual arousal in women include clitoral strain gauges (Karacen *et al.* 1970), measuring vaginal surface oxygen tension (Wagner and Levin 1978*a*), recording transvaginal potential difference (Wagner and Levin 1978*b*), detecting local temperature changes by thermistors embedded in vaginal diaphragms (Shapiro *et al.* 1972) or applied to the labia (Henson and Rubin 1978), or by thermography (Abramson *et al.* 1981). Fugl-Meyer *et al.* (1984) devised a radiotelemetric vaginal temperature-recording device so that sexual arousal could be recorded without the volunteer being constrained by wires. The design of the device permitted intercourse to occur without disrupting the recordings.

Vaginal blood flow has been monitored by film anemometry using a heated oxygen electrode, maintained at constant temperature, which is held against the vaginal surface by a suction device (Wagner and Levin 1978*a*). This method has been used to study the effect of atropine on sexual arousal (Wagner and Levin 1980). Vaginal blood flow during sexual arousal has also been studied by the method of washout of radioactive xenon after intra-epithelial injection (Wagner and Ottesen 1980). The most widely used method for monitoring sexual arousal in women is vaginal photoplethys-mography (Geer *et al.* 1974). The two commonly employed indices of sexual arousal derived from vaginal photoplethysmography are the vaginal blood volume and the vaginal pulse amplitude. The latter has been found to be a more sensitive and informative measure of sexual arousal than vaginal blood volume (Osborn and Pollack 1977; Korff and Geer 1983). The data output from a vaginal photoplethysmograph can be recorded directly on a 'Medilog' miniature analogue tape recorder to enable studies to be undertaken in the security of the volunteer's own home (Sarrel *et al.* 1977).

An important feature of sexual arousal in women is increased production of vaginal lubricating fluid. Although this can be assessed subjectively by using rating scales (Wincze *et al.* 1976; Riley and Riley 1986), it has also been measured gravimetrically by collecting the fluid on pre-weighed pieces of filter paper (Semmens and Wagner 1982) or tampons (Riley and Riley 1983).

Orgasm

When studying the effects of drugs on orgasm it is necessary to consider orgasmic latency (the time between onset of stimulation and attainment of orgasm), and the sensation or pleasure component. Some workers have also included 'satisfaction' or 'relief from sexual tension' following orgasm (Riley and Riley 1986). Although orgasm in both sexes is generally associated with somatic manifestations, such as muscle spasm, these do not correlate with subjective pleasure/sensations and therefore can not be used as objective parameters. Hence orgasmic pleasure can only be assessed subjectively by the use of either rating scales or questions. Wagner and Levin (1980) in their study of the effects of atropine on female sexual arousal graded orgasms on a five point scale: poor or weak (1), fair or moderate (2), strong or good (3), very good (4), and most powerful or excellent (5). Ordinal rating scales from 1 (very weak) to 5 (extremely strong), with an addition category (zero) for no orgasm have been used in several studies of the effects of drugs on sexual response in women (Riley and Riley 1983, 1986). In contrast, in a study of the effects of alcohol, Malatesta *et al.* (1982) employed a scale of just three categories, in which orgasm was less intense (1), no different (2), or more intense (3).

Objective measures can be used to record orgasmic latency. Riley and Riley (1983) used a blinded stop clock which the subjects started when stimulation was commenced and stopped at the onset of orgasm. In a similar vein, orgasmic latency has been measured by the use of a response button connected to a polygraph which the subject activates to signal the beginning of sexual stimulation, the onset of orgasm, and the end of orgasm (Malatesta *et al.* 1982). In women, the onset of orgasm is characterized by a dramatic decrease in vaginal blood volume as recorded by plethysmography (Geer and Quartararo 1976). This, probably resulting from movement rather than an actual change in vasocongestion, provides a means of measuring orgasmic latency.

Study design and standardization

Since expectation plays a role in determining sexual response to erotic stimuli (Wilson and Lawson 1976; Heiman 1977) studies must be undertaken under at least single- and preferably double-blind conditions. There are large interpersonal differences in volunteers' sexual responding in laboratory studies whether measured physiologically or assessed subjectively. To control for this variance, very large numbers of volunteers need to be studied if the parallel group design is used. This is usually impractical.

Cross-over study design reduces the variance caused by interpersonal differences in response but creates other difficulties. Well controlled studies require at least two experimental sessions, one with active and one with placebo. It is sometimes useful to have a familiarization session before the randomized treatment sessions and often more sessions are needed, such as when looking for dose-related effects. An important consideration in the design of such studies is the possibility of habituation to the stimulus. Studies have shown that repeated exposures to the same sexual stimuli result in decreased responsiveness (Howard *et al.* 1970; O'Donohue and Geer 1985). These changes may complicate the interpretation of treatment-induced effects in cross-over studies.

Another possible complicating factor in laboratory studies is distraction. Geer and Fuhr (1976) showed that sexual arousal in male volunteers, as measured by changes in penile tumescence, varied directly as a function of the complexity of simultaneously applied distracting and interfering cognitive operations. Hence study procedures must not be too complicated or distracting so as to interfere with sexual responding.

Every attempt must be made to standardize the experimental conditions. While some conditions can be controlled, others, such as fantasy, are impossible to control. It seems prudent to control the interval between the subject's previous orgasmic experience and the study session as this could influence sexual responding, although there are no convincing data to support this.

For studies in women, the influence of the menstrual cycle should be taken into account. Masters and Johnson (1966) observed higher levels of sexual-arousal-induced vaginal vasocongestion during the pre-menstrual phase than at other times in the menstrual cycle. Schreiner-Engel *et al.*

(1981*b*) found that subjective reports of sexual arousal induced in the laboratory did not differ significantly between follicular, ovulatory, and luteal phases of the menstrual cycle whereas an objective measure of sexual arousal, vaginal vasocongestion, did vary significantly with higher mean levels occurring during the follicular and luteal phases than during the ovulatory phase. They also found that correlation between subjective and objective measures of sexual arousal was higher during the luteal phase than at other times in the menstrual cycle (Schreiner-Engel *et al.* 1981*a*). Hence changes in sexual responding or subjective assessment of sexual response resulting from the influence of the menstrual cycle may confound the interpretation of results of studies undertaken in different phases of the cycle.

CLINICAL TRIALS

Whereas volunteers may be reluctant to participate in laboratory studies of sexual function, patients experiencing sexual difficulties are often extremely willing to take part in clinical trials evaluating pharmacotherapeutic approaches to their difficulties. It follows their need to explain their difficulties in terms of physical factors.

Early trials frequently involved patients with all types of sexual problems, with little attempt being made to classify the patients according to principal presenting symptom. It is now appreciated that the majority of patients complaining of sexual difficulties fall into well defined diagnostic categories, such as those described by the American Psychiatric Association (American Psychiatric Association 1980). Such diagnostic categories can be used as inclusion criteria for clinical trials. Whether patients with different sexual diagnoses are recruited to a trial or recruitment is restricted to one diagnostic category will depend on the pharmacological properties of the drug under test and the objectives of the study. In either case it is essential to make and record the actual sexual diagnosis before the patient enters the trial.

In the case of many sexual dysfunctions it is assumed that the patient included in the trial has potential to improve. Indeed, in many cases it is impossible to explore this potential before entry to the study. However, in the case of erectile dysfunction it is known that some men, such as those with severe pelvic arterial occlusive disease, may not have the potential for improvement in response to drug treatment. It would therefore be desirable to exclude such patients from clinical trials, but at the present state of knowledge it is not always possible to identify patients who lack capacity for improvement. Erectile response to intracorporeally administered vasoactive drugs (e.g. prostaglandin E_1 or papaverine), monitoring nocturnal tumescence, and recording response to visual erotic stimuli are useful screening tests for different aspects of erectile function (Bancroft *et al.* 1991).

Primary measures of outcome in clinical trials usually involve subjective assessments. In some trials of drug treatments for erectile dysfunction the outcome is assessed in terms of ability to satisfactorily complete sexual intercourse. Likewise, in trials of drugs for the treatment of premature ejaculation the outcome is generally assessed in terms of ejaculatory control during intercourse. When the outcome assessment is based on sexual behaviour with a partner, consideration must be given to the quality of the relationship and the presence of any sexual difficulties in the partner. A drug may well improve erections but this improvement will not be detected if the patient's partner has vaginismus and the only outcome criterion is attainment of vaginal penetration. It is also important to consider that the patient's sexual partner may have a latent sexual difficulty which only becomes manifest when the patient's sexual function improves. The emerging sexual difficulty in the partner could obscure any improvement in the patient. Questionnaires such as the 'Locke-Wallace marital adjustment scale' (Locke and Wallace 1959) are available which assess the quality of sexual and non-sexual components of relationships, and it would be prudent to include such a questionnaire in the pre-trial assessment of patients so that those found to have significant disharmony which might interfere with or obscure the patient's improvement can be excluded from the trial.

It is essential to record baseline data before the patient enters the treatment phase of the trial. This is usually collected in two ways, first by assessment in the consulting room using either questionnaires or by structured interview, and secondly by the patient keeping a daily record of his sexual activity over the course of four or more weeks. Data collected in this way will depend on the diagnosis and the objectives of the study but since it is not always known precisely what aspect of sexual functioning the drug under test will affect at the outset of the study, it is useful to collect data on most aspects of sexual activity. This may include frequency of sexual thoughts, masturbation and lovemaking as indices of sexual drive, awakening erections, spontaneous daytime erections, erections in response to sexual stimulation, and intercourse as measures of erectile function, occurrence of ejaculation, and/or orgasm, whether it is premature or delayed, and its quality. The daily record should be easy for the patient to complete and should be in a format that does not cause embarrassment if seen by other family members or friends.

There may be some benefit in the patient taking placebo under single (patient) blind conditions during the baseline data-collection phase. Firstly, placebo responders can be identified and excluded from the treatment phase of the trial thereby reducing the total number of patients required in the trial and, secondly, as a test of the patient's compliance. Patients who do not comply with taking the treatment or in completing the daily record of their sexual activity should be excluded from the trial.

During the course of the study treatment the patient should continue to complete the same daily record of sexual activity. Whether there is any value in the patient's partner keeping a similar record is debatable. In most studies where this has been done (e.g. Riley and Riley 1979) there is a high level of concordance between the patient's and his partner's data, and the question whether collusion occurred must be asked.

CONCLUSION

Pharmacotherapy will play an increasingly important role in the management of sexual difficulties. It is essential that we continue to develop and improve methods for the evaluation of drugs on human sexual functioning, both in normal volunteers during the early phases of drug development and for use in clinical trials in patients. The limitation of volunteer studies has been described and no potential drug should be rejected entirely on the absence of good effect in volunteers.

REFERENCES

Abramson, P.R., Perry, L.B., Seeley, T.T., Seeley, D.M., and Rothblatt, A.B. (1981). Thermographic measures of sexual arousal: a discriminant validity analysis. *Archives of Sexual Behaviour*, **10**, 171–6.

American Psychiatric Association (1980). *Diagnostic and statistical manual of mental disorders*. APA, Washington DC.

Baker, W.J. and Perlman, D. (1975). Volunteer bias and personality traits in sexual standards research. *Archives of Sexual Behaviour*, **4**, 161–71.

Bancroft, J. (1974). *Deviant sexual behaviour: modification and assessment*. Clarendon, Oxford.

Bancroft, J. and Bell, C. (1985). Simultaneous recording of penile diameter and penile arterial pulse during laboratory based erotic stimulation in normal subjects. *Journal of Psychosomatic Research*, **29**, 303–13.

Bancroft, J. and Wu, F.C.W. (1983). Changes in erectile responsiveness during androgen replacement therapy. *Archives of Sexual Behaviour*, **12**, 59–66.

Bancroft, J., Smith, G., Munoz, M., and Ronald, P. (1991). Erectile response to visual erotic stimuli before and after intracavernosal papaverine and its relationship to nocturnal penile tumescence and psychometric assessment. *British Journal of Urology*, **68**, 629–38.

Bradley, W.E., Timm, G.W., Gallagher, J.H., and Johnson, B.K. (1985). New method for continuous measurement of nocturnal penile tumescence and rigidity. *Urology*, **26**, 4–9.

Butler, C.A. (1976). New data about female sexual response. *Journal of Sex and Marital Therapy*, **2**, 40–6.

Costa, F., Abrosioni, E., and Magnani, B. (1979). Side effects of antihypertensive drugs: incidence and methods of collection. *International Journal of Pharmacology and Biopharmacology*, **17**, 405–9.

Dekker, J., Everaerd, W., and Verhelst, N. (1985). Attending to stimuli or to images of sexual feelings: effects on sexual arousal. *Behavioural Research and Therapy*, **23**, 139–49.

Fisher, C., Gross, J., and Zuch, J. (1965). Cycle of penile erection synchronous with dreaming (REM) sleep. *Archives of General Psychiatry*, **12**, 29–45.

Fox, C. (1970). Reduction in the rise of systolic blood pressure during coitus of the beta adrenergic blocking agent propranolol. *Journal of Reproduction and Fertility*, **22**, 587–90.

Fugl-Meyer, A., Sjogren, K., and Johansson, K. (1984). A vaginal temperature registration system. *Archives of Sexual Behaviour*, **13**, 247–60.

Geer, J.H. and Fuhr, R. (1976). Cognitive factors in sexual arousal: the role of distraction. *Journal of Consulting and Clinical Psychology*, **44**, 238–43.

Geer, J. and Quartararo, J. (1976). Vaginal blood volume responses during masturbation. *Archives of Sexual Behaviour*, **5**, 403–13.

Geer, J.H., Morokoff, P., and Greenwood, P. (1974). Sexual arousal in women: the development of a measuring device for vaginal blood volume. *Archives of Sexual Behaviour*, **3**, 559–64.

Gillman, M.A. and Lichtigfeld, F.J. (1983). The effects of nitrous oxide and naloxone on orgasm in human females: a preliminary report. *Journal of Sex Research*, **19**, 49–57.

Goldstein, J.A. (1986). Erectile function and naltrexone. *Annals of Internal Medicine*, **105**, 799.

Griffitt, W. (1975). Sexual experience and sexual responsiveness: sex differences. *Archives of Sexual Behaviour*, **4**, 529–40.

Hall, K.S., Binik, Y., and Tomasso, E.D. (1985). Concordance between physiological and subjective measures of sexual arousal. *Behavioural Research and Therapy*, **23**, 297–303.

Heiman, J.R. (1977). A psychophysiological exploration of sexual arousal patterns in females and males. *Psychophysiology*, **14**, 266–74.

Henson, D. and Rubin, H. (1978). A comparison of two objective measures of sexual arousal in women. *Behavioural Research and Therapy*, **16**, 143–51.

Hoon, P., Wincze, J., and Hoon, E.F. (1976). Physiological assessment of sexual arousal in women. *Psychopharmacology*, **13**, 196–204.

Howard, J.L., Reifler, C.B., and Liptzin, M.B. (1970). Effects of exposure to pornography. *Technical Report of the Commission on Obscenity and Pornography* (Vol. B). US Government Printing Office, Washington DC.

Kaats, G. and Davis, K. (1971). Effects of volunteer biases in studies of sexual behaviour and attitudes. *Journal of Sex Research*, **7**, 26–34.

Karacen, I., Rosenbloom, A.L., and Williams, R.L. (1970). The clitoral erection cycle during sleep. *Psychopharmacology*, **7**, 338–42.

Korff, J. and Geer, J.M. (1983). The relationship between sexual arousal experience and genital response. *Psychopharmacology*, **20**, 121–7.

Kowalski, A., Stanley, R.O., Dennerstein, L., Burrows, G., and Maguire, K.P. (1985). The sexual side effects of antidepressant medication: a double-blind comparison of two antidepressants in a non-psychiatric population. *British Journal of Psychiatry*, **147**, 413–18.

Kwan, M., Greenleaf, W.J., Mann, J., Crapo, L., and Davidson, J.M. (1983). The nature of androgen action on male sexuality: a combined laboratory self report study in hypogonadal men. *Clinical Endocrinology and Metabolism*, **57**, 557–67.

Lasagna, L. and von Felsinger, J.M. (1954). The volunteer subject in research. *Science*, **120**, 359–61.

Locke, H.J. and Wallace, K.M. (1959). Short marital adjustment and prediction tests: their reliability and validity. *Marriage and Family Living*, **21**, 252–5.

Malatesta, V.J., Pollack, R.H., Crotty, T.D., and Peacock, L.J. (1982). Acute alcohol intoxication and female orgasmic response. *Journal of Sex Research*, **18**, 1–17.

Masters, W.H. and Johnson, V.E. (1966). *Human sexual response*. Churchill Livingstone, London.

Masters, W.H. and Johnson, V.E. (1970). *Human sexual inadequacy*. Churchill Livingstone, London.

Nirenberg, T.D., Wincze, J.P., Bansal, S., Liepman, M.R., Engle-Friedman, M., and Begin, A. (1991). Volunteer bias in a study of male alcoholics' sexual behaviour. *Archives of Sexual Behaviour*, **20**, 371–9.

O'Carroll, R.E., Shapiro, C., and Bancroft, J. (1985). Androgens, behaviour and nocturnal erection in hypogonadal men: the effects of varying the replacement dose. *Clinical Endocrinology*, **23**, 527–38.

O'Donohue, W.T. and Geer, J.H. (1985). The habituation of sexual arousal. *Archives of Sexual Behaviour*, **14**, 233–46.

Osborn, C.A. and Pollack, R.H. (1977). The effects of two types of erotic literature on physiologic and verbal measures of female sexual arousal. *Journal of Sex Research*, **13**, 250–6.

Pollin, W. and Perlin, S. (1958). Psychiatric evaluation of 'normal control' volunteers. *American Journal of Psychiatry*, **115**, 129–33.

Pritchard, B.N.C., Johnston, A., Hill, I., and Rosenheim, M. (1968). Bethanidine, guanethidine and methyldopa in treatment of hypertension: a within patient comparison. *British Medical Journal*, **i**, 135–44.

Renshaw, D.C. (1978). Sex and drugs. *South African Medical Journal*, **54**, 323–6.

Riley, A.J. (1990). Are women who volunteer for sexual response studies representative of women in general? *Sexual and Marital Therapy*, **5**, 131–40.

Riley, A.J. and Riley, E.J. (1979). Amitriptyline–perphenazine and the squeeze technique in premature ejaculation. *Journal of Pharmacotherapy*, **2**, 136–40.

Riley, A.J. and Riley, E.J. (1981). The effect of labetalol and propranolol on the pressor response to sexual arousal in women. *British Journal of Clinical Pharmacology*, **12**, 341–4.

Riley, A.J. and Riley, E.J. (1983). Cholinergic and adrenergic control of human sexual responses. In *Psychopharmacology and sexual disorders* (ed. D. Wheatley). Oxford University Press.

Riley, A.J. and Riley, E.J. (1986). The effect of single dose diazepam on female sexual response induced by masturbation. *Sexual and Marital Therapy*, **1**, 49–53.

Riley, A.J., Riley, E.J., and Davies, H.J. (1982). A method for monitoring drug effects on male sexual response. The effect of single dose labetalol. *British Journal of Clinical Pharmacology*, **14**, 695–700.

Riley, A.J., Steiner, J.A., Cooper, R., and McPherson, C.K. (1987). The prevalence of sexual dysfunction in male and female hypertensive patients. *Sexual and Marital Therapy*, **2**, 131–8.

Sarrel, P.M., Foddy, J., and McKinnon, J.B. (1977). Investigation of human sexual response using a cassette recorder. *Archives of Sexual Behaviour*, **6**, 341–8.

Schreiner-Engel, P., Schiavi, R.C., and Smith, H. (1981a). Female sexual arousal: relation between cognitive and genital assessment. *Journal of Sex and Marital Therapy*, **7**, 256–67.

Schreiner-Engel, P., Schiavi, R.C., Smith, H., and White, D. (1981b). Sexual arousability and the menstrual cycle. *Psychosomatic Medicine*, **43**, 199–214.

Semmens, J.P. and Wagner, G. (1982). Estrogen deprivation and vaginal function in postmenopausal women. *Journal of the American Medical Association*, **248**, 445–8.

Shapiro, A., Cohen, H., DiBiancho, P., and Rosen, G. (1972). Vaginal blood flow during sleep and sexual arousal. *Psychopharmacology*, **4**, A394.

Silva, J.P., Coelho-Moos, E., Vaz, F., Gomez, C., and Lencastre, J. (1990). Real time rigidometry with RigiScan and its accuracy. In *Diagnosing impotence* (ed. D. Pozza and G.M. Colpi). Masson, Milan.

Stock, W. and Geer, J. (1982). A study of fantasy-based arousal in women. *Archives of Sexual Behaviour*, **11**, 33–47.

Wagner, G. and Levin, R. (1978a). Oxygen tension of the vaginal surface during sexual stimulation in the human. *Fertility and Sterility*, **30**, 50–3.

Wagner, G. and Levin, R. (1978b). Vaginal fluid. In *The human vagina* (ed. E.S.E. Hafez), pp. 121–37. Elsevier, Amsterdam.

Wagner, G. and Levin, R. (1980). Effect of atropine and methylatropine on human vaginal blood flow, sexual arousal and climax. *Acta Pharmacologica and Toxicologica*, **46**, 321–5.

Wagner, G. and Ottesen, B. (1980). Vaginal blood flow during sexual stimulation. *Obstetrics and Gynaecology*, **56**, 621–4.

Wilson, G.T. and Lawson, D. (1976). Effects of alcohol on sexual arousal in women. *Journal of Abnormal Psychology*, **85**, 489–97.

Wincze, J.P., Hoon, E.F., and Hoon, P.W. (1976). Physiological responsivity of normal and sexually dysfunctional women during erotic stimulus exposure. *Journal of Psychosomatic Research*, **20**, 445–51.

Wincze, J.P., Hoon, P., and Hoon, E.F. (1977). Sexual arousal in women: a comparison of cognitive and physiological responses by continuous measurement. *Archives of Sexual Behaviour*, **6**, 121–33.

Wolchick, S.A., Spencer, S.L., and Lisi, I.S. (1983). Volunteer bias in research employing vaginal measures of sexual arousal. *Archives of Sexual Behaviour*, **12**, 399–408.

Zuckerman, M. (1971). Physiological measures of sexual arousal in the human. *Psychological Bulletin*, **75**, 297–329.

6

The nature of human sexual desire and its modification by drugs

John Kellett

INTRODUCTION

There are various ways of classifying sexual desire, and even more ways of attempting to measure it. Intrapsychically it is manifest by a sensitivity to sexual stimuli, preoccupation with sexual fantasies, and/or a longing to be with the preferred partner. Physiologically there is a lowered threshold for genital engorgement which may only be relieved by orgasm. The relation between physical and psychological changes is complex, which prevents one making any clear assessments of the libido from physical arousal. Certainly the physical and psychological changes react with each other in the manner of a feedback loop, the feeling of genital engorgement leading to psychic arousal and vice versa. There are several difficulties in assessing sexual desire.

First, there are likely to be differences in the degree to which an individual will perceive a stimulus as erotic. This is obvious if one is giving a heterosexual stimulus to a homosexual but even within the heterosexual community there are big differences in choice of eroticism. Second, there are physical changes which reduce the physiological response independent of libido. A good example is age changes where the level of sexual physical arousal may show little relation to psychic sexual desire. Third is the opposite phenomenon in which erections may occur without sexual stimulation such as during REM sleep. Fourth is the response of the individual to physical arousal. Some young women, for example, misinterpret vaginal lubrication as a discharge, a source of discomfort which inhibits further arousal.

Animal research has long distinguished between proceptive and receptive sexuality, typifying the response of the male and female respectively. As Leiblum and Rosen (1988) have observed 'men have a more insistent and constant sexual appetite . . . whilst women have more sporadic sexual desires which they are more likely to suppress if a host of conditions are not met'. More specifically the female can respond quickly to a desired advance but will not seek that contact as actively as the male. There is some evidence that only proceptive sexuality is androgen dependent (Herbert 1978).

The image of the hunter, aroused by visual stimuli from afar, igniting the desire of his partner by an embrace, has been dented by evidence of similar arousal in women by visual stimuli (Rubinsky *et al.* 1987). Nevertheless, there does appear to be a difference in the choice of pornography, men preferring pictures of 'pin-ups' and explicit descriptions of coitus, whilst women choose accounts of courting behaviour (Faun 1981). Even visual images are processed differently, with men imagining they are making love to the girl in the picture of a couple whereas women imagine they are that girl (Money and Erhardt 1972). The naked male seems to have much less effect on the male and female heterosexual, which may account for the decision of *Playgirl* to give up the example of *Playboy* in displaying photographs of the opposite sex nude. (Another explanation may be the ambiguity of the female nude's state of sexual arousal compared with frontal views of the male, which would generally invite censorship if such magazines portrayed the aroused male.) Some would argue that these sexual differences are largely cultural in origin, it being less acceptable for women to express sexual interest. Either way it leaves comparative measurement of male and female libido in difficulties.

In many ways the search for an effective aphrodisiac is the philosopher's stone of psychopharmacology. However, the outcome of that search has been equally fruitless. Drugs to suppress libido are available in abundance, but the true aphrodisiac remains elusive. In part this is because it is also expected to be the elixir of youth, and in part because of man's suggestibility, that many such remedies have been found, accepted, and then rejected (from cocoa to honey, hence honeymoon—a month of honey). A strong appetite for food and sex is the mark of health, and drugs which promote well-being, such as Ginseng, not surprisingly gain a reputation in this area.

HORMONES

The natural stimulant of male sexuality is testosterone. This is demonstrated by surgical (Heim 1981) and chemical (Money 1970; Bancroft *et al.* 1974) castration, which first causes a loss of sexual drive and later of activity. However, such subjects still show normal physical arousal to erotic films (Bancroft and Wu 1983) and some remain sexually active (Bremer 1959). Though it may be tempting to attribute the loss of sexual activity with age to the decline in circulating testosterone levels, Davidson *et al.* (1983) found that in a sample of 220 males aged 41 to 93 only three per cent of the variance in libido (sexual thoughts) was explained by the levels of free testosterone whilst age accounted for 16 per cent. Testosterone exerts its masculinizing effects largely through its metabolite, dihydrotestosterone, which raises the question as to which is most active on the brain. In apes, dihydrotestosterone seems inactive (Herbert 1978) in this regard, but in humans Bancroft (1989) quotes two studies suggesting that they are equally effective, one showing that those with 5-α-reductase deficiency, who cannot produce dihydrotestosterone, develop normal libido, whilst the other indicated that men given the latter for androgen deficiency recover their libido equally well.

Though testosterone restores sexual activity in the hypogonad (Davidson *et al.* 1979), this effect disappears as one approaches normal testosterone levels (Davidson *et al.* 1982; Carani *et al.* 1990). However, O'Carroll and Bancroft (1984) found testosterone increased sexual thoughts but not activity in men with inhibited desire and normal testosterone levels. The role of testosterone in the female is far less clear. Attempts to relate female sexuality to her levels of testosterone have in general been unsuccessful. Sanders and Bancroft (1982) found a significant correlation between levels of testosterone in mid-cycle and frequency of masturbation. There is a trend for higher levels of circulating testosterone in women who work full time, and Sanders and Bancroft (1982) postulate that this may have an androgenizing effect on offspring during gestational development. A larger study by the same group investigated the effect of hormones on the sexuality of 55 female undergraduates taking and 53 not taking the contraceptive pill. Pill users had lower levels of free testosterone but it was only in this group that correlations emerged, namely a positive correlation with interest and activity, but, on this occasion not with masturbation. The effects were small and the authors conclude that psychosocial factors overwhelm the slight effects of testosterone in women (Bancroft *et al.* 1991*b*).

Anecdotal accounts of the effect of testosterone given to women in the 1940s and 50s suggest it causes a marked increase in libido. For example, Kennedy and Nathanson (1953) reported that there was such an increase in libido, when testosterone was given for cancer, that treatment had to be stopped. The dose given was a male replacement dose which would be virilizing if not combined with oestrogens. Carney *et al.* (1978) found that sublingual testosterone increased the effect of psychotherapy for low libido when compared with diazepam. Theoretically, as anxiety inhibits sexual arousal, benzodiazepines should be helpful, but as explained below this is not the case. In a subsequent study, Mathews *et al.* (1983) found that testosterone had no more effect than placebo, and the previous results were probably due to the libido-suppressing effect of diazepam. Nevertheless, there are several reports of an increase in libido when testosterone is added to female sex hormones given after the menopause (Greenblatt *et al.* 1950; Studd *et al.* 1977; Sherwin and Gelfand 1984). Sherwin and Gelfand (1987) noted that the addition of 150 mg of testosterone to oestrogen replacement in 44 women with a surgical menopause significantly increased ratings of sexual desire, fantasies, sexual activity, and orgasms per coitus. Surprisingly the only double-blind study in this area (Dow *et al.* 1983) did not reach significance. The role of suggestion in this subject is well illustrated by a sensible and happily married middle-aged lady with whom I entered into a double-blind study of 100 mg of Sustanon (testosterone ester), i.m. three weekly. After five years of distressingly low libido, the first injection produced a dramatic change, with a nocturnal spontaneous orgasm and regular enjoyable coitus for the first two weeks. The second injection had no effect, though as we eventually discovered it was this second injection which was the active preparation.

Welling *et al.* (1990) have suggested that testosterone may have a place in treating women who have had a menopause due to oophorectomy but is probably unnecessary in those whose menopause is natural.

Oestrogens and progesterone

There is little evidence that either of these hormones have much effect on female libido, not least because of the various studies on the effect of the contraceptive pill (Bancroft *et al.* 1991*a*) and the relatively little effect of the menopause (Hallstrom and Samuelsson 1990). In males, both oestrogens and progesterone can reduce libido. Oestrogen is certainly necessary for priming genitalia, an effect which is antagonized by progesterone. Female rhesus monkeys given both hormones become more proceptive, arguably because of the failure of oestrogens to increase attention from the male, rather than any direct effect of progesterone on libido (Herbert 1978).

Prolactin

High levels of prolactin appear to inhibit sexual drive in both men (Marrama *et al.* 1984) and women (Riley 1984) which is restored by treatment with bromocriptine (Sobrinho *et al.* 1987) (though this could be a direct dopaminergic or antidepressant effect). Though in males there seems to be an association between low libido and moderately raised levels of prolactin (Weizman *et al.* 1983), which could be stress related, lactating women do not appear to show such an effect (Robson *et al.* 1981). Elliott and Watson (1985) and Alder and Bancroft (1988) report a reduction of pleasure derived from coitus in lactating women. It has been suggested that this effect of prolactin is due to a reduction in testosterone production, though this is not an invariable effect of increased prolactin (Brown *et al.* 1981), which initially stimulates testosterone secretion (Rubin *et al.* 1976). The finding of Oseko *et al.* (1988) that testosterone falls with sulpiride-induced hyperprolactinaemia, while the response to human gonadotrophin is not affected, would suggest that any effect is not directly on the testes.

Other neuropeptides

Dornan and Malsbury (1989) in a recent review of the subject conclude that LHRH, oxytocin, α-MSH, and substance P stimulate male sexual behaviour whilst the three stress-related peptides CRF, β-endorphin, and prolactin are inhibitory.

DRUGS

Alcohol

Alcohol is the most widely used aphrodisiac in our society. There is, however, little doubt that alcohol has a dose-related effect in reducing penile engorgement as measured by diameter, when watching erotic films (Farkas and Rosen 1976; Rubin and Henson 1976). The loss of erection cannot, of course, be taken to equate to a reduction in libido. There are also many reports of a reduction in drive and erectile ability in chronic alcoholics (e.g. Mandell and Miller 1983; Forrest 1983).

Fahrner (1987) reported on sexual dysfunction in 101 male chronic alcoholics finding that 47 per cent suffered low libido, 42 per cent erectile failure, and 72 per cent some form of sexual dysfunction. Surprisingly, after four months treatment as an in-patient and a nine-month follow-up in the community, 66 per cent continued to have sexual problems which affected the 73 per cent who remained abstinent as much as those who relapsed. Levels of testosterone remained within the normal range throughout. The feminization of male alcoholics is not due to a failure of the liver to break down oestrogens, as was once thought, but to an increase in their production from testosterone, as well as changes in oestrogen-receptor-site sensitivity and in binding proteins (Lieber 1989). Though reducing libido, alcohol also appears to broaden the range of erotic stimuli to which a man may respond, thus increasing the development of sexual deviance (Langevin *et al.* 1988).

Sexual arousal in women, as measured by vaginal pulse amplitude when watching an erotic film, was also reduced in a dose-related manner (Wilson and Lawson 1976), but unlike the men, women reported greater psychological arousal after alcohol. This can be attributed to disinhibition, which can occur with any sedative drug, but this may be an oversimplification, and alcohol may indeed have mild aphrodisiac qualities. However, the effect in the alcoholic is the same as in the male, namely 64 per cent complaining of loss of libido, and of anorgasmia (Covington 1983).

Marijuana

Most studies of drug users find that marijuana increases sexual pleasure and responsiveness, though this may not extend to proceptive sexuality (Koff

1974). In their study of 345 undergraduates, males were more likely to report an increase in pleasure and females an increase in desire. Gay *et al.* (1973) interviewed long-term drug users in San Francisco and noted that 80 per cent reported an enhancement of sexual pleasure from marijuana. Such surveys suffer from problems of selection but it is of interest that practically no subject reported a damaging effect on sexuality. There have been no penile tumescence and vaginal pulse studies on this drug. Curiously, animal studies have failed to demonstrate any aphrodisiac effect of marijuana (Taylor-Segraves 1988). Though Kolodney *et al.* (1974) concluded that marijuana reduces testosterone production in males (through reduction in LH levels) and sperm count, Mendelson *et al.* (1974) could not confirm changes in testosterone.

Cocaine

This is also reported to heighten sexual pleasure (Gay *et al.* 1982) and desire, though it is difficult to separate sexual enjoyment from desire. Chronic use, however, leads to the opposite effect (Taberner 1985). Street drugs go through the same processes as prescription ones—a honeymoon period of uncritical use, the occasional report of bad 'trips', followed by transfer to the next drug of addiction. Cocaine is still in this first period, at least as far as 'crack' is concerned.

Amphetamine

This is also associated with sexual enhancement, as noted by Gay *et al.* (1973) who found subjects reporting an immediate erection on intravenous injection of methylamphetamine and increased desire, though the same group (Gay *et al.* 1982) found less enhancement in later studies. The amphetamine effect may be due to general arousal within the CNS perhaps mediated by enhanced catecholamine release.

Tobacco

Nicotine is also a stimulant but there is no evidence of any effect on libido. Tobacco does, however, reduce fertility in women and hastens the menopause (Abel 1985).

Opiates

These are generally associated with a reduction in both desire and performance (Cushman 1972). At one time the delay in ejaculation with heroin was used therapeutically. Further evidence for this effect of opiates is the increased sexual drive on withdrawal of the drug and the spontaneous erections and ejaculation which occur with naltrexone, an opiate antagonist (Charney *et al.* 1986). Since endorphins appear to be the major rewarding neurotransmitters, they may well be released at orgasm, their effect being diminished as the brain becomes tolerant of exogenous opiates.

Minor tranquillizers

Though originally recommended for sexual dysfunction there is no doubt that these drugs reduce libido. Riley and Riley (1986) studied the effect of different doses of diazepam or placebo given blind to eight women who masturbated two hours later. Using subjective ratings there was a dose-related reduction in arousability, lubrication, and speed and sensation of orgasm, but there was no consistent effect on ratings of satisfaction, probably because of a euphoriant action of the diazepam making up for any loss of sexual pleasure. This could of course, be a simple process of inhibition of physical arousal without affecting libido, as has been suggested for alcohol. Against this was the finding by Carney *et al.* (1978) that testosterone was better than diazepam at stimulating libido, and the later finding by Mathews *et al.* (1983) that testosterone had no more effect than placebo, leading the authors to suggest that diazepam reduced the efficacy of the behavioural programme through a reduction in libido. An alternative explanation is that benzodiazepines interfere with all psychological procedures to reduce anxiety (Sartory 1983). A reduction in male libido caused by benzodiazepines has been noted by Magnus *et al.* (1977). If valid these results must bring into question the effects of giving benzodiazepines as night sedatives.

Buspirone is a 5-HT agonist, from which one might predict that it would inhibit libido like other 5-HT agonists. However, it is a fairly specific 1A agonist which stimulates male sexual behaviour in animals. Othmer and Othmer (1987) describe its effects when given to three men and seven women with an anxiety state and sexual dysfunction. After four weeks treatment in an open trial all but one reported that their sexual function had returned to normal. Apart from one patient who dropped out of the trial, the others reported a uniform and significant improvement in all four scales (interest, arousability, performance, and sexual contact). There was no record of hypersexuality. They did not rule out the effects of withdrawal from other psychotropic medication two to three weeks before starting buspirone, or a placebo effect. The only other sedative suspected of affecting sexual function is methaqualone which was reported as aphrodisiac (Gay *et al.* 1982; Abel 1985) more effective in women than men.

Major tranquillizers

These have in common the capacity to block dopamine transmission at D_2 receptors, thereby increasing levels of prolactin. They also have antihistamine, anticholinergic, and antiadrenergic effects, some of which may affect function if not libido (Laughren *et al.* 1981). Dopamine, if given in the form of L-dopa for the treatment of Parkinson's disease has been noted to increase libido (see below). The antilibidinal effect of the major tranquillizers may be therefore a direct effect of dopamine blockade. Benperidol has been promoted for its antilibidinal effect (Tennant *et al.* 1974), but there is no reason to think that it differs from other neuroleptics in this capacity. Now there are neuroleptics available which seem to be more specific in acting on D_3 receptors (Lancet 1990) whose effect on libido is unknown.

Antidepressants

Loss of libido is one of the most fundamental symptoms of depression mirroring the hypersexuality of mania. One would therefore predict that antidepressants would increase libido, but such is not the case. Some antidepressants like clomipramine and phenelzine impair ejaculation and have a useful role in treating a premature response. This has probably nothing to do with their antidepressant action since the effect is immediate, whilst the antidepressant effects take several days to appear. I have recently reviewed antidepressants on their effect on the genital item of the Hamilton scale for depression. Sadly, despite the widespread use of this scale, many studies have not retained this individual rating. From the little data available, phenelzine and imipramine were less effective than placebo (Harrison *et al.* 1985), as were amitriptyline and fluvoxamine, which in the fourth week actually reduced the already impaired libido (Bohacek *et al.* 1976; Lapierre *et al.* 1984; Amin *et al.* 1984). Murphy and Bridgeman (1978) compared mianserin with amitriptyline and imipramine, respectively, and noted negligible change in sexual desire despite recovery of depression. Similar results were obtained with lithium (Delandale Laboratories, private report), flupenthixol, and nortriptyline (Johnson 1983). Only two antidepressants have been shown to increase libido independent of mood: viloxazine (De Leo and Magni 1983) and trazodone (Gartrell 1986; Sullivan 1988). Other drugs which may stimulate libido include lofepramine (Kimura *et al.* 1978), doxepin (Renshaw 1975), and tranylcypromine (Simpson *et al.* 1965). All these drugs appear to be noradrenergic except trazodone whose effects are still little understood. Its effects on depression may indicate a serotonergic action but it may also have antagonist activity especially on 5-HT$_2$ receptors. These results are therefore consistent with the view that, in general, serotonin (5-HT) reduces libido, whilst dopamine, and possibly noradrenaline stimulate libido. Mention must be made of a syndrome of apparently excessive proceptive sexuality noted after clomipramine and other 5-HT specific antidepressants (McLean *et al.* 1983). This syndrome is not the result of mania, but gives rise to irresistible sexual feelings, leading to impulsive sexual assaults on others; this hypersexuality is far from an exaggeration of normal sexual drive. Fenfluramine, another serotonergic agent, has been reported to increase (Stevenson and Solyom 1990) and decrease libido (Hughes 1971), which may relate to its ability to first release and then deplete serotonin levels, and/or its α_2-blocking action may be involved as well.

Non-psychotropic drugs

Many drugs have the effect of reducing erections though it is usually assumed that these effects are direct, and do not operate through a reduction in libido. These include thiazides and β blockers (Taylor *et al.* 1981). Some drugs may antagonize the effects of testosterone, such as spironolactone and cimetidine, both of which cause gynaecomastia in males (Clark 1965; Fave *et al.* 1977). Toxic drugs are likely to reduce libido simply because of malaise, though cytotoxic drugs also have hormonal effects (Chapman *et al.* 1979). Similarly, chronic digoxin therapy lowers libido and reduces testosterone and LH levels in males (Neri *et al.* 1980). Clofibrate is also reported to reduce libido (Coronary Drug Project Research Group 1975).

Many of the drugs used to treat epilepsy are likely to reduce libido because of their ability to increase levels of sex-hormone-binding globulin, and reduce levels of free testosterone (Fenwick *et al.* 1985). Barbiturates are rated by addicts as one of the least effective at improving sexual function and generally appear to reduce libido (Abel 1985). The low libido of epileptic patients noted by Fenwick *et al.* (1985) may be related to drug treatment; carbamazepine and phenytoin having less effect than phenobarbitone and primidone (Mattson and Cramer 1985). On the other hand, low libido is a feature of temporal-lobe epilepsy (Gastaut and Collomb 1954), whether or not the patient was taking anticonvulsants (Hierons and Saunders 1966). Spark *et al.* (1984) reported on a study of 16 hyposexual men, 11 of whom were found to have temporal-lobe epilepsy. Despite hormonal deficits, the libido did not respond to hormonal therapy until the fits had been brought under control, suggesting that anticonvulsants are more likely to *increase* than decrease the libido of epileptic patients.

Dopamine

Though the increase in libido noted in patients receiving L-dopa for Parkinson's disease has been attributed to non-specific factors such as the effect of general clinical improvement, hypomania, or disinhibition associated with confusion, most reports suggest that the increase in libido is relatively specific (Barbeau 1969; Hyppa *et al.* 1970; O'Brien *et al.* 1971; Harvey 1988), although only a minority are affected (25 per cent of men and women). There are even suggestions that testosterone may exert its effect through altering levels of dopamine, at least in the rat (Hyppa *et al.* 1970) where castration causes a drop in levels of hypothalamic dopamine, which is not elevated by L-dopa but by testosterone.

This raises the question as to whether dopamine has a threshold effect, like testosterone, or is dose related, and whether it is an appropriate treatment for those presenting with low libido where testosterone is contra-indicated as in cases of prostatic cancer, or menopausal women. Taylor-Segraves (1988) quotes three studies of L-dopa in males with declining potency, all of which showed positive effects. Animal studies provide supporting evidence that dopamine has a stimulatory role in the control of male sexual arousal and activity (see Chapter 1). As a result, several dopaminergic drugs are being used to improve sexual function, including selegiline, L-dopa combined with a decarboxylase inhibitor, and bromo-criptine. The latter has helped restore the sexual function of those on renal dialysis (Weizman *et al.* 1983) but in other conditions it seems ineffective, and it has no effect on libido in man (Cooper 1977).

Antilibidinal drugs

Though aphrodisiacs are in greatest demand, an effective suppressant of sexual desire can be a valuable treatment for those whose sexual inclinations are too deviant to be tolerated. They fall into two groups: dopamine antagonists, and drugs which antagonize or reduce the secretion of testosterone. Testosterone antagonists include cyproterone acetate, oestrogens, flutamide, progesterone, and LHRH agonists (buserelin and gosrelin). It would appear that the latter produce most effective suppression of libido (Labrie *et al.* 1985). Not surprisingly, they have only been used therapeutically to reduce libido in males, though antiandrogens have been used to treat hirsutism in women, without an obvious effect on their sexuality. Their supposedly greater effect than cyproterone acetate and benperidol may be due to their ability to block secretion of LH and LHRH as well as testosterone.

CONCLUSION

It might be expected that it would be difficult to alter the libido of man in view of the importance of this particular drive in the procreation and survival of the species. In Darwinian terms this would appear to be the primary purpose of our life on earth, a capacity with which man is at present obviously well endowed. However, the ability of drugs to reduce sexual drive is not necessarily by an ability to increase it beyond natural levels. For so long an area of superstition and myth, the psychopharmacology of human sexual desire has been given a fillip by the discovery of the aphrodisiac effects of dopamine. Even the stimulant effects of cocaine can be explained through this mechanism. This discovery may well be the spark to light the way to effective scientific study.

REFERENCES

Abel, E.L. (1985). *Psychoactive drugs and sex*. Plenum Press, New York.

Alder, E. and Bancroft J. (1988). The relationship between breast feeding persistence, sexuality and mood in the post-partum woman. *Psychological Medicine*, **18**, 384–96.

Amin, M.M., Ananth, J.V., Coleman, B.S., Darcourt, G., Farkas, T., and Goldstein, B. (1984). Fluvoxamine: antidepressant effects confirmed in a placebo-controlled international study. *Clinical Neuropharmacology*, **7** (Suppl. 1), 580–1.

Bancroft, J. (1989). *Human sexuality and its problems*. Churchill Livingstone, Edinburgh.

Bancroft, J. and Wu, F.C.W. (1983). Changes in erectile response during androgen replacement therapy. *Archives of Sexual Behaviour*, **12**, 59–66.

Bancroft, J., Tennant, G., Loucas, K., and Cass, J. (1974). The control of deviant sexual behaviour by drugs: 1. Behavioural changes following oestrogens and antiandrogens. *British Journal of Psychiatry*, **125**, 310–5.

Bancroft, J., Sherwin, B.B., Alexander, G.M., Davidson, D.W., and Walker, A. (1991*a*). A comparison of sexual experience, sexual attitudes and gender role in oral contraceptive users and non-users. *Archives of Sexual Behaviour*, **20**, 105–20.

Bancroft, J., Sherwin, B.B., Alexander, G.M., Davidson, D.W., and Walker, A. (1991*b*). Oral contraceptives, androgens and the sexuality of young women II: The role of androgens. *Archives of Sexual Behaviour*, **20**, 121–36.

Barbeau, A. (1969). L-dopa therapy in Parkinson's Disease: a critical review of nine year's experience. *Canadian Medical Association Journal*, **101**, 59–68.

Bohacek, N., Mihovilovic, J., and Bakran, I. (1976). Terapijsko djelovanje i nuspojave triciklickih i tetracickih antidepresiva. Usporedni dvostruke slijepi pokus emitriptilina i mianserina. (Org GB 94). *Acta Medica Iugoslavica*, **30**, 425–40.

Bremer, J. (1959). *Asexualisation: a follow-up study of 244 cases*. Macmillan, New York.

Brown, W.A., Laughren, T.P., and Williams, B. (1981). Differential effects of neuroleptic agents on the pituitary gonadal axis in men. *Archives of General Psychiatry*, **38**, 1270–2.

Carani, C., Zini, D., Baldini, A., Della Casa, L., Ghizzani, A., and Marrama, P. (1990). Effects of androgen treatment in impotent men with normal and low levels of free testosterone. *Archives of Sexual Behaviour*, **19**, 223–9.

Carney, A., Bancroft, J., and Mathews, A. (1978). Combination of hormonal and psychological treatment for female sexual unresponsiveness in a comparative study. *British Journal of Psychiatry*, **132**, 339–46.

Chapman, R.M., Rees, L.H., Sutcliffe, S.B., Edwards, C.R.W., and Malpas, J.S. (1979). Cyclical combination chemotherapy and gonadal function. *Lancet*, **ii**, 285–9.

Charney, D.S., Heninger, G.R., and Kleber, H.D. (1986). The combination of clonidine and naltrexone as a rapid, safe, and effective treatment of abrupt withdrawal from methadone. *American Journal of Psychiatry*, **143**, 831–7.

Clark, E. (1965). Spironolactone therapy and gynaecomastia. *Journal of the American Medical Association*, **193**, 163–4.

Cooper, A.J. (1977). Bromocriptine in impotence. *Lancet*, **ii**, 567.

Coronary Drug Project Research Group (1975). Clofibrate and niacin in coronary heart disease. *Journal of the American Medical Association*, **231**, 360–81.

Covington, S. (1983). Sex and alcohol. What do women tell us? *6th World Congress of Sexology*, Washington DC.

Cushman, P. (1972). Sexual behaviour in heroin addiction and methadone maintenance. *Journal of Medicine*, **72**, 1261–5.

Davidson, J.M., Caamargo, C.A., and Smith, E.R. (1979). Effects of androgen on sexual behaviour in hypogonadal men. *Clinics in Endocrinology and Metabolism*, **48**, 955–8.

Davidson, J.M., Kwan, M., and Greenleaf, W. (1982). Hormonal replacement and sexuality in men. *Clinics in Endocrinology and Metabolism*, **11**, 599–623.

Davidson, J.M., Chen, J.J., Crapo, L., Gary, G.D., Greenleaf, W.J., and Catania, J.A. (1983). Hormonal changes and sexual function in ageing men. *Journal of Clinical Endocrinology and Metabolism*, **57**, 71–7.

De Leo, D. and Magni, G. (1983). Sexual side effects of antidepressant drugs. *Psychosomatics*, **24**, 1076–82.

Dornan, W.A. and Malsbury, C.W. (1989). Neuropeptides and male sexual behaviour. *Neuroscience and Biobehavioural Reviews*, **13**, 1–15.

Dow, M.G.T., Hart, D.M., and Forrest, C.A. (1983). Hormonal treatment of sexual unresponsiveness in postmenopausal women: a comparative study. *British Journal of Obstetrics and Gynaecology*, **90**, 361–6.

Elliott, S.A. and Watson, J.P. (1985). Sex during pregnancy and the first post-natal year. *Journal of Psychomatic Research*, **29**, 541–8.

Fahrner, E. (1987). Sexual dysfunction in male alcoholics: prevalence and treatment. *Archives of Sexual Behaviour*, **16**, 247–57.

Farkas, G.M. and Rosen, R.C. (1976). The effects of ethanol on male sexual arousal. *Journal of Studies on Alcohol*, **37**, 265–72.

Faust, F. (1981). *Women, sex and pornography*. Penguin, London.

Fave, G.F.D., Tamburrono, G., Magistria, L.D., Natoli, C., Santoro, M.LO., Carratu, R., and Torsoli, A. (1977). Gynaecomastia with cimetidine. *Lancet*, **i**, 1319.

Fenwick, P.B.C., Toone, B.K., Wheeler, M.J., Nanjee, M.N., Grant, R., and Brown, D. (1985). Sexual behaviour in a centre for epilepsy. *Acta Neurologica Scandinavica*, **71**, 428–35.

Forrest, G.G. (1983). *Alcoholism and human sexuality*. Springfield, Illinois.

Gartrell, N. (1986). Increased libido in women receiving trazodone. *American Journal of Psychiatry*, **143**, 781–2.

Gastaut, H. and Collomb, H. (1954). Etude du compatment sexuel chez les epileptiques psychomoteurs. *Annanales Medico-Psychologiques*, **2**, 657–96.

Gay, G.R., Sheppard, C.W., Inaba, D.S., and Newmeyer, J.A. (1973). Cocaine in perspective: 'Gift from the sun god' to 'The rich man's drug'. *Drug Forum*, **2**, 409–30.

Gay, G.R., Newmeyer, J.A., Perry, M., Johnson, G., and Kurland, M. (1982). Love and hate, the sensuous hippie revisited. Drug/sex practices in San Francisco. *Journal of Psychoactive Drugs*, **14**, 111–23.

Greenblatt, R.B., Barfield, W.E., Garner, J.F., Calk, G.L., and Harrod, J.P. (1950). Evaluation of an oestrogen, androgen, oestrogen–androgen combination, and placebo in the treatment of the menopause. *Journal of Clinical Endocrinology*, **10**, 1547–58.

Hallstrom, T. and Samuelsson, S. (1990). Changes in womens' sexual desire in middle life; the longitudinal study of women in Gothenburg. *Archives of Sexual Behaviour*, **19**, 259–68.

Harrison, W.M., Stewart, J., Ehrhardt, A.E., Rabkin, J., McGrath, P., and Liebowitz, M. (1985). A controlled study on the effect of antidepressants on sexual function. *Psychopharmacology*, **21**, 85–8.

Harvey, O.N.S. (1988). Serial cognitive profiles in levadopa-induced hypersexuality. *British Journal of Psychiatry*, **153**, 833–6.

Heim, N. (1981). Sex behaviour of castrated offenders. *Archives of Sexual Behaviour*, **8**, 281–305.

Herbert, J. (1978). Neurohormonal integration of sexual behaviour in female primates. In *Biological determinants of sexual behaviour* (ed. J.B. Hutchinson), pp. 467–92. Wiley, Chichester.

Hierons, R. and Saunders, R. (1966). Impotence in patients with temporal lobe lesions. *Lancet*, **ii**, 761–4.

Hughes, B.D. (1971). Reports on the use of Ponderax in mentally disturbed patients. *South African Medical Journal*, **45**, 37.

Hyppa, M.T., Rinne, V.K., and Sonninen, V. (1970). The activating effect of L-dopa treatment on sexual function and its experimental background. *Acta Neurologica Scandinavica*, **43** (Suppl. 43), 232–4.

Johnson, D.A.W. (1983). Symptom response in a double blind comparison of flupenthixol, nortriptyline, and diazepam in neurotic depression. *Journal of International Biomedical Information and Data*, **4**, 19–28.

Kennedy, B.J. and Nathanson, I.T. (1953). Effects of intensive sex steroid hormone therapy in advanced breast cancer. *Journal of the American Medical Association*, **152**, 1135–41.

Kimura, M., Ferkamachi, T., Ono, T., Makawaga, T., Aoki, H., Ago, A., and Kono, T. plus seven collaborators (1978). Clinic evaluation of lofepramine a new antidepressant. Comparison with amitryptyline by double blind trial. *Basic Pharmacology and Therapeutics*, **6**, 64–78.

Koff, W.C. (1974). Marihuana and sexual activity. *Journal of Sex Research*, **10**, 194.

Kolodney, R.C., Masters, W.H., Kolodney, R.M., and Toro, G. (1974). Depression of plasma testosterone levels after chronic intensive marihuana use. *New England Journal of Medicine*, **290**, 872–4.

Labrie, F., Dupont, A., Belanger, A., Lachance, R., and Giguere, M. (1985). Long term treatment with luteinising hormone releasing hormone agonists and maintenance of serum testosterone to castration concentration. *British Medical Journal*, **291**, 369–70.

Lancet (1990). Now we understand antipsychotics (editorial, pp. 1222–3).

Langevin, R., Bain, J., Wortzman, G., Hucker, S.M., Dickey, R., and Wright, P. (1988). Sexual sadism: brain, blood and behaviour. *New York Academy of Science*, **528**, 163–71.

Lapierre, Y.D., Paykel, E., and Wakelin, J.S. (1984). Fluvoxamine: antidepressant effects confirmed in a placebo-controlled international study. *Clinical Neuropharmacology*, **7** (Suppl. 1), 580–1.

Laughren, W.A. and Williams, B. (1981). Differential effects of neuroleptic agents on the pituitary–gonadal axis in men. *Archives of General Psychiatry*, **38**, 1270–2.

Leiblum, S.R. and Rosen, R.C. (1988). *Sexual desire disorders*. Guildford Press, New York.

Lieber, C.S. (1989). Toxic and metabolic changes induced by ethanol. In *Alcoholism, biomedical and genetic aspects* (ed. H. Werner Goedde and D.P. Agarwal), pp. 57–84. Pergamon, New York.

Magnus, R.V., Dean, B.C., and Curry, S.H. (1977). Clorazepate: double blind crossover comparison of a single nightly dose with diazepam thrice daily in anxiety. *Diseases of the Nervous System*, **38**, 819–21.

Mandell, W. and Miller, C.M. (1983). Male sexual dysfunction as related to alcohol consumption: a pilot study. *Alcoholism*, **7**, 65–9.

Marrama, P., Carini, C., Montamini, V.M., Baraghini, G.R., Tridenti, A., and Pederzini, R.M. (1984). Gonadal function: sexual behaviour in bromocriptine-treated men with prolactinoma. In *Emerging dimensions of sexology* (ed. T.T. Segraves and E.J. Haeberle). Praeger, New York.

Mathews, A., Whitehead, A., and Kellett, J. (1983). Psychological and hormonal factors in the treatment of female sexual dysfunction. *Psychological Medicine*, **13**, 83–92.

Mattson, R.H. and Cramer, J.A. (1985). Epilepsy, sex hormones and antiepileptic drugs. *Epilepsia*, **26** (Suppl. 1), 540–51.

McLean, J.D., Forsythe, R., and Kapkin, I.A. (1983). Unusual side effects of clomipramine associated with yawning. *Canadian Journal of Psychiatry*, **28**, 569–70.

Mendelson, J.H., Kuehnle, J., and Ellingboe, J. (1974). Plasma testosterone levels before, during and after chronic marihuana smoking. *New England Journal of Medicine*, **291**, 1051–5.

Money, J. (1970). Use of an androgen-depleting hormone in the treatment of male sex offenders. *Journal of Sex Research*, **6**, 165–72.

Money, J. and Ehrhardt, A.A. (1972). *Man and woman, boy and girl. Differentiation and dimorphism of gender identity from conception to maturity*, Johns Hopkins University Press, Baltimore.

Murphy, J.E. and Bridgeman, K.M. (1978). A comparative clinical trial of mianserin (Norval) and amitryptyline in the treatment of depression in general practice. *Journal of International Medical Research*, **6**, 199–206.

Neri, A., Aygen, M., Zukerman, Z., and Bahary, C. (1980). Subjective assessment of sexual dysfunction of patients on long-term administration of digoxin. *Archives of Sexual Behaviour*, **9**, 343–7.

O'Brien, C.P., Di Giancomo, J.N., Fahn, S., and Schwartz, G.A. (1971). Mental effects of high-dosage levodopa. *Archives of General Psychiatry*, **24**, 61–4.

O'Carroll, R.F. and Bancroft, J. (1984). Testosterone for low sexual interest and erectile dysfunction in men. *British Journal of Psychiatry*, **145**, 146–51.

Oseko, F. Nobuyukioka, Furuya, H., and Morikawa. (1988). Effects of chronic sulpiride-induced hyperprolactinaemia on plasma testosterone and its response to hCG in normal men. *Journal of Andrology*, **9**, 231–3.

Othmer, E. and Othmer, S.C. (1987). Effect of buspirone on sexual function in patients with generalised anxiety disorder. *Journal of Clinical Psychiatry*, **48**, 201–3.

Renshaw, D.C. (1975). Doxepin treatment of sexual dysfunction associated with depression. In *A monograph of recent clinical studies* (ed. J. Mendels), pp. 23–31.

Riley, A.J. (1984). Prolactin and female sexual function. *British Journal of Sexual Medicine*, **11**, 14–17.

Riley, A.J. and Riley, E.J. (1986). The effect of single dose diazepam on female sexual response induced by masturbation. *Sexual and Marital Therapy*, **1**, 49–53.

Robson, K.M., Brant, H.A., and Kumar, R. (1981). Maternal sexuality during first pregnancy and after childbirth. *British Journal of Obstetrics and Gynaecology*, **88**, 882–9.

Rubin, H.B. and Henson, D.E. (1976). Effects of alcohol on male sexual responding. *Psychopharmacology*, **47**, 123–4.

Rubin, R.T., Poland, R.E., and Tower, B.B. (1976). Prolactin related testosterone secretion in normal adult men. *Journal of Clinical Endocrinology and Metabolism*, **24**, 211–34.

Rubinsky, H., Eckerman, D., Rubinsky, E., and Hoover, C. (1987). Early phase physiological response patterns to psychogenic stimuli; comparison of male and female patterns. *Archives of Sexual Behaviour*, **16**, 45–56.

Sanders, D. and Bancroft, J. (1982). Hormones and the sexuality of women. *Clinics in Endocrinology and Metabolism*, **11**, 639–59.

Sartory, G. (1983). Benzodiazepines and behavioural treatment of phobic anxiety. *Behavioural Psychotherapy*, **11**, 204–17.

Sherwin, B.B. and Gelfand, M.M. (1984). Effects of parenteral administration of oestrogen and androgen on plasma hormone levels and hot flushes in the surgical menopause. *American Journal of Obstetrics and Gynaecology*, **148**, 552–7.

Sherwin, B.B. and Gelfand, M.M. (1987). The role of androgen in the maintenance of sexual functioning in oopherectomized women. *Psychosomatic Medicine*, **49**, 397–409.

Simpson, G.M., Blair, J.H., and Amuso, D. (1965). Effects of antidepressants on genito-urinary function. *Diseases of the Nervous System*, **26**, 787–9.

Sobrinho, L.G., Sa-Melo, P., Nunes, M.C.P., Barrocco, L.E., Calhaz-Jorge, C., Oliveira, L.C., and Santos, M.A. (1987). Sexual dysfunction of hyperprolactinaemic women, effects of bromocriptine. *Journal of Psychosomatic Obstetrics and Gynaecology*, **6**, 43–8.

Spark, R.F., Wills, C.A., and Royal H. (1984). Hypogonadism hyperprolactinaemia and temporal lobe epilepsy in hyposexual men. *Lancet*, **i**, 413–17.

Stevenson, R.W.D. and Solyom, L. (1990). The aphrodisiac effect of fenfluramine: two case reports of a possible side effect to the use of fenfluramine in the treatment of bulimia. *Journal of Clinical Psychopharmacology*, **10**, 69–71.

Studd, J.W., Collins, W.P., Charkrauarti, S., Newton, J.R., Oram, D., and Parson, A. (1977). Oestradiol and testosterone implants in the treatment of psychosexual problems in the post-menopausal women. *British Journal of Obstetrics and Gynaecology*, **84**, 314–16.

Sullivan, G. (1988). Increased libido in three men treated with trazodone. *Journal of Clinical Psychiatry*, **49**, 202–3.

Taberner, P.V. (1985). *Aphrodisiacs: the science and the myth*. Croom Helm, London.

Tagliamonte, A., Taglimonte, P., Gessa, G.L., and Brodie, B.B. (1969). Compulsive sexual activity induced by *p*-chlorophenylalanine in normal and pinealectomised male rats. *Science*, **166**, 1433–5.

Taylor, R.G., Crisp, A.J., Hoffbrand, B.I., Maguyire, A., and Jacobs, H.S. (1981). Plasma sex hormone concentrations in men with hypertension treated with methyl dopa and/or propranolol. *Postgraduate Medical Journal*, **57**, 425–6.

Taylor-Segraves, R. (1988). Hormones and libido. In *Sexual desires and disorders* (ed. S.R. Lieblum and R.C. Rosen). Guildford Press, New York.

Tennent, G., Bancroft, J., and Cass, J. (1974). The control of deviant sexual behaviour by drugs: a double blind controlled study of benperidol, chlorpromazine, and placebo. *Archives of Sexual Behaviour*, **3**, 261–71.

Weizman, A., Weizman, R., Hart, J., Maoz, B., Wijeseneek, H., and Ben David M. (1983). The correlation of increased serum prolactin levels with decreased sexual desire and activity in elderly men. *Journal of the American Geriatric Society*, **31**, 485–8.

Welling, M., Andersen, B.L., and Johnson, S.R. (1990). Hormonal replacement therapy for postmenopausal women: A review of sexual outcomes and related gynaecological effects. *Archives of Sexual Behaviour*, **19**, 119–37.

Wilson, G.T. and Lawson, D.M. (1976). The effects of alcohol on sexual arousal in women. *Journal of Abnormal Psychology*, **85**, 489–97.

7

Antihypertensive medication and sexual problems

Rhodri Huws

INTRODUCTION

Cardiovascular disease has become a common cause of morbidity and mortality in the western world. Over the past twenty years the mortality has been dropping due to a combination of early detection, improved treatment, and a general change in lifestyle. It is more common in men, with the incidence increasing with age, but in women the increase starts at the menopause. Certain factors lead to an increased risk of disease and some of these are amenable to modification (Levy and Kannel 1988). Hypertension is a risk factor, with an increased risk even with blood pressure that would be considered in the upper limit of the normal range. Other risk factors include cigarette smoking, obesity, and a high level of cholesterol. These risk factors are cumulative, with a low incidence of cardiovascular disease in their absence.

It is well established that there is an association between sexual dysfunction and cardiac disease. Wabrek and Burchell (1980) found that two-thirds of male patients hospitalized after a myocardial infarct had a significant sexual problem predating the myocardial infarct. Abramov (1976) found similar findings in women admitted with a myocardial infarct. Before the infarct, sexual dissatisfaction was found in 65 per cent compared with 24 per cent in a control group. A study of post-infarct sexual function (Dhabuwala *et al.* 1986) found sexual dysfunction in 76 per cent of 50 males, with erectile dysfunction in 42 per cent. However, in a control group matched for age, hypertension, diabetes, and smoking, there was sexual dysfunction in 68 per cent and erectile dysfunction in 48 per cent. This suggests that the sexual dysfunction after a myocardial infarct is due to the effects of the risk factors rather than the effect of the infarct *per se*. Other work lends support to this view. Virag *et al.* (1985) investigated 440 men with erectile failure. They looked at the four main arterial risk factors (diabetes, smoking, hypertension, and hyperlipidaemia) as well as the presence of an organic cause for the impotence. The frequency of organic erectile dysfunction increased from 49 per cent in those without risk factors to 100 per cent in those with three or four risk factors.

There are other associations between hypertension and sexual problems with both conditions sharing some aetiological factors, including sustained stressful life situations, obesity, cigarette smoking, and excessive alcohol intake. Hypertension also increases the risk of damage to the vasculature and the peripheral autonomic nervous system, which can lead to an organic sexual dysfunction.

DRUG TREATMENT OF HYPERTENSION

Due to the morbidity associated with hypertension, its treatment is of some importance and medication is often used to reduce the blood pressure. Whilst drugs are effective in lowering blood pressure their mode of action is often unclear. Out of 1180 men attending a medical out-patient clinic, 401 (34 per cent), with a mean age of 59.4 years, were impotent (Slag *et al.* 1983). Hypertension was more common in the group with erectile dysfunction and medication was felt to be the likely cause of erectile dysfunction in 25 per cent, particularly antihypertensives and diuretics. In many cases the erectile dysfunction led to non-compliance, as the patients were unwilling to discuss the problem with their doctors. Another study of 88 hypertensive patients found that 50 had impaired erectile function and 40 of these attributed it to their drug therapy (Laver 1974). Bulpitt *et al.* (1976) compared patients with treated and untreated hypertension and found a higher incidence of sexual dysfunction in untreated hypertension which increased even further with diagnosis and treatment (Table 7.1). Two studies looking at the general side-effects of antihypertensive medication found that in women, treatment was not associated with arousal or orgasmic dysfunction or a decrease in the frequency of intercourse (Riley *et al.* 1987; Bulpitt *et al.* 1989) and even though another placebo-controlled study (Table 7.1, Bauer *et al.* 1978) did not find such an increase, the issue of whether treatment can increase morbidity has received much attention.

The increased sexual dysfunction in the untreated group is likely to be organic in origin, but many factors could influence the treated group. Studies have shown that simply diagnosing hypertension leads to a worsening of psychological well-being and also leads to increased absenteeism from work (Haynes *et al.* 1978). Hypertension is known by laypeople to be associated with an increased risk of myocardial infarcts and strokes and a fear of this can lead to depression as well as apprehension of dying during intercourse. Similar fears can be produced in the non-hypertensive partner. In women a diagnosis of hypertension may lead to a change from the use of oral contraception to other means of contraception and this may lead to a change in the sexual practices for both male and female. The reduction in

Table 7.1   Studies reporting sexual side-effects of antihypertensive drugs

MRC (1981)

	Prevalence of impotence (%)	
	Three months	Two years
Bendrofluazide	16	23 (*)
Propranolol	14	13
Placebo	9	10

Bulpitt et al. (1976)

	Control	Hypertensive (untreated)	Hypertensive (treated)
Impotence (%)	7	17	24 (**)
Frequency of coitus per year	50	50	27 (NS)

Bauer et al. (1978)

	Control	Hypertensive (untreated)	Placebo treatment	Active treatment
Impotence (%)	10	20	14	19 (NS)
Failed ejaculation (%)	6	10	5	9 (NS)

TAIM (1991)

	Chlorthalidone	Atenolol	Placebo
Problems with erection (%)	28	11	3 (***)
Female sexual problems (%)	18	20	15 (NS)

* $p < 0.05$; ** $p < 0.001$; *** $p < 0.006$; NS, not significant.

morbidity due to drug treatment is not impressive (Medical Research Council 1985) and it has been suggested that the ill-effects of diagnosing mild hypertension outweighs the benefits of treatment.

Before embarking on a major study of the effects of antihypertensive drugs the Medical Research Council looked at the effect of diagnosis and treatment in a pilot study (Mann 1986). Patients were given regular counselling which led to an improvement in psychological well-being that was independent of drug treatment. It would be seen that there are a number of possible reasons for an increase in sexual dysfunction after treatment and a great deal of interest surrounds whether antihypertensive medication plays a part. From our knowledge of the physiology of sexual functioning, this would be expected, but unfortunately much of the research is of poor quality, being subject to several methodological deficiencies. Due to a lack of consensus on terminology, different studies cannot be compared. The definition used is rarely stated and a term such as 'impotence' may be defined so widely as to encompass all male erectile abnormalities. Under-reporting can occur due to embarrassment by both patient and professional. When screening for impotence, Slag *et al.* (1983) found 401 cases, but only six of these had previously volunteered their problem to their doctor and in a study of the sexual side-effects of methyldopa, seven per cent volunteered to the doctor that they suffered erection failure. When the same population were given a questionnaire, 53 per cent admitted to the problem (Alexander and Evans 1975). The research is almost exclusively on males with little mention of female dysfunction. Even in males most research concentrates on the presence or absence of an erection with sexuality in general not studied. Many of the reports are case histories with very few controlled studies. Mild hypertension tends to fall with time even without treatment, rendering the interpretation of uncontrolled trials difficult. Erectile dysfunction is known to increase with age, which may account for the higher reported incidence of dysfunction on drugs in some studies (Bauer *et al.* 1978) and, as stated previously, the illness itself may cause dysfunction. The high incidence of sexual dysfunction in those with cardiovascular disease means that uncontrolled studies are of no more value than case histories. Many of the controlled studies do not even control for alcohol intake or smoking, both of which can cause erectile dysfunction. Unfortunately, well conducted controlled studies have been performed on relatively few drugs, with most of the work being case reports or uncontrolled studies (Table 7.2). The commonly used drugs will be discussed further.

Thiazide diuretics

Thiazide diuretics lead to an initial reduction in blood pressure by decreasing sodium reabsorption in the kidney, leading to a reduction in plasma volume. In the long term, they reduce blood pressure by a reduction in peripheral resistance. The mechanism for this effect is unclear. They are the first-line drug treatment for mild hypertension and are also used for the treatment of cardiac failure. A single-blind, placebo-controlled study of 23 582 patients on bendrofluazide or propranolol (Medical Research Council 1981) showed that after two years, use of bendrofluazide was significantly associated with erectile dysfunction (Table 7.1). Withdrawal from the study due to erectile dysfunction was significantly associated with both drugs ($p < 0.001$). Other studies have also shown that thiazide diuretics are more likely to cause erectile dysfunction than propranolol (Veterans Administration Cooperative Study Group 1982). In another double-blind

Table 7.2 Sexual dysfunction due to cardiovascular drugs

Drug	Impotence	Impaired ejaculation	Decreased libido	Priapism	Gynaecomastia
Thiazide diuretic	+	−	?		
β Blockers	+	−	?		
ACE inhibitors	−	−	−		
Calcium-channel blockers	?				
Methyldopa	+	?	?		?
Vasodilators	?			?	
α Blockers		+		?	
Spironolactone	?		?		?
Digoxin	+		+		?

+, Controlled studies showing dysfunction; −, controlled studies showing no dysfunction; ?, case reports or uncontrolled studies showing dysfunction.

study (Croog *et al.* 1988) the addition of a diuretic caused a significant deterioration of erectile function in patients taking propranolol or methyldopa, but not in a group taking captopril. The American 'Treatment of mild hypertension study' (TOMHS) has followed the progress of 900 men over two years and the results single out diuretics as causing sexual dysfunction (Mason 1991). The Medical Research Council study used higher doses of diuretics that are currently used for hypertension, and as not all studies have shown dysfunction (Bauer *et al.* 1978), it may be that the problems caused are minimal. A recent study (the TAIM study) of various treatments for mild hypertension found that while diuretics caused erection-related problems (Table 7.1) they did not differ from placebo in terms of sexual functioning in general and indeed led to a general improvement in quality of life (Wassertheil-Smoller *et al.* 1991). It is not clear why thiazide diuretics should cause dysfunction, but reduction of peripheral vascular resistance could play a part.

β-Blocking drugs

β Blockers are used for hypertension, angina, and for the prevention of myocardial infarct. If they are not effective by themselves they should be used in combination with a diuretic. They block peripheral adrenoceptors leading to arteriolar dilatation. They also reduce heart rate, contractility, and metabolism. This leads to a lowered blood pressure with decreased cardiac output. Some also inhibit renin release from the kidney leading to a reduction in arteriolar pressure. Many studies have shown that propranolol causes erectile dysfunction, but to a lesser degree than diuretics (Medical Research Council 1981; Veterans Administration Cooperative Study Group 1982). In the double-blind study by Croog *et al.* (1988) propranolol caused a significant deterioration in the ability to maintain an erection. The dysfunction is dose related (Burnett and Chanine 1979) and may depend on the specificity of the drug. There have been case reports of erectile dysfunction associated with propranolol being relieved when atenolol, a less lipophilic, β_1-selective drug was substituted (Bathen 1978). Atenolol has been shown to cause dysfunction in a controlled study (Wassertheil-Smoller *et al.* 1991) but the TOMH study shows acebutolol (a relative β_1-selective drug) to be free of side-effects. It could be that decreased β_2 vasodilation produces unopposed α_1 vasoconstriction of the corpus cavernosum and erectile dysfunction, explaining why β_1-selective drugs appear to cause fewer problems. There have been reports of propranolol causing decreased libido (Hollifield *et al.* 1976), but the Croog (1988) study did not find this. Cases of Peyronie's disease in patients taking propranolol have been reported (Osborne 1977; Wallis *et al.* 1977) but with relative infrequency, so the association may be a coincidence. In the patient with cardiovascular disease, angina and palpitations can occur during intercourse. β Blockers can reduce or even eliminate these complications and lead to an increase in sexual activity (Jackson 1980).

Angiotensin-converting enzyme (ACE) inhibitors

These drugs block the conversion of angiotensin I to angiotensin II, a powerful vasoconstrictor. This leads to a drop in blood pressure. They are also used as adjuncts to diuretics in the treatment of heart failure. They have fewer side-effects than diuretics and β blockers and have been recommended as first-line treatment in the elderly (Kligman and Higbee 1989). In a double-blind study Croog *et al.* (1988) found no reported sexual dysfunction in patients taking captopril and the TOMH study has found no dysfunction with enalapril.

Calcium-channel blocking drugs

These drugs inhibit calcium entry into the smooth muscle of the arterial system, thus reducing its contractility. This leads to a dilatation of the peripheral arterioles, reducing systemic vascular resistance thus leading to a drop in blood pressure. Nifedipine is used for angina and hypertension and verapamil for angina, supraventricular arrhythmias, and occasionally for hypertension. They are not first-line treatments for hypertension and are used when other drugs are ineffective or not tolerated. Nifedipine can be used in conjunction with a β blocker. As they act by direct relaxation of smooth muscle and have no effect on the autonomic nervous system, erectile difficulties would not be expected and although cases of erectile dysfunction have been reported with verapamil (King *et al.* 1983) they are not commonly thought to cause sexual dysfunction. The TOMH study appears to confirm this but there has not been adequate research on the issue.

Other antihypertensive drugs

Other treatment options are available if the above mentioned drugs fail to work or are not tolerated. They are used in patients with moderate or severe hypertension who have an increased risk of having a sexual dysfunction. This makes it more difficult to attribute sexual difficulties to the drug.

Vasodilators

These act by decreasing smooth muscle tone leading to a fall in arteriolar resistance and blood pressure. They would not therefore be expected to cause erectile dysfunction and in spite of a few case reports (Ahmad 1980) they appear free of sexual side-effects. However, they cause a reflex stimulation of the heart so that tachycardia and palpitations often occur, which limit their usefulness.

Centrally acting drugs

Methyldopa used to be commonly used as an antihypertensive but treatment with it is now rarely initiated. Its antihypertensive action is due to its metabolite acting as a false neurotransmitter, stimulating α receptors in the brain. The reduced adrenergic stimulation from the brain leads to a drop in blood pressure. Due to its inhibition of the sympathetic nervous system, sexual dysfunction would be expected and indeed methyldopa is commonly cited as a cause of dysfunction which is dose dependent (Kolodny 1978). It also causes increased prolactin secretion, which can cause amenorrhoea and galactorrhoea (Arze *et al*. 1981). Most of the research was done in the 1960s and 1970s and is of poor quality with some contradictory reports. The same is true for clonidine, where some studies have shown it to cause erectile dysfunction (Onesti *et al*. 1971; Hogan *et al*. 1981) but others have not (Saunders and Kong 1980; Pentland *et al*. 1981).

α-Receptor blocking drugs

These reduce blood pressure in association with a fall in peripheral resistance. α-Receptor blockers (such as prozosin and indoramine) do not appear to cause impotence and they have been used as antihypertensive agents in patients with diabetes where other drugs are either contraindicated or have caused sexual problems (Lipson 1984). Intracavernosal penile injections of α blockers have been used in the treatment of impotence and surprisingly the TOMH study found that oral doxazocin produced less dysfunction than placebo. It remains to be seen whether this is a therapeutic effect, but phenoxybenzamine has been used as an adjunct to the behavioural treatment of impotence (Riley and Riley 1984). Unfortunately, with the medication, delayed ejaculation occurs (Pentland *et al*. 1981). Indeed phenoxybenzamine at a high enough dose will invariably cause failure of ejaculation (Homonnai *et al*. 1984). There have also been reports of priapism (Bhalla *et al*. 1979).

Other cardiovascular drugs

Digoxin

This glycoside increases the force of cardiac contractions and reduces conduction. It is used mainly for supraventricular arrhythmias and sometimes for heart failure. It has chemical similarities to oestrogen. In a controlled study, Neri *et al*. (1987) showed a significant decrease in sexual desire, erection, and frequency of sexual activity in the digoxin group. The digoxin group had significantly lower testosterone levels, which may be the cause of the dysfunction.

Spironolactone

This diuretic is an aldosterone antagonist that inhibits its action at the distal tubule of the kidney. This causes potassium retention and loss of sodium and water. It is used for the treatment of congestive cardiac failure as well as rare cases of hypertension caused by hyperaldosteronism. Gynaecomastia, loss of libido, menstrual abnormalities, and erectile dysfunction have been reported (Loriaux *et al.* 1976) which may be dose related, with a higher incidence at doses above 400 mg per day (Spark and Melby 1968). It is postulated that these are mediated hormonally, probably as a result of progestational activity.

NON-PHARMACOLOGICAL TREATMENT OF HYPERTENSION

A sexual problem will affect the partner and it is important to consider the effect that the treatment of hypertension will have on them. Jachuck *et al.* (1982) compared patients', doctors', and relatives' perception of quality of life (including sexual activity) following the use of antihypertensive drugs. The doctors felt that all 75 participants had improved, 35 of the patients thought that things had improved, but relatives of 74 of the patients felt that things had deteriorated. The impact on the family must be taken into account when evaluating the benefit of drug treatment.

For many years a number of alternatives to the drug treatment of hypertension have been proposed, including diet and salt reduction, relaxation or meditation techniques, assertiveness training, psychotherapy, and marital counselling. Unfortunately most of the research is uncontrolled, with similar methodological problems as the work on drugs. Both relaxation therapy and simple counselling are known to reduce blood pressure in mild hypertension with long-lasting effects (Chesney *et al.* 1987), but the reduction is not as great as when drugs are used (Jacob *et al.* 1986). Weight reduction and weight counselling are also beneficial and can have long-term benefit (Stamler *et al.* 1987) with weight reduction not only improving sexual function but also ameliorating the detrimental effects of medication (Wassertheil-Smoller *et al.* 1991). Reducing smoking and alcohol intake is also of benefit.

CONCLUSION

Hypertension and sexual problems are both common and both can affect day-to-day functioning. They interact in many ways. Similar psychological and physical factors can predispose to both and the physical effects of hypertension can cause sexual dysfunction. Unless adequate counselling is provided at the time of giving a diagnosis of hypertension then this event can be harmful to the individual and could even outweigh the benefits of treatment. It is also important to remember the impact of the diagnosis on the family as a whole.

Pharmacological treatment of mild hypertension is common. Studies have shown that non-pharmacological treatment can be as effective and these options should not be neglected, especially as the drugs used are not free from side-effects. Diuretics have been most often found to cause erectile dysfunction, which also occurs with β blockers, but the problem is reduced when a β_1-selective drug is used. ACE inhibitors appear to be free of sexual side-effects. Despite information being available about the side-effects of drugs, the patient might be unwilling to talk about any sexual dysfunction caused and could present with non-compliance. Clarification of these issues could improve compliance.

The following suggestions are made regarding the management of hypertension.

1. Before treatment, take a psychosexual history noting current sexual functioning. If there is a sexual problem try to ascertain how much is physical and how much is psychological in origin.

2. Provide simple education to patient and partner, and if necessary simple counselling.

3. If a change in contraception is required, be aware that this may either bring to light or produce sexual dysfunction.

4. Before embarking on drug therapy for mild hypertension, wait for three to six months as the blood pressure may fall either of its own accord or secondary to the measures above.

5. If using medication note that
   (a) thiazide diuretics are more likely than other drugs to cause sexual dysfunction and should be avoided if a sexual dysfunction is already present;
   (b) if problems occur with a β blocker then a change to a β_1-specific blocker might be beneficial;
   (c) ACE inhibitors are not known to cause sexual dysfunction and should be considered if other drugs are causing problems. Indeed, there is a case for considering these drugs as first-line pharmacological treatment for sexually active men.

6. Remember that patients will often not volunteer that there is a sexual problem and might present with inexplicable non-compliance.

REFERENCES

Abramov, L.A. (1976). Sexual life and sexual frigidity in women developing acute myocardial infarction. *Psychosomatic Medicine*, **38**, 418–25.

Ahmad, S. (1980). Hydralazine and male impotence. *Chest*, **78**, 358.

Alexander, W.D. and Evans, J.I. (1975). Side effects of methyldopa. *British Medical Journal*, **2**, 501.

Arze, R.S., Ramos, J.M., Rashid, H.U., and Kerr, D.N.S. (1981). Amenorrhoea, galactorrhoea, and hyperprolactinaemia induced by methyldopa. *British Medical Journal*, **283**, 194.

Bathen, J. (1978). Propranolol erectile dysfunction relieved. *Annals of Internal Medicine*, **88**, 716–17.

Bauer, G.E., Baker, J., Hunor, S.N., and Marshall, P. (1978). Side effects of anti hypertensive treatment: a placebo controlled study. *Clinical Science and Molecular Medicine*, **55**, 341s–344s.

Bhalla, A.K., Hoffbrand, B.I., Phatak, P.S., and Reuben, S.R. (1979). Prazosin and priapism. *British Medical Journal*, **2**, 1093.

Bulpitt, C.J., Dollery, C.T., and Carne, S. (1976). Change in the symptoms of hypertensive patients after referral to hospital clinic. *British Heart Journal*, **38**, 121–8.

Bulpitt, C.J., Beevers, D.G., Butler, A., Coles, E.C., Munroe-Faure, A.D., Newson, R.B., O'Riodan, P.W., Petrie, J.C., Rajagopalan, B., Rylance, P.B., Twallin, G., Webster, J., and Dollery, C.T. (1989). The effects of antihypertensive drugs on sexual function in men and women: a report from the DHSS hypertension care computing project (DHCCP). *Journal of Human Hypertension*, **3**, 53–6.

Burnett, W.C. and Chanine, R.A. (1979). Sexual dysfunction as result of propranolol therapy in men. *Cardiovascular Medicine*, **4**, 811–15.

Chesney, M., Black, G., Swan, G.E., and Ward, M. (1987). Relaxation training for essential hypertension at the workshop. The untreated mild hypertensive. *Psychosomatic Medicine*, **49**, 250–63.

Croog, S.H., Levine, S., Sudilovski, A., Baume, R., and Clive, J. (1988). Sexual symptoms in hypertensive patients. A clinical trial of antihypertensive medication. *Archives of Internal Medicine*, **148**, 788–94.

Dhabuwala, C.B., Kumar, A., and Pierce, J.M. (1986). Myocardial infarct and its influence on male sexual function. *Archives of Sexual Behaviour*, **15**, 499–504.

Haynes, B., Sackett, D., Taylor, W., Gibson, E., and Johnson, A. (1978). Increased absenteeism from work after detection and labelling of hypertensive patients. *New England Journal of Medicine*, **299**, 741–4.

Hogan, M.J., Wallin, J.D., and Baer, R.M. (1981). Antihypertensive therapy and male sexual dysfunction. *Psychosomatics*, **21**, 234–7.

Hollifield, J.W., Sherman, K., Vander, Zwagg, R., and Shand, D.G. (1976). Proposed mechanism of propranolol's antihypertensive effect in essential hypertension. *New England Journal of Medicine*, **295**, 68–73.

Homonnai, Z.T., Shilon, M., and Paz, G.F. (1984). Phenoxybenzamine—an effective male contraceptive pill. *Contraception*, **29**, 479–91.

Jachuck, S., Brierly, H., Jachuck, S., and Willcox, P. (1982). The effect of hypotensive drugs on the quality of life. *Journal of the Royal College of General Practitioners*, **32**, 103–5.

Jackson, G. (1980). Sexual intercourse and angina pectoris. *International Rehabilitation Medicine*, **3**, 35–7.

Jacob, R.G., Shapiro, A.P., Reeves, R., Johnsen, A., McDonald, R.H., and Coburn, C. (1986). Relaxation therapy for hypertension. *Archives of Internal Medicine*, **146**, 2335–40.

King, B.D., Pitchon, R., Stern, E.H., Schweitzer, P., Schneider, R.R., and Weiner, I. (1983). Impotence during therapy with verapamil. *Archives of Internal Medicine*, **143**, 1248–9.

Kligman, E.W. and Higbee, M.D. (1989). Drug therapy for hypertension in the elderly. *Journal of Family Practice*, **28**, 81–7.

Kolodny, R.C. (1978). Effects of alpha-methyldopa on male sexual function. *Sexuality and Disability*, **1**, 223–7.

Laver, M.C. (1974). Sexual behaviour patterns in male hypertensives. *Australian and New Zealand Journal of Medicine*, **4**, 29–31.

Levy, D. and Kannel, W.B. (1988). Cardiovascular risks: new insights from Framingham. *American Heart Journal*, **116**, 266–72.

Lipson, L.G. (1984). Treatment of hypertension in diabetic men: problems with sexual dysfunction. *American Journal of Cardiology*, **53**, 46A–50A.

Loriaux, D.L., Menard, R., Taylor, A., Pita, J., and Santem, R. (1976). Spironolactone and endocrine dysfunction. *Annals of Internal Medicine*, **85**, 630–6.

Mann, A.H. (1986). The psychological aspects of essential hypertension. *Journal of Psychosomatic Research*, **30**, 527–41.

Mason, I. (1991). Antihypertensives and sexual function. *Prescriber*, 19 September, 69–70.

Medical Research Council (1981). Adverse reaction to bendraflurazide and propranolol for the treatment of mild hypertension. *Lancet*, **ii**, 539–43.

Medical Research Council (1985). MRC trial of mild hypertension: principal results. *British Medical Journal*, **291**, 97–104.

Neri, A., Zukerman, Z., Aygen, M., Lidor, Y., and Kaufman, H. (1987). The effect of long term administration of digoxin on plasma androgens and sexual dysfunction. *Journal of Marital and Sex Therapy*, **13**, 58–63.

Onesti, G., Bock, K.D., Heimsoth, V., Kim, K.E., and Merguet, P. (1971). Clonidine: a new antihypertensive agent. *American Journal of Cardiology*, **28**, 74–83.

Osborne, D.R. (1977). Propranolol and Peyronie's disease. *Lancet*, **i**, 1111.

Pentland, B., Anderson, D.A., and Critchley, J.A.J.H. (1981). Failure of ejaculation with indoramine. *British Medical Journal*, **282**, 1433–4.

Riley, A.J. and Riley, E.J. (1984). Alpha-blockade and impotence. *British Journal of Psychiatry*, **144**, 215–16.

Riley, A.J., Steiner, J.A., Cooper, R., and McPherson, C.K. (1987). The prevalence of sexual dysfunction in male and female hypertensive patients. *Sexual and Marital Therapy*, **2**, 131–8.

Saunders, E. and Kong, B.W. (1980). Sexual activity in male hypertensives while taking clonidine. *Urban Health*, **9**, 22–6.

Slag, M.F., Morley, J.E., Elson, M.K., Trence, D.L., Nelson, C.J., Nelson, A.E., Kinlaw, W.B., Beyer, S., Nuttal, F.Q., and Shafer, R.B. (1983). Impotence in medical clinic outpatients. *Journal of the American Medical Association*, **249**, 1736–40.

Spark, R.F. and Melby, J.C. (1968). Aldosteronism in hypertension—the spironolactone response test. *Annals of Internal Medicine*, **69**, 685–91.

Stamler, R., Stamler, J., Grimm, R., Gosch, F., Elmer, P., Dyer, A., Berman, R., Fishman, J., Heel, N., Civinelli, J., and McDonald, A. (1987). Nutritional therapy for high blood pressure. Final report of a four year randomized controlled trial. *Journal of the American Medical Association*, **257**, 1484–91.

Veterans Administration Cooperative Study Group (1982). Comparison of propranolol and hydrochlorothiazide for the initial treatment of hypertension. Results of long term therapy. *Journal of the American Medical Association*, **248**, 2004–11.

Virag, R., Bouilly, P., and Frydman, D. (1985). Is impotence an arterial disorder? *Lancet*, **i**, 181–4.

Wabrek, A.J. and Burchell, R.C. (1980). Male coronary dysfunction associated with coronary heart disease. *Archives of Sexual Behaviour*, **9**, 69–75.

Wallis, A.A., Bell, R., and Sutherland, P.W. (1977). Propranolol and Peyronie's disease. *Lancet*, **ii**, 980.

Wassertheil-Smoller, S., Blaufox, M.D., Oberman, A., Davis, B.R., Swencionis, C., O'Connell Knerr, M., Hawkins, C.M., and Lansford, H.G. (1991). Effect of antihypertensives on sexual function and quality of life: the TAIM study. *Annals of Internal Medicine*, **1148**, 613–20.

8

The effect on sexual function of anticonvulsant, antiparkinsonian, and other miscellaneous drugs

Malcolm Peet and Janice Gillow

INTRODUCTION

Erectile and other sexual dysfunctions are relatively common in the general population. The prevalence of sexual problems increases with age and is higher in populations with medical or psychiatric illness than in the general population. Sexual dysfunction which is presumed to be drug related must be assessed against this background prevalence. Drug treatment can be associated with non-specific effects on sexual function, for example due to anxiety produced by medical diagnosis and treatment. Side-effects such as sedation can lead to a general non-specific lowering of interest and drive, including libido. Conversely, sexual dysfunction associated with illness can in some cases be improved by successful drug treatment of that illness. It follows that anecdotal reports of sexual effects from medication in individual patients are highly unreliable. The effect of drugs on sexual function can be assessed only in the setting of a randomized placebo-controlled trial with careful psychosexual assessment. Unfortunately, virtually all medication trials depend on self-reporting of sexual side-effects and this is very unreliable. There is thus a serious dearth of adequate research in this field, and the present chapter must be set in that context.

ANTICONVULSANTS

Any attempt to assess the effects of anticonvulsant drugs on sexual function is confounded by observations that epilepsy itself is associated with sexual dysfunction. Gastaut and Collomb (1954) focused attention on the high frequency of global hyposexuality in institutionalized patients with severe temporal-lobe epilepsy (TLE). Several more recent surveys have suggested a high rate of erectile dysfunction and global hyposexuality in epileptic patients (Shukla *et al.* 1979; Toone *et al.* 1989; Demerdash *et al.* 1991). Some have reported that erectile dysfunction and hyposexuality are particularly prevalent amongst patients with TLE (Hierons and Saunders 1966; Taylor 1969; Saunders and Rawson 1970; Shukla *et al.* 1979; Demerdash *et al.* 1991). Thus, in a comparative study, Shukla *et al.* (1979) found hyposexuality in 63 per cent of males with TLE, compared with 12 per cent of a control group with generalized epilepsy of *grand mal* type. Hierons and Saunders (1966) reported three cases in which erectile dysfunction preceded the development of TLE by more than six months, during which time no drugs were being taken. However, recent work has called into question the specific association between TLE and hyposexuality. Thus, Jensen *et al.* (1990) carried out a particularly careful study in which patients with severe psychopathology, mental handicap, and serious physical illness including neurological disease were all excluded. They found no relationship between type of epilepsy and sexual dysfunction. Indeed, the rate of sexual dysfunction amongst the uncomplicated epileptic patients did not significantly differ from that in a normal control group. Toone *et al.* (1989) also found no differences in sexual dysfunction between temporal-lobe and non-temporal-lobe epileptic patients, but those with focal epilepsy (that is, including both temporal and non-temporal-lobe foci) were more impaired sexually than those with primary generalized epilepsy. The observation that sexual dysfunction is particularly related to seizures which begin prior to or during puberty (Blumer and Walker 1967; Taylor 1969), and the reported correlation between sexual dysfunction and global social adjustment (Taylor 1969), implies that psychosocial as well as biological factors should be considered when assessing the effect of epilepsy on sexual function.

It has been suggested that anticonvulsants might affect sexual functioning through their effects on sex hormone levels. For example, there are consistent reports of increased sex-hormone-binding globulin and decreased free testosterone levels in patients treated with anticonvulsant drugs (Dana-Haeri *et al.* 1982; Toone *et al.* 1989). This appears to be a drug effect, since similar changes have been reported in normal volunteers treated prospectively with carbamazepine (Connell *et al.* 1984). A relationship between reduced free testosterone levels and hyposexuality has been reported (Toone *et al.* 1983; Fenwick *et al.* 1985). These workers found a small but statistically significant reduction in free testosterone in epileptic patients with low sex drive, as measured by frequency of sexual activity culminating in orgasm and frequency of early morning erections. The same group (Fenwick *et al.* 1986) reported that nocturnal penile tumescence was significantly less in five epileptic patients with low total-serum testosterone levels than in a control group of five patients with high levels. However, there is no way of ascertaining whether anticonvulsant medication was the primary determinant of low serum testosterone in this selected group of patients. Others have found no such relationship between hormone levels and sexual dysfunction, and have suggested that slight decreases of plasma concentrations of free testosterone seen in both male and female epileptic patients are unlikely to be of clinical importance (Jensen *et al*. 1990). Studies of other sex hormones, such as luteinizing hormone and prolactin in drug-treated epileptic patients have not produced consistent findings (Toone *et al*. 1989; Jensen *et al*. 1990).

Direct evidence relating sexual function to particular anticonvulsant medication is sparse. Few studies have directly addressed this issue. Commonly, patients studied have been taking more than one anticonvulsant drug, and other patients have been taking a variety of different medications, so that direct comparisons between different drugs have not been possible. When attempts have been made to relate sexual function to drug treatment, little or no association has been found. Thus, Jensen *et al*. (1990) found no relationship between sexual dysfunction and type of anticonvulsant medication amongst patients mostly treated with a single drug. Fenwick *et al*. (1985), in another group of patients treated mostly with monotherapy, reported that patients taking carbamazapine had more sexual dreams, and that sexually active patients taking valproate were more able to get an erection, but there were no other apparent associations with specific drug treatment. Saunders and Rawson (1970), in a series of 100 patients, could find only one subject in whom there was any good evidence that sexuality had been adversely affected by drug treatment. This was a male who apparently suffered reduced libido whilst taking phenobarbitone, which returned to normal when treatment was altered to hydantoin sodium. They suggested that anticonvulsants cause erectile dysfunction as part of the general obtunding which occurs with excessive dosage, but that clinical doses are unlikely to have this effect. There is some evidence that erectile dysfunction associated with epilepsy improves when adequate seizure control has been achieved (Hierons and Saunders 1966). Spark *et al*. (1984) identified a group of hyposexual men with previously unrecognized TLE. In four men with low serum-testosterone levels, treatment with testosterone alone did not increase libido or potency. After treating the epilepsy, hormonal levels and sexual function normalized in two patients, without requiring hormonal treatment.

In summary, there is evidence that patients with epilepsy have an excess of sexual dysfunction, particularly erectile dysfunction and global hyposexuality. It is not well established whether this sexual dysfunction is primarily related to the epilepsy *per se* or whether it is due to other related factors. An excess of erectile dysfunction and sexual disinterest has been claimed particularly in TLE though not confirmed by all workers, and there is some limited evidence that erectile dysfunction associated with epilepsy can be improved by adequate seizure control. Anticonvulsant drugs induce hormonal changes, including reduced free testosterone levels which could, in theory, have effects upon sexual behaviour, but adequate evidence to support the existence of any clinically meaningful effect of non-toxic doses of anticonvulsant drugs upon sexual functioning is as yet lacking.

ANTIPARKINSONIAN DRUGS

Dopaminergic pathways are important in the modulation of sexuality (see Chapter 1). Therefore it is not surprising that changes in sexual interest and performance have been reported during treatment of parkinsonian patients with drugs which enhance dopaminergic function.

A 'clear cut, visually evident increase in libido' during treatment with L-dopa was first noted by Barbeau (1969) in at least four out of 62 male patients. The reported frequency with which L-dopa treatment enhances sexual interest and activity depends on the method by which this is ascertained. In studies where patients were directly questioned about this aspect of behaviour, increased sexual interest and performance occurred in approximately one-third of patients treated with L-dopa (Hyppa *et al.* 1970; Bowers *et al.* 1971; O'Brien *et al.* 1971; Brown *et al.* 1978). Studies which did not specifically question about sexuality but relied on spontaneous reports have given lower estimates of the incidence of this side-effect. There is a distinct male preponderance with a sex ratio of perhaps three to one, so that increased sexuality in males during L-dopa treatment approaches 50 per cent (Brown *et al.* 1978).

Untreated Parkinson's disease is associated with reduced sexual interest and function. It has therefore been suggested that increased sexuality during L-dopa treatment simply represents a return to normal functioning (Duvoisin and Yahr 1972; De Ajuriaguerra *et al.* 1972). However, others have shown clear evidence of frank hypersexuality occurring in a small number of patients treated with L-dopa. Goodwin (1971) reviewed the literature on side-effects amongst 908 reported patients' treatment with L-dopa. He found that restoration of normal sexual interest was frequent with L-dopa treatment, but that frank hypersexuality occurred in only 0.9 per cent. He opined that this occurred in the setting of a more generalized hypomanic syndrome. Hypomania is a recognized complication of L-dopa treatment (Goodwin 1971) which gives rise to overactive and disinhibited behaviour, including sexual excesses. However, there are clear reports of hypersexuality occurring in the absence of hypomania or other psychiatric disturbance (O'Brien *et al.* 1971; Brown *et al.* 1978; Quinn *et al.* 1983; Harvey 1988; Uitti *et al.* 1989). Also, there is no general correlation between improved locomotor function and enhanced sexuality following L-dopa treatment. Brown *et al.* (1978) conducted a prospective study in seven men with Parkinson's disease who were rated for sexual interest, sexual behaviour, affect, and locomotor function before and after treatment with L-dopa. Four out of the seven men showed increased sexual interest, though one of these showed the same phenomenon during the initial placebo phase of treatment. No relationship was found between ratings of locomotor function and sexual interest or activity in this small group of patients.

Others have made the same observation (O'Brien *et al.* 1971; Uitti *et al.* 1989). Bowers *et al.* (1971) divided their patients into three groups: those whose sexual drive increased proportionately to their mobility, those whose sexual drive increased independently of motor improvement, and those who developed hypersexuality as part of an acute psychiatric disturbance with agitation and overactivity. The occurrence of hypersexuality has been reported to be dose dependent by several investigators (Jenkins and Groh 1970; Uitti *et al.* 1989).

Hypersexuality as a side-effect of L-dopa occurs not only in parkinsonian patients, but has also been described in psychiatric patients. Angrist and Gershon (1976) gave L-dopa to a group of schizophrenic and non-schizophrenic psychiatric patients. Four out of ten schizophrenic patients developed increased severity of sexually related delusions. Three out of six male, non-schizophrenic subjects reported sexual effects including inappropriate erections, reversal of long-standing erectile dysfunction, and compulsive masturbation unaccompanied by evidence of hypomania.

The hypersexuality attributed to L-dopa has included both increased sexual interest and increased frequency of erection. Thus, O'Brien *et al.* (1971) reported spontaneous penile erections in six of nine males given 4–6 g per day of L-dopa. Three of the men had been impotent for up to ten years. In general, the erections were not related to a sexual object and were not accompanied by sexual fantasies. Attempts to use L-dopa as a treatment for impotence have produced questionable and, at best, only transitory improvement (Benkert *et al.* 1972). Cases of enhanced sexual interest accompanied by continuing erectile dysfunction have also been reported (Uitti *et al.* 1989). Sexual deviation can also become overt during L-dopa treatment. Quinn *et al.* (1983) reported deviations including sadomasochism and bondage in patients taking L-dopa together with other antiparkinsonian drugs. Both the patients described had experienced an attraction to these forms of sexual behaviour prior to their illness and its treatment. The drugs can thus enhance sexuality in whatever mode the individual is predisposed to: most reports have related to heterosexual behaviour, but sexual deviations and homosexual behaviour can also occur. There is evidence that administration of dopamine-receptor blocking drugs can reverse the hypersexuality induced by antiparkinsonian drugs (Quinn *et al.* 1983), though this carries the risk of impairing the antiparkinsonian effect of the drugs. Similar findings of hypersexuality with L-dopa and its reversal by the dopamine-receptor blocking drug, pimozide, have been reported in animals (Malmnas 1976). Failure of ejaculation has also been reported during L-dopa treatment (Hallstrom and Persson 1970).

Less information is available regarding other antiparkinsonian agents. Bromocriptine has been reported to increase sexual desire and activity and to reverse impotence in hyperprolactinaemic men (Bommer *et al.* 1979; Marsch 1979; Buckmann and Kellner 1985) but has little effect on erectile dysfunction in men who are not hyperprolactinaemic (Cooper 1977; Ambrosi *et al*. 1977). There are no data suggesting improvement of erectile dysfunction in patients with Parkinson's disease treated with bromocriptine, and indeed there is a report of four men with idiopathic Parkinson's disease and no history of sexual difficulty who spontaneously complained of impotence associated with bromocriptine treatment which was reversed following partial substitution with L-dopa (Cleeves and Findley 1987). Uitti *et al*. (1989) report two cases in which bromocriptine treatment appeared to be associated with an undue increase in sexual interest and behaviour. One of the cases of deviant hypersexuality reported by Quinn *et al*. (1983) may have been related to bromocriptine. Cases of hypersexuality which may have been related to treatment with deprenyl, pergolide, and amantadine have also been reported (Quinn *et al*. 1983; Uitti *et al*. 1989). In a larger study of pergolide, seven out of eighteen male patients reported increased erections and spontaneous ejaculation (Jeanty *et al*. 1984).

In summary, parkinsonism is associated in some with diminished sexual interest and erectile dysfunction. Treatment with L-dopa can restore sexual functioning towards normal. Frank hypersexuality, including both enhanced sexual interest and increased frequency of erections, occurs in about one per cent of parkinsonian patients treated with L-dopa, and this can be seen as a direct effect of L-dopa upon sexuality which is not necessarily associated with a hypomanic mood swing. The object of the sexual behaviour depends upon previous sexual inclinations, so that covert sexual deviation can become manifest during L-dopa treatment. There are individual case reports implicating other antiparkinsonian drugs in the production of hypersexuality.

HISTAMINE H$_2$-RECEPTOR BLOCKERS

There is evidence from animal studies that cimetidine is an antiandrogen (Winters *et al*. 1979). In man, endocrine changes consistent with antiandrogen activity have been reported (Peden and Wormsley 1982). Thus, there are several reports of significantly elevated serum testosterone levels with cimetidine treatment (Van Thiel *et al*. 1979; Peden *et al*. 1981; Wang *et al*. 1982) though others have found no significant effect (Valk *et al*. 1979; Carlson *et al*. 1981; Stubbs *et al*. 1983). Furthermore, there is evidence that ranitidine does not have antiandrogen effects. Peden *et al*. (1981) reported that cimetidine treatment was associated with increased basal levels of serum testosterone in males treated for duodenal ulcer, but that ranitidine had no such effect. Cimetidine is also capable of stimulating increased serum prolactin levels, but this occurs primarily with large bolus doses given intravenously (Carlson *et al*. 1981) whereas oral administration has little or no effect (Majumdar *et al*. 1978; Spiegel *et al*. 1978; Van Thiel *et al*. 1979; Valk *et al*. 1979; Carlson *et al*. 1981).

There are numerous reports, mostly anecdotal, of erectile dysfunction and gynaecomastia during treatment with cimetidine. Wolfe (1979) reported a male patient who lost sexual interest and developed erectile dysfunction whilst taking cimetidine, returning to normal within two weeks of stopping the drug. Peden *et al.* (1979) reported three cases of reduced libido and erectile dysfunction during cimetidine treatment, and two of these did not regain normal sexual functioning after stopping the drug. Reversible reduction of libido, which disappeared after re-challenge with cimetidine and which appeared to be dose related, was reported by Biron (1979). In contrast, Webster (1979) reported a sustained increase in libido associated with improvement in ulcer symptoms during treatment with cimetidine. The post-marketing surveillance programme in the USA suggested a very low incidence of sexual dysfunction in only four patients out of 9907 treated (Gifford *et al.* 1980). Flind *et al.* (1982) summarized UK long-term placebo-controlled studies with cimetidine which showed a very low incidence of erectile dysfunction not differing from the placebo-treated group. The Committee on Safety of Medicines continues to receive reports of reversible erectile dysfunction not only with cimetidine but also with ranitidine and the newer agents, nizatidine and famotidine (Kassianos 1989). Gynaecomastia was reported in 18 out of 9907 patients surveyed by Gifford *et al.* (1980), and an incidence of approximately 0.1–0.2 per cent was cited by Flind *et al.* (1982). In a survey of 61 cases of Zollinger–Ellison syndrome and other hypersecretory states treated with cimetidine, there were five cases of gynaecomastia (in the absence of raised prolactin levels) but no reported sexual dysfunction (McCarthy 1978).

Anecdotal reports and uncontrolled observations are not an adequate basis from which to assess possible associations between the drug and erectile dysfunction. However, more systematic work has been carried out. Jensen *et al.* (1983) investigated 22 patients given high-dose cimetidine for hypersecretory states. Sexual side-effects were sought by questionnaire. Nine of these patients reported erectile dysfunction, nine suffered breast changes, and seven had both. The time of onset of erectile dysfunction and breast changes was similar, in most cases within two months of starting treatment. The patients with these side-effects were taking, on average, around 5 g per day of cimetidine. Nine patients were changed to an equally potent dose of ranitidine which led to the disappearance of these side-effects, with erectile dysfunction reversing usually within a month. Nocturnal penile tumescence studies were carried out in three patients, who showed impaired tumescence during cimetidine treatment, which returned to normal after ranitidine had been substituted. Peden and Wormsley (1982) also reported cases in which gynaecomastia and erectile dysfunction associated with 1 g daily of cimetidine resolved when the treatment was changed to ranitidine. In conclusion, erectile dysfunction and gynaecomastia occur as relatively rare side-effects of cimetidine at normal therapeutic dosages but become much more frequent at the high dosages used in hyper-secretory states. These side-effects are probably due to the antiandrogen effect of cimetidine and may be relieved by changing treatment to ranitidine, which appears to lack antiandrogen effects.

ANAESTHETIC AGENTS

It is well recognized that sedation with anaesthetic agents can give rise to fantasies of a sexual nature (Brahams 1989). Dundee (1990*a*, *b*) reported 35 cases of fantasies experienced during benzodiazepine sedation. Of these, 27 were female and 21 had a sexual content to the fantasy which they generally found unpleasant. Such fantasies have led to allegations of sexual impropriety on the part of the person administering the drug. However, sexual trespass was impossible in all but a few cases, usually because of the presence of others at the time of drug administration. Nevertheless, dental practitioners have been struck off by the General Dental Council as a result of such allegations (Dundee 1990*b*). Midazolam has been particularly implicated and there seems to be a dose relationship. Dundee (1990*a*) reported no incidence of fantasy with doses up to 0.1 mg kg^{-1} but an incidence of about 0.5 per cent with higher dosages. Often the content of the fantasy could be related to misinterpretation of a real event. Thus, the use of dental suckers and oral endoscopy has been associated with complaints of oral sex, and placing a swab between the legs has been associated with a complaint of sexual assault. The intravenous agent propofol, usually in combination with other agents, has also been implicated in the production of sexual fantasy and amorous behaviour, especially during the recovery period (Hunter *et al.* 1987; Young 1988; Smyth and Collins-Howgill 1988; Bricker 1988; Schaefer and Marsch 1989). This has led to accusations of sexual assault in the recovery room (Schaefer and Marsch 1989), and amorous advances towards staff members by both male and female patients. Bricker (1988) reported that disinhibited amorous behaviour did not occur after laparoscopy under propofol anaesthesia, but occurred in as many as 12 per cent of 130 propofol/alfentanil anaesthetics for procedures involving the urogenital region such as dilation and curettage, cystoscopy, and cervical biopsy. Nitrous oxide, particularly in concentrations greater than 50 per cent, can have psychic effects including hallucinations, paranoid ideas, and emotional changes (Rosenberg 1974), and this has included sexual experiences (Jastak and Malamed 1984). In a study of female volunteers, Gillman and Lichtigfeld (1983) gave nitrous oxide in a dose which caused a tingling sensation but minimal effect on consciousness. The women were asked to sexually fantasize during nitrous oxide administration and to rate their level of sexual arousal. For comparative purposes, control periods of oxygen administration were included in a cross-over design. Nitrous oxide clearly enhanced the sexual arousal resulting from sexual fantasy. Because of these events occurring during sedation with anaesthetic agents it has been recommended that a third party should always be present (Jastak and Malamed 1984; Schaefer and Marsch 1989). It has been suggested that patients should also be forewarned about the possibility of this unwanted effect (Boheimer and Thomas 1990), but Schaefer and Marsch (1991) considered this to be inappropriate.

Penile erection can occur during anaesthesia, either spontaneously or secondary to penile manipulation in the cause of surgical procedures such as cystoscopy or circumcision, and this prevents continuation with the surgical procedure. It has been reported that the intravenous anaesthetic agent, ketamine, is effective in preventing penile erection during anaesthesia and for detumescence once erection has occurred (Gale 1972) though success has not been universal (Benzon *et al.* 1983). Baraka and Sibai (1988) report small series of patients in whom detumescence during anaesthesia was achieved using intravenous diazepam or midazolam, and there is a single case report of the successful use of amyl nitrite (Welti and Brodsky 1980).

OTHER DRUGS

Cytotoxic drugs

Cytotoxic drugs cause dose-related gonadal damage (Shalet 1980). Chapman *et al.* (1979*a*) reported a retrospective study of clinical chemotherapy (MVPP: nitrogen mustard, vinblastine, procarbazine, and prednisolone) in 74 males treated for Hodgkin's disease. All men tested were azoospermic during treatment. Of the 54 men who completed a questionnaire on sexual performance, 74 per cent reported a decrease of libido and sexual performance. In 59 per cent there was little or no sexual activity and in 46 per cent decreased libido was persistent after completion of treatment. Testosterone levels were generally normal and did not correlate with decreased libido. Only six men suffered erectile dysfunction. This antedated the illness in three cases; a psychological origin was considered likely in four cases and the other two had low testosterone levels. A similar study of MVPP chemotherapy for Hodgkin's disease in 41 young women was reported by Chapman *et al.* (1979*b*); 92 per cent of the women reported strong or moderate libido prior to therapy but 73 per cent reported little or no libido after completion of treatment. Only 12 per cent continued to have regular menstrual cycles. Other symptoms, such as hot flushes, irritability, sleep disturbance, dry vagina, and painful intercourse were common. The separation and divorce rate was four times higher than in the general population. Hormonal replacement resulted in marked relief of symptoms and usually return of normal libido.

Erectile dysfunction has also been reported in individuals treated with methotrexate for rheumatoid arthritis (Blackburn and Alarcon 1989). Small doses used to treat psoriasis appear to have little effect on gonadal function (Grunnet *et al.* 1977).

Adverse effects on sexual function are so common with large doses of cytotoxic drugs that patients should be counselled about these effects.

Carbonic anhydrase inhibitors

Epstein and Grant (1977) reported a symptom complex of malaise, fatigue, weight loss, depression, anorexia, and often loss of libido in 44 of 92 patients taking acetazolamide or methazolamide. They felt that this was related to acidosis and some patients were relieved when sodium bicarbonate was administered. Wallace *et al.* (1979) reported 39 cases of decreased libido in patients with glaucoma treated with carbonic anhydrase inhibitors, of whom 33 were male. It appeared that at least two weeks of treatment was required before decreased libido occurred. Five patients also had erectile dysfunction though only three were thought to be drug related. Libido returned in all cases after discontinuing the drug. In 12 patients that were re-challenged, libido again decreased. Four cases of erectile dysfunction without disturbance of libido or general malaise were reported by Epstein *et al.* (1987).

Disulfiram

Disulfiram is used in the treatment of alcoholism. The drug inhibits liver aldehyde dehydrogenase, so that ingestion of alcohol leads to high circulating levels of acetaldehyde and consequent unpleasant symptoms which are a disincentive for drinking. The drug is reported to cause alterations in hypothalamic–pituitary–gonadal function (Van Thiel *et al.* 1979). Sexual difficulties including erectile dysfunction are relatively common in chronic alcoholics (see Chapter 10). This must therefore be balanced against reports that disulfiram can cause erectile dysfunction. However, direct evidence that disulfiram causes erectile dysfunction comes from a study by Snyder *et al.* (1981): 30 abstinent alcoholics were treated at random with either disulfiram, 250 mg daily, or placebo for seven days, and nocturnal penile tumescence was measured. There was a significant decrease in frequency and duration of full erections in the disulfiram group relative to the placebo-treated group.

Etretinate

Etretinate is used in the management of treatment-resistant psoriasis. It is very teratogenic, and can have an effect on the fetus for up to two years after the course has been completed. There are case reports of erectile dysfunction associated with etretinate treatment (Halkier-Sorensen 1988; Reynolds 1990) but a causal relationship has not been established.

Lipid-lowering agents

There are case reports of erectile dysfunction occurring in patients taking lipid-lowering agents. Schneider and Kaffarnik (1975) reported three cases of erectile dysfunction occurring in patients on long-term treatment with clofibrate. Two patients who chose to stop taking the drug regained potency, and re-exposure led to recurrence of erectile dysfunction. The patient who continued on the drug remained dysfunctional. In a major multicentre study of clofibrate (Coronary Drug Project Research Group 1975) in which over 1000 patients were treated with the drug, the percentage of patients complaining of 'decreased libido or potentia' at some point during five years of treatment was 14.1 per cent in the clofibrate group and 10 per cent in the placebo group, a small but statistically significant difference. Pizarro *et al.* (1990) reported a case of erectile dysfunction in a patient taking another lipid-lowering agent, gemfibrozil, together with propranolol. The erectile dysfunction appeared related in time to the introduction, withdrawal, and re-challenge with gemfibrozil.

Sulphasalazine

Sulphasalazine is used to treat ulcerative colitis and Crohn's disease and can cause oligospermia (Birnie *et al.* 1981). There is a case report of erectile dysfunction in a man on long-term sulphasalazine treatment (Ireland and Jewell 1989) which resolved after six to eight months off the drug and recurred two to three months after re-challenge, but did not occur with olsalazine which is used in patients intolerant of sulphasalazine (Ireland and Jewell 1987).

Heparin

Duggan and Morgan (1970) first proposed an association between heparin treatment and priapism by presenting four case reports. Since then there have been frequent reports of heparin-related priapism (Klein *et al.* 1972; Clark *et al.* 1981; Burke *et al.* 1983; Bergmann *et al.* 1987; Adjiman *et al.* 1988). It has been suggested that heparin-induced priapism has a particularly poor outcome (Adjiman *et al.* 1988). The mechanism of this adverse effect is poorly understood, though abnormal spontaneous platelet aggregation has been suggested as an aetiological factor (Burke *et al.* 1983).

Miscellaneous agents

Zorgniotti and Rossman (1987) report 16 cases of erectile dysfunction apparently associated with chronic use of nasal vasoconstrictors for sinusitis. They note that there are histopathological similarities between the corpus cavernosum and the nasal turbinate, and that in some men nasal congestion develops with sexual excitation.

Dose-related erectile dysfunction with baclofen is reported by Hedley *et al.* (1978) in one of 35 patients with multiple sclerosis treated with this drug. Erectile dysfunction and constipation (as well as marked relief of spasticity) occurred with a dose of 30 mg daily and potency was restored by a dose reduction to 15 mg daily.

Non-steroidal anti-inflammatory drugs have also been implicated in male sexual dysfunction. Wei and Hood (1980) reported a case in whom ejaculatory failure coincided with naproxen treatment, resolved on stopping the drug, and returned on re-challenge with naproxen. Miller *et al.* (1989) reported a case of decreased libido and erectile dysfunction after two to three weeks treatment with indomethacin, which resolved with drug discontinuation and did not recur during subsequent treatment with naproxen.

Ketoconazole, an antifungal agent, causes a transient fall in serum testosterone levels (Schurmeyer and Nieschlag 1982), though testosterone levels are not generally depressed with chronic usage. Gynaecomastia can occur rarely with this drug (Cohen 1982), but effects on sexual function are not well documented.

Fenfluramine has been reported to cause reduced libido in women treated for obesity, especially when large doses are used (Sproule 1971). This effect has been said to be unrelated to the sedation produced by the drug. In contrast, there are also case reports of increased libido during fenfluramine treatment of bulimia (Stevenson and Solyom 1990), in one case associated with a euphoriant and stimulant effect (Rosenvinge 1975). Fenfluramine is used much less frequently in males, though erectile dysfunction was reported in two out of 36 obese men given the drug (Hollingsworth and Amatruda 1969).

CONCLUSION

There is a substantial variation in the validity of available information regarding the sexual side-effects of drugs. Sexual side-effects are under-reported, and the importance of such effects to patients is commonly unrecognized by prescribers. Few drugs have been evaluated with the vigour described by Riley and Riley (Chapter 5): data on individual drugs should be judged against the methodological standards proposed by these authors.

REFERENCES

Adjiman, S., Fava, P., Bitker, M.O., and Chatelain, C. (1988). Priapisme induit par l'heparine. *Annales de Urologie*, **22**, 125–8.

Ambrosi, B., Bara, R., and Faglia, G. (1977). Bromocriptine in impotence. *Lancet*, **ii**, 987.

Angrist, B. and Gershon, S. (1976). Clinical effects of amphetamine and L-dopa on sexuality and aggression. *Comprehensive Psychiatry*, **17**, 715–22.

Baraka, A. and Sibai, A.N. (1988). Benzodiazepine treatment of penile erection under general anaesthesia. *Anaesthesia and Analgesia*, **67**, 596–606.

Barbeau, A. (1969). L-dopa therapy in Parkinson's disease: A critical review of nine years experience. *Canadian Medical Association Journal*, **101**, 59–101.

Benkert, O., Crombach, G., and Kockott, G. (1972). Effect of L-dopa on sexually impotent patients. *Psychopharmacologia*, **23**, 91–5.

Benzon, H.T., Leventhal, J.B., and Ovassapian, A. (1983). Ketamine treatment of penile erection in the operating room. *Anaesthesia and Analgesia*, **62**, 457–8.

Bergmann, J.F., Fava, P., Bitker, M.O., Chatelain, C., Caulin, C., and Segrestaa, J.M. (1987). Priapisme au cours d'un traitement par heparinate de calcium. *Therapie*, **42**, 250–1.

Birnie, G.G., McLeod, T.I.F., and Watkinson, G. (1981). Incidence of sulphasalazine-induced male infertility. *Gut*, **22**, 452–5.

Biron, P. (1979). Diminished libido with cimetidine therapy. *Canadian Medical Association Journal*, **121**, 404–5.

Blackburn, W.D. and Alarcon, G.S. (1989). Impotence in three rheumatoid arthritis patients treated with methotrexate. *Arthritis and Rheumatism*, **32**, 1341–2.

Blumer, D. and Walker, A.E. (1967). Sexual behaviour in temporal lobe epilepsy. *Archives of Neurology*, **16**, 37–43.

Boheimer, N.O. and Thomas, J.S. (1990). Amorous behaviour and sexual fantasy following anaesthesia or sedation. *Anaesthesia*, **45**, 699.

Bommer, J., Del Pozo, E., Ritz, E., and Bommer, G. (1979). Improved sexual function in male haemodialysis patients on bromocriptine. *Lancet*, **ii**, 496–7.

Bowers, M.B., Van Woert, M., and Davis, L. (1971). Sexual behaviour during L-dopa treatment for parkinsonism. *American Journal of Psychiatry*, **127**, 127–9.

Brahams, D. (1989). Benzodiazepine sedation and allegations of sexual assault. *Lancet*, **i**, 1339–40.

Bricker, S.R.W. (1988). Hallucinations after propofol. *Anaesthesia*, **43**, 171.

Brown, E., Brown, G.M., Kofman, O., and Quarrington, B. (1978). Sexual function and effect in parkinsonian men treated with L-dopa. *American Journal of Psychiatry*, **135**, 1552–5.

Buckmann, M.T. and Kellner, R. (1985). Reduction of distress in hyperprolactinaemia with bromocriptine. *American Journal of Psychiatry*, **142**, 242–4.

Burke, B.J., Scott, G.L., Smith, P.J.B., and Wakerley, G.R. (1983). Heparinassociated priapism. *Postgraduate Medical Journal*, **59**, 332–3.

Carlson, H.E., Ippoliti, A.F., and Swerdloff, R.S. (1981). Endocrine effects of acute & chronic cimetidine administration. *Digestive Diseases and Sciences*, **26**, 428–32.

Chapman, R.M., Rees, L.H., Sutcliffe, S.B., Edwards, C.R.W., and Malpas, J.S. (1979*a*). Cyclical combination chemotherapy and gonadal function: a retrospective study in males. *Lancet*, **i**, 285–9.

Chapman, R.M., Sutcliffe, S.B., and Malpas, J.S. (1979*b*). Cytotoxic-induced ovarian failure in Hodgkin's Disease II: Effects on sexual function. *Journal of the American Medical Association*, **242**, 1882–4.

Clark, S.K., Tremann, J.A., Sennewald, F.R., and Donaldson, J.A. (1981). Priapism: an unusual complication of heparin therapy for sudden deafness. *American Journal of Otolaryngology*, **2**, 69–72.

Cleeves, L. and Findley, I.J. (1987). Bromocriptine induced impotence in Parkinson's Disease. *British Medical Journal*, **295**, 367–8.

Cohen, J. (1982). Antifungal chemotherapy. *Lancet*, **ii**, 532–7.

Connell, J.M.C., Rapeport, W.G., Beastall, G.H., and Brodie, M.J. (1984). Changes in circulating androgens during short-term carbamazepine therapy. *British Journal of Clinical Pharmacology*, **17**, 347–51.

Cooper, A.J. (1977). Bromocriptine in impotence. *Lancet*, **ii**, 567.

Coronary Drug Project Research Group (1975). Clofibrate and niacin in coronary heart disease. *Journal of the American Medical Association*, **231**, 360–81.

Dana-Haeri, J., Oxley, J., and Richens, A. (1982). Reduction of free testosterone by antiepileptic drugs. *British Medical Journal*, **284**, 85–6.

De Ajuriaguerra, J., Constantinides, J., Eisenring, J.J., Yanniotis, J., and Tissot, R. (1972). Behaviour disorders and L-dopa therapy in Parkinson's syndrome. In *Parkinson's disease. Proc. IV Int. Symp.* (ed. Siegfried J.) Bern: Hans Huber,

Demerdash, A., Shaalan, M., Midania Kamel, F., and Bahri, M. (1991). Sexual behaviour of a sample of females with epilepsy. *Epilepsia*, **32**, 82–5.

Duggan, M.L. and Morgan, C. (1970). Heparin: a cause of priapism? *Southern Medical Journal*, **63**, 1131–5.

Dundee, J.W. (1990*a*). Complaints of sexual fantasies following benzodiazepine sedation in women. *Anaesthesiology*, **73**, A27.

Dundee, J.W. (1990*b*). Unpleasant sequelae of benzodiazepine sedation. *Anaesthesia*, **45**, 336.

Duvoisin, R.C. and Yahr, M.D. (1972). Behavioural abnormalities occurring in parkinsonism during treatment with L-dopa. In *L-dopa and behaviour* (ed. S. Malitz). Raven Press, New York.

Epstein, D.L. and Grant, W.M. (1977). Carbonic anhydrase inhibitor side-effects. *Archives of Ophthalmology*, **95**, 1378–82.

Epstein, R.J., Allen, R.C., and Lunde, M.W. (1987). Organic impotence associated with carbonic anhydrase inhibitor therapy for glaucoma. *Annals of Ophthalmology*, **19**, 48–50.

Flind, A.C., Jenkinson, S.I., and Rowley-Jones, D. (1982). Is cimetidine a clinically important anti-androgen? *Scandinavian Journal of Gastroenterology*, **17** (Suppl. 78), 240.

Fenwick, P.B.C., Toone, B.K., Wheeler, M.J., Nanjee, M.N., Grant, R., and Brown, D. (1985). Sexual behaviour in a centre for epilepsy. *Acta Neurologica Scandinavica*, **71**, 428–35.

Fenwick, P.B.C., Mercer, S., Grant, R., Wheeler, M., Nanjee, N., Toone, B., and Brown, D. (1986). Nocturnal penile tumescence and serum testosterone levels. *Archives of Sexual Behaviour*, **15**, 13–21.

Gale, B. (1972). Ketamine prevention of penile turgescence. *Journal of the American Medical Association*, **219**, 1629.

Gastaut, H. and Collomb, H. (1954). Etude du comportement sexuel chez les epileptiques psychomoteurs. *Annales Medico Psychologiques*, **112**, 223–59.

Gifford, L.M., Aeugle, M.E., Myerson, R.M., and Tannenbaum, P.J. (1980). Cimetidine postmarket outpatient surveillance program. *Journal of the American Medical Association*, **243**, 1532–5.

Gillman, M.A. and Lichtigfeld, F.J. (1983). The effects of nitrous oxide and naloxone on orgasm in human females—a preliminary report. *Journal of Sex Research*, **19**, 49–57.

Goodwin, F.K. (1971). Psychiatric side effects of levodopa in man. *Journal of the American Medical Association*, **218**, 1915–20.

Grunnet, E., Nyfors, A., and Hansen, K.B. (1977). Studies on human semen in topical corticosteroid-treated and methotrexate-treated psoriatics. *Dermatologica*, **154**, 78–84.

Halkier-Sorensen, L. (1988). Sexual dysfunction in a patient treated with etretinate. *Acta Dermato Venereologica*, **68**, 90–1.

Hallstrom, T. and Persson, T. (1970). L-dopa and non-emission of semen. *Lancet*, **i**, 1231–2.

Harvey, N.S. (1988). Serial cognitive profiles in levodopa-induced hypersexuality. *British Journal of Psychiatry*, **153**, 853–6.

Hedley, D.W., Marovn, J.A., and Espir, M.L.E. (1978). Evaluation of baclofen (Lioresal) for spasticity in multiple sclerosis. *Postgraduate Medical Journal*, **51**, 615–18.

Hierons, R. and Saunders, M. (1966). Impotence in patients with temporal lobe lesions. *Lancet*, **ii**, 761–3.

Hollingsworth, D.R. and Amatruda, T.T. (1969). Toxic and therapeutic effects of EMTP in obesity. *Clinical Pharmacology and Therapeutics*, **10**, 540–2.

Hunter, D.N., Thorvily, A., and Whitburn, R. (1987). Arousal from propofol. *Anaesthesia*, **42**, 1128–9.

Hyppa, M., Rinne, V.K., and Sonninen, V. (1970). The activating effect of L-dopa treatment on sexual functions and its experimental background. *Acta Neurologica Scandanavica*, **43** (Suppl.), 223–4.

Ireland, A. and Jewell, D.P. (1987). Olsalazine in patients intolerant of sulphasalazine. *Scandanavian Journal of Gastroenterology*, **22**, 1038–40.

Ireland, A. and Jewell, D.P. (1989). Sulfasalazine-induced impotence: a beneficial resolution with olsalazine. *Journal of Clinical Gastroenterology*, **11**, 71.

Jastak, J.T. and Malamed, S.F. (1984). Nitrous oxide sedation and sexual phenomena. *Dental Anaesthesia and Sedation*, **13**, 70–3.

Jeanty, P., Van Den Kerchove, M., Lowenthal, A., and De Bruyne, H. (1984). Pergolide therapy in Parkinson's Disease. *Journal of Neurology*, **231**, 148–52.

Jenkins, R.B. and Groh, R.H. (1970). Mental symptoms in parkinsonian patients treated with L-dopa. *Lancet*, **ii**, 177–80.

Jensen, R.T., Collen, M.J., Pandol, S.J., Allende, H.D., Ravfman, J.P., Bissonnette, B.M., Duncan, W.C., Durgin, P.L., Gillin, J.C., and Gardner, J.D. (1983). Cimetidine-induced impotence and breast changes in patients with gastric hypersecretory states. *New England Journal of Medicine*, **308**, 883–7.

Jensen, P., Jensen, S.B., Sorensen, P.S., Bjerre, B.D., Rizzi, D.A., Sorenson, A.S., Klysner, R., Brinch, K., Jespersen, B., and Nielson, H. (1990). Sexual dysfunction in male and female patients with epilepsy: a study of 86 outpatients. *Archives of Sexual Behaviour*, **19**, 1–14.

Kassianos, G.C. (1989). Impotence and nizatidine. *Lancet*, **i**, 963.

Klein, L.A., Hall, R.L., and Smith, R.B. (1972). Surgical treatment of priapism with a note on heparin-induced priapism. *Journal of Urology*, **108**, 104–6.

Majumdar, S.K., Thomson, A.D., and Shaw, G.K. (1978). Cimetidine and serum prolactin. *British Medical Journal*, **1**, 409.

Malmnas, C.O. (1976). The significance of dopamine versus other catecholamines for L-dopa induced facilitators of sexual behaviour in the castrated male rat. *Pharmacology, Biochemistry and Behaviour*, **4**, 521–6.

Marsch, C.M. (1979). Bromocriptine in the treatment of hypogonadism and male impotence. *Drugs*, **17**, 349–58.

McCarthy, D.M. (1978). Report on the United States experience with cimetidine in Zollinger–Ellison syndrome and other hypersecretory states. *Gastroenterology*, **74**, 453–8.

Miller, L.G., Rogers, J.C., and Swee, D.E. (1989). Indomethacin associated sexual dysfunction. *Journal of Family Practice*, **29**, 210–11.

O'Brien, C.P., Di Giacomo, J.N., Fahn, S., and Schwarz, G.A. (1971). Mental effects of high dose levodopa. *Archives of General Psychiatry*, **24**, 61–4.

Peden, N.R. and Wormsley, K.G. (1982). Effect of cimetidine on gonadal function in man. *British Journal of Clinical Pharmacology*, **13**, 791–4.

Peden, N.R., Boyd, E.J.S., Browning, M.C.K., Saunders, J.H.B., and Wormsley, K.G. (1981). Effects of two histamine H$_2$-receptor blocking drugs on basal levels of gonadotrophins, prolactin, testosterone and oestradiol during treatment of

Peden, N.R., Boyde, E.J.S., Browning, M.C.K., Saunders, J.H.B., and Wormsley, K.G. (1981). Effects of two histamine H$_2$-receptor blocking drugs on basal levels of gonodotrophins, prolactin, testosterone and oestradiol during treatment of duodenal ulcers in male patients. *Acta Endocrinologica*, **96**, 564–8.

Pizarro, S., Bargay, J., and D'Agosto, P. (1990). Gemfibrozil-induced impotence. *Lancet*, **ii**, 1135.

Quinn, N.P., Toone, B., Lang, A.E., Marsden, C.D., and Parkes, J.D. (1983). Dopa dose-dependent sexual deviation. *British Journal of Psychiatry*, **142**, 296–8.

Reynolds, O.D. (1990). Erectile dysfunction in a patient treated with etretinate. *Acta Dermato Venereologica*, **68**, 90–1.

Rosenberg, P. (1974). The effect of nitrous oxide oxygen inhalation on subjective experiences in healthy young adults. *Annales Chirurgiae Gynaecologiae*, **63**, 504.

Rosenvinge, H.P. (1975). Abuse of fenfluramine. *British Medical Journal*, **1**, 735.

Saunders, M. and Rawson, M. (1970). Sexuality in male epileptics. *Journal of Neurological Sciences*, **10**, 577–83.

Schaefer, H.G. and Marsch, S.C.U. (1989). An unusual emergence after total intravenous anaesthesia. *Anaesthesia*, **44**, 928–9.

Schaefer, H.G. and Marsch, S.C.U. (1991). Forewarning patients of sexual arousal during anaesthesia. *Anaesthesia*, **46**, 238–9.

Schneider, J. and Kaffarnik, H. (1975). Impotence in patients treated with clofibrate. *Atherosclerosis*, **21**, 455–7.

Schurmeyer, T. and Nieschlag, E. (1982). Ketoconazole-induced drop in serum and saliva testosterone. *Lancet*, **ii**, 1098.

Shalet, S.M. (1980). The effects of cancer chemotherapy on gonadal function in patients. *Cancer Treatment Reviews*, **7**, 141–52.

Shukla, G.D., Srivastava, O.N., and Katiyar, B.C. (1979). Sexual disturbances in temporal lobe epilepsy: a controlled study. *British Journal of Psychiatry*, **134**, 288–92.

Smyth, D.G. and Collins-Howgill, P.J. (1988). Hallucinations after propofol. *Anaesthesia*, **43**, 170.

Snyder, S., Karacan, I., and Salis, P.J. (1981). Disulfiram and nocturnal penile tumescence in the chronic alcoholic. *Biological Psychiatry*, **16**, 399–406.

Spark, R.F., Wills, C.A., and Royal, H. (1984). Hypogonadism, hyperprolactinaemia and temporal lobe epilepsy in hypersexual men. *Lancet*, **i**, 413–16.

Spiegel, A.M., Lopatin, R., Peikin, S., and McCarthy, D. (1978). Serum prolactin in patients receiving oral cimetidine. *Lancet*, **i**, 881.

Sproule, B.C. (1971). Treatment of the grossly obese with a high dose of fenfluramine. *South African Medical Journal*, **45** (Suppl.), 46–7.

Stevenson, R.W.D. and Solyom, L. (1990). The aphrodisiac effect of fenfluramine: two case reports of a possible side-effect to the use of fenfluramine in the treatment of bulimia. *Journal of Clinical Psychopharmacology*, **10**, 69–71.

Stubbs, W.A., Delitala, G., Besser, G.M., Edwards, C.R.W., Labrooy, S., Taylor, R., Misiewicz, J.J., and Alberti, K.G.M.M. (1983). The endocrine and metabolic effects of cimetidine. *Clinical Endocrinology*, **18**, 167–78.

Taylor, D.C. (1969). Sexual behaviour and temporal lobe epilepsy. *Archives of Neurology*, **21**, 510–16.

Toone, B.K., Wheeler, M., Nanjee, M., Fenwick, P., and Grant, R. (1983). Sex hormones, sexual activity and plasma anticonvulsant levels in male epileptics. *Journal of Neurology, Neurosurgery and Psychiatry*, **46**, 844–6.

Toone, B.K., Edeh, J., Nanjee, M.N., and Wheeler, M. (1989). Hyposexuality and epilepsy: a community survey of hormonal and behavioural changes in male epileptics. *Psychological Medicine*, **19**, 937–43.

Uitti, R.J., Tanner, C.M., Rajput, A.H., Goetz, C.G., Klawans, H.L., and Thiessen, B. (1989). Hypersexuality with antiparkinsonian therapy. *Clinical Neuropharmacology*, **12**, 375–83.

Valk, T.W., England, B.G., and Marshall, J.C. (1979). Pituitary function on oral cimetidine therapy. *Clinical Research*, **27**, 681.

Van Thiel, D.H., Gavaler, J.S., Smith, W.I., and Paul, G. (1979). Hypothalamic–pituitary–gonadal dysfunction in men using cimetidine. *New England Journal of Medicine*, **300**, 1012–15.

Wallace, T.R., Fraunfelder, F.T., Petursson, G.J., and Epstein, D.L. (1979). Decreased libido: a side-effect of carbonic anhydrase inhibitors. *Annals of Ophthalmology*, **ii**, 1563–6.

Wang, C., Lai, C.L, Lam, K.C., and Yeung, K.K. (1982). Effect of cimetidine on gonadal function in man. *British Journal of Clinical Pharmacology*, **13**, 791–4.

Webster, J. (1979). Male sexual dysfunction and cimetidine. *British Medical Journal*, **i**, 889.

Wei, N. and Hood, J.C. (1980). Naproxen and ejaculatory dysfunction. *Annals of Internal Medicine*, **93**, 933.

Welti, R.S. and Brodsky, J.B. (1980). Treatment of intraoperative penile tumescence. *Journal of Neurology*, **124**, 925–6.

Winters, S.J., Banks, J.L., and Loriavx, D.L. (1979). Cimetidine is an antiandrogen in the rat. *Gastroenterology*, **76**, 504–8.

Wolfe, W.M. (1979). Impotence on cimetidine treatment. *New England Journal of Medicine*, **300**, 94.

Young, P.N. (1988). Hallucinations after propofol. *Anaesthesia*, **43**, 170.

Zorgniotti, A.W. and Rossman, B. (1987). Possible role of chronic use of nasal vasoconstrictors in impotence. *Urology*, **30**, 594.

9

Psychiatric drugs and sexuality

Thomas R.E. Barnes and Carol A. Harvey

INTRODUCTION

Knowledge about the effects of psychiatric drugs on sexual function is relevant for two main reasons. First, familiarity with the possible sexual side-effects of a particular drug is necessary if the adverse effects are to be adequately monitored in an individual patient or clinical trial. Second, if a patient presents with a sexual dysfunction, information on drug-induced sexual problems is required in order to assess the possible contribution of their current medication and drug history.

Unfortunately, the data available on the prevalence and severity of sexual difficulties related to psychotropic drugs are 'inaccurate and contradictory' (Hugues 1989) and relate predominantly to male problems. Drug effects on human female sexuality have been studied far less than effects on male sexuality, and are generally less acknowledged and understood. Appreciation of the impact of drug treatment on sexual behaviour and function is limited by the variety of factors involved, the scarcity of epidemiological data, and the difficulties of assessment, which include the lack of agreement on specific terms for the various dysfunctions (Barnes 1984; Vanelle and Poirier 1989). There is often a lack of clarity about the specific nature of the sexual dysfunction being reported; for example, a distinction is rarely made between ejaculation and orgasm in males. Such imprecision is a hindrance to elucidation of the mechanism by which drugs produce their sexual side-effects.

A further issue is the difficulty attributing sexual problems to drug treatment rather than the psychiatric illness for which it was prescribed. For example, Friedman and Harrison (1984) found that 40 per cent of a sample of schizophrenic women reported a general lack of interest in sexual activity before receiving treatment with antipsychotic drugs. Mitchell and Popkin (1983) pointed out that it seemed likely that patients with depression who developed sexual dysfunction secondary either to their illness or their antidepressant medication would consequently develop changes of libido.

For many drugs used in psychiatric practice, the information on sexual side-effects must be culled from a variety of sources, such as isolated case reports and comments in reviews of the area. The published reports of drug trials may provide a list of side-effects, including sexual problems, but the methods for monitoring these vary widely. If sexual side-effects are missing from the list, it may not be clear whether sexual problems were absent or the investigators failed to enquire about them. Very few such studies have been set up specifically to investigate drug effects on sexual function. Sexual side-effects are probably commonly under-reported in drug trials because they are so easily missed. Monteiro *et al.* (1987) noted that most patients report sexual side-effects only when asked directly and specifically, and not in response to simple questionnaires. Thus, the published data do not allow us to make confident statements about the prevalence or incidence of particular drug-induced sexual dysfunctions.

Pharmacological treatment in psychiatric practice is largely limited to three categories: antipsychotic, antidepressant, and anxiolytic drugs. Although each of the categories contains drugs from a number of different classes, most clinicians would regularly prescribe only a few of these. In large studies, anxiolytics have not emerged as an important cause of sexual dysfunction, although isolated case reports suggest that benzodiazepines such as chlordiazepoxide, lorazepam, alprazolam, and diazepam may interfere with ejaculation and achievement of orgasm (Hughes 1964; Morley 1986; McWaine and Procci 1988). This chapter will cover the two groups of drugs most commonly implicated in sexual problems: the antidepressant and antipsychotic drugs.

ANTIPSYCHOTIC DRUGS

Antipsychotic, or neuroleptic, drugs are effective in the treatment of acute psychotic episodes, and when administered in the long term play a role in the prevention of psychotic relapse. The majority of patients receiving these drugs will have a diagnosis of schizophrenia. The common pharmacological action of antipsychotic drugs is dopamine receptor blockade, but many also possess anticholinergic and antiadrenergic activity. These drugs are associated with a wide range of side-effects, including sedation, postural hypotension, weight gain, and movement disorders such as parkinsonism, dystonia, akathisia, and tardive dyskinesia. They also cause a number of sexual dysfunctions, although Nestoros *et al.* (1980) considered the possibility that certain schizophrenic patients might function better sexually when receiving medication. They surmised that the drugs might alleviate symptoms that would otherwise interfere with sexual functioning, such as psychotic anxiety, thought disorganization and fear of physical intimacy with potential sexual partners.

These postulated beneficial effects might help to explain the definite increase in the reproductive rates of schizophrenic patients associated with the introduction of antipsychotic drugs, reported by Erlenmeyer-Kimling *et al.* (1969). This increase is apparent when fertility rates in the pre-neuroleptic era (Essen-Moller 1935) are compared with those in the post-neuroleptic (Slater *et al.* 1971) era. Nestoros *et al.* (1980) attribute this increase to the therapeutic effects of the drugs which allow schizophrenic patients 'more years of community life as well as more opportunities for marriage and reproduction.'

Sexual dysfunction with antipsychotic drugs

Antipsychotic drugs have been reported to cause loss of sexual interest and drive, erectile and ejaculatory difficulties, priapism, and inhibition of orgasm. However, the prevalence and severity of these drug-induced sexual dysfunctions are not clearly documented in the literature (Smith and Talbert 1986; Barnes 1984; Segraves 1988*a*). Although these problems are potentially reversible if the drugs are stopped, most patients receiving these drugs do so long term. Thus, drug-induced sexual dysfunctions will tend to be persistent, with the potential for serious secondary adverse affects on patients and their relationships.

The sexual problems may go unrecognized, partly because doctors do not always enquire systematically about the presence of such difficulties and partly because patients may be reluctant to talk about them, particularly if they do not perceive them as related to drug treatment. This lack of communication about sexual problems is reflected in the scarcity of the research literature on sexual dysfunction in schizophrenia, the condition most commonly treated with antipsychotic drugs. Nevertheless, Verhulst and Schneidman (1981) found that reliable data on sexual problems could be obtained at interview from patients with schizophrenia. In their small sample of 12 females and 8 males, four males reported decreased sexual interest when they took antipsychotic drugs, three had occasional erectile problems, and one patient, receiving thioridazine, 'failed to ejaculate'. Three of the women described reduced sexual interest on medication and five reported delay in vaginal lubrication or reaching orgasm. The investigators considered the incidence of sexual dysfunction, other than that related to antipsychotic medication, to be low.

Assessment of sexual dysfunction associated with antipsychotic medication is confounded in most patient samples by the co-administration of other drugs such as anticholinergics and antidepressants, and by the presence of the psychotic illness, most often schizophrenia, for which the drugs were originally prescribed. While certain specific dysfunctions such as retrograde ejaculation and priapism are known effects of antipsychotic drugs, psychotic illness may be responsible for some of the sexual problems, such as low drive, that are identified. Loss of volition, social withdrawal, and anhedonia are negative symptoms of schizophrenia which will tend to militate against having a regular sexual partner. Many schizophrenic patients have poor, immature social skills. In some cases this may be related to the illness developing in the late teenage years before adult social skills have been learned and the personality has matured. The illness may also delay the acquisition of appropriate social skills by causing patients to spend long periods in hospital away from family and friends, denying them a range of normal social experience. Buddeberg *et al.* (1988) recommended that increased attention should be paid to sexual counselling in schizophrenic patients.

Loss of sexual interest and drive

A common problem in both females and males receiving antipsychotic drugs is loss of sexual interest and desire, or loss of libido. Low drive has been reported with phenothiazines (Pomme *et al.* 1965; Mitchell and Popkin 1982) and butyrophenones (Brambilla *et al.* 1974). Withdrawal of antipsychotic drugs may be associated with the reappearance of sexual activity (Leconte *et al.* 1960).

Theoretical mechanisms All antipsychotic drugs currently available have dopamine-antagonist properties, and many have serotonin antagonism to a greater or lesser extent. Increased dopaminergic activity may enhance sexual behaviour while inhibition of central dopaminergic systems may reduce sexual activity (Gessa and Tagliamonte 1974; Everett 1975). The evidence for this comes chiefly from animal studies, observations of patients with Parkinson's disease receiving L-DOPA, and studies of L-DOPA on human sexual functioning. Thus central dopamine-blockade associated with antipsychotic drugs might serve to suppress sexual interest and activity (Mitchell and Popkin 1983). On the other hand, Wein and Van Arsdalen (1988) noted that agents which increase central serotonergic activity have been found to decrease sexual activity in laboratory animals, while serotonin antagonists have been reported to produce hypersexuality.

Aside from the neurotransmitter and neuroendocrine explanations for this problem, a number of other factors such as weight gain, sedation, and parkinsonism might be relevant in patients with chronic psychotic illnesses treated with antipsychotic drugs.

Erectile dysfunction

Difficulties achieving and maintaining erection have been reported with a variety of antipsychotic drugs such as thioridazine, chlorpromazine, thiothixene, fluphenazine, haloperidol, and benperidol (Barnes 1984; Mitchell and Popkin 1982).

Two clinical studies, by Ghadirian and colleagues (1982) and Kotin and co-workers (1986) explored the extent to which erectile problems occurred in male psychiatric patients receiving long-term treatment with antipsychotic drugs. Kotin *et al.* (1976) analysed 121 episodes of drug prescription among 87 male psychiatric patients (age range 21–68 years, median 49 years): 23 treated with thioridazine alone, 30 who had taken antipsychotics other than thioridazine, and 34 who had received thioridazine and other antipsychotics (included in both groups). They found what they referred to as 'erectile insufficiency' in 44 per cent of a sample of patients who had been on thioridazine for a minimum of two weeks, a figure significantly greater than the 19 per cent found in the comparison sample of patients receiving other antipsychotics.

Ghadirian *et al.* (1982) studied a sample of 26 male schizophrenic outpatients (age range 24–57 years, median 34 years) receiving maintenance treatment with fluphenazine, either oral or depot preparations. The investigators assessed changes in sexual functioning since antipsychotic drug treatment had been started. Difficulties in achieving and maintaining erection were found in 38 and 42 per cent, respectively. There was a significant partial correlation coefficient (eliminating the effect of age) between log plasma prolactin and sexual dysfunction score.

Theoretical mechanisms   The physiological mechanisms involved in penile erection are not clearly understood (Segraves 1989). The general view is that erection is a consequence of stimulation of sacral parasympathetic vasodilator fibres, although sympathetic fibres from the thoracolumbar outflow may also be involved in the vascular response. Blood is shunted to the erectile tissue, the two corpora cavernosa, and the corpus spongiosum, to produce an erection. The sympathetic system may also contribute further by mediating the constriction of veins in erectile tissue to reduce venous outflow. Antipsychotic drugs have both anticholinergic and α-adrenergic blocking activity which presumably disturbs this neurophysiological control of erection via the parasympathetic and sympathetic systems.

Ejaculatory dysfunction

Ejaculatory dysfunction has been considered the most frequent adverse effect on sexual function (Smith and Talbert 1986). Ejaculatory problems, most typically retrograde ejaculation, have been reported with thioridazine, chlorpromazine, mesoridazine, chlorprothixene, perphenazine, trifluoperazine, butaperazine, and haloperidol (Barnes 1984; Segraves 1988*a*). Thioridazine seems to be the most culpable, on the basis of its potent peripheral α-adrenergic blocking action. Blair and Simpson (1966) estimated that 30 per cent of one group of patients taking thioridazine experienced ejaculatory dysfunction. Similarly, in the study by Kotin *et al.* (1976), a third of the patient group treated with thioridazine suffered specifically from retrograde ejaculation compared with none of the patients receiving other antipsychotics.

In the study by Ghadirian *et al.* (1982) of schizophrenic out-patients receiving fluphenazine, decreased quantity of ejaculate was reported by 46 per cent of the sample. Changes in quality of orgasm and a decreased ability to achieve orgasm were each complained of by 58 per cent.

Theoretical mechanisms Knowledge of the neurophysiology of ejaculation is even less certain than that of erection (Segraves 1989). Ejaculation is thought to occur in three phases: emission; bladder neck closure, and true (anterograde) ejaculation. Emission involves the contraction of the smooth muscle of the vas deferens, seminal vesicles, and prostate to release semen into the posterior urethra. There is closure of the bladder neck and the internal urethral sphincter, probably mediated via α-adrenergic stimulation. Anterograde ejaculation is then produced by clonic contractions of the striated bulbocavernosus, ischiocavernosus, and urethral muscles, possibly mediated via the parasympathetic sacral outflow and somatic efferents.

There is little evidence to implicate dopaminergic systems in the ejaculatory response, and antipsychotics probably interfere with ejaculatory function via α-adrenergic blockade and possibly their anticholinergic action. The α-adrenergic action affects the vas deferens, seminal vesicles, ejaculatory ducts, and bladder neck, and leads to a reduction in ejaculate volume. Thioridazine seems to be particularly prone to cause retrograde ejaculation into the bladder because of failure of closure of the internal sphincter, a consequence of its relatively potent anti-adrenergic effects (Nininger 1979). It has been reported that urine passed after retrograde ejaculation may be milky due to the presence of semen. However, Kedia and Markland (1975) found no evidence of sperm in the post-masturbation urine samples of men taking thioridazine. Wein and Van Arsdalen (1988) concluded that the relevant action was likely to be one of inhibition of seminal emission. Antipsychotic drugs can also cause partial ejaculatory incompetence where emission is unimpaired but the true ejaculatory phase is lacking.

Gould *et al.* (1984) proposed calcium antagonist activity as a possible explanation for the relatively high frequency of ejaculatory difficulties with thioridazine. These authors argued that this side-effect of the drug was not adequately explained in terms of α-adrenergic or muscarinic receptor blockade as other antipsychotics had similar potency at these receptors. Compared with other antipsychotic drugs, thioridazine is one of the most potent calcium antagonists, exerting effects at plasma levels obtained with therapeutic doses. Further, these investigators found that thioridazine blocked calcium-dependent contractions of the vas deferens in the rat, while a potent α-adrenergic blocker (phentolamine) had no effect. However, as Opler and Feinberg (1991) pointed out, pimozide possesses calcium antagonist activity (being structurally similar to the calcium-channel blocker, verapamil) yet only a relatively low incidence of sexual dysfunction has been reported for this drug.

Priapism

Priapism has been described as a 'prolonged and painful erection of the penis which may occur without sexual stimulation, [which] is usually painful and becomes self-perpetuating' (Becker and Mitchell 1965). The condition '. . . should be regarded as a medical emergency requiring prompt urological consultation if permanent physiological impotence is to be avoided' (Mitchell and Popkin 1982). In their survey of the literature, Mitchell and Popkin (1982) found 19 case reports of priapism with antipsychotic drugs, with chlorpromazine and thioridazine being the most common ones implicated. Priapism has been reported with a host of other antipsychotic drugs (Griffith and Zil 1984; Kogeorgos and de Alwis 1986) including fluphenazine hydrochloride, pericyazine, mesoridazine, molindone, chlorprothixene, and perphenazine. Priapism seems to be more frequently reported in association with phenothiazines than butyrophenone drugs such as haloperidol (Banos *et al.* 1989).

Theoretical mechanisms   Two reports (Osborne 1974; Fishbain 1985) suggest that intravenous anticholinergic medication can reverse priapism associated with antipsychotic medication. Fishbain (1985) hypothesized that the α-adrenergic blockade with antipsychotic drugs inhibits the sympathetically innervated detumescence, so cholinergic dominance persists leading to prolongation of the erection. Anticholinergic agents presumably reverse this cholinergic dominance, facilitating sympathetically innervated detumescence and reversing the priapism.

The argument that drug-induced priapism is related to α-adrenergic antagonism, and thus blockade of the thoracolumbar sympathetic tone, is supported by case reports of priapism with the antidepressant, trazodone, which is a potent α-adrenergic antagonist but has minimal anticholinergic activity. Further, priapism has been produced after intracorporeal injection of drugs with α-blocking properties such as phenoxybenzamine, trazodone, and chlorpromazine (Brindley 1983, 1984; Abber *et al.* 1987). These erections could be reversed with the α-adrenoceptor agonist, metaraminol.

However, overall there is a low reported incidence of priapism in psychiatric patients treated with antipsychotics. This may be because several factors are required for the condition to manifest: for example, increased sensitivity to α-adrenergic receptor blockade (at polster level) and possibly a history of alcohol or marijuana abuse (Winter 1981; Banos *et al.* 1989). Further, the condition may not be reported by patients if it remits spontaneously in a short time. Griffith and Zil (1984) suggest that when patients present with priapism, half will give a history of delayed penile detumescence.

Neuroendocrine mechanisms

As antipsychotics consistently elevate plasma prolactin levels and may also reduce testosterone levels, it has been suggested that these neuroendocrine drug effects may result in loss of libido and changes in sexual functioning (Ghadirian *et al.* 1982). Hyperprolactinaemia due to other causes, such as prolactin-secreting tumours, may cause hypogonadism, with symptoms such as impotence, gynaecomastia, and galactorrhoea presenting relatively late (Carter *et al.* 1978).

Out of 850 'clinically idiopathic' cases of erectile impotence referred for treatment, Buvat *et al.* (1985) found marked hyperprolactinaemia in ten (six of whom were found to have pituitary adenomas). None of the patients referred with other sexual dysfunctions showed elevation of plasma prolactin to this degree, although two per cent of the impotent patients and ten per cent of the patients with premature ejaculation showed mild hyperprolactinaemia. Other neuroendocrine studies of samples of men presenting with erectile problems have reported similar results, with hyperprolactinaemia only found in a relatively small proportion (Schwartz *et al.* 1982; El-Beheiry *et al.* 1988). However, the results of one such study led the authors, Cunningham *et al.* (1982), to conclude that testosterone deficiency and/or hyperprolactinaemia occurred often enough in association with abnormal nocturnal penile tumescence to warrant their routine measurement. All antipsychotic drugs (with the exception of clozapine) cause a relatively prolonged elevation of plasma prolactin levels, although how long these levels remain raised with continued administration of antipsychotics remains uncertain.

Further, hyperprolactinaemia in males is often associated with low plasma testosterone, and it has been suggested that the low testosterone levels may be responsible for the sexual dysfunctions seen. However, Buvat *et al.* (1985) concluded that impotence in hyperprolactinaemic males cannot be only a consequence of low plasma testosterone, as seven of their 16 impotent men had normal testosterone values. Further, when plasma prolactin was lowered by a dopamine agonist, bromocriptine, potency returned before plasma testosterone was markedly increased.

Arato *et al.* (1979) examined the relationship between prolactin, testosterone, LH, and FSH in schizophrenic patients on long-term therapy with antipsychotic drugs. One sample comprised 17 married, schizophrenic males receiving regular depot injections of fluphenazine decanoate, all of whom had sexual problems, either a substantially reduced level of sexual activity or erectile or ejaculatory dysfunction. There was a second sample of 10 schizophrenic patients with no evidence of sexual problems and a control group of 15 healthy men, not receiving drug treatment, also with no sexual problems. Both drug-treated groups had higher mean prolactin levels than the control group, but there was no statistically significant difference between the two patient groups. Testosterone and FSH levels showed no significant differences between the groups, but in the patients with normal sexual activity, the increase in LH was greater. The authors speculated that normal sexual behaviour, despite antipsychotic treatment and hyperprolactinaemia, is related to high plasma LH concentration. Contradictory data have been provided by Meco *et al.* (1985) in a similar study. These researchers found that male patients with sexual disturbance, principally erectile dysfunction and loss of sexual interest, had significantly higher plasma prolactin levels than their non-dysfunctional fellows.

In another relevant clinical study, Martin-du-Pan *et al.* (1979) investigated the neuroendocrine effects of the chronic administration of antipsychotic drugs in a sample of 20 psychiatric patients. They found testosterone levels were in the normal range, and prolactin levels were elevated only in those patients receiving anticholinergic drugs. These studies suggest that the relationship between drug dose, prolactin, and testosterone plasma levels and sexual side-effects in schizophrenic patients remains unclear.

Female sexual dysfunction

For females, there is very limited documented evidence of sexual dysfunction associated with antipsychotic drugs (Barnes 1984). Orgasmic disturbances have been reported with thioridazine (Shen and Park 1982), trifluoperazine (Degen 1982) and fluphenazine (Ghadirian *et al.* 1982). However, no double-blind studies have addressed the nature or extent of antipsychotic effects on female orgasm.

One of the few studies to systematically examine antipsychotic-induced female sexual dysfunctions was conducted by Ghadirian *et al.* (1982). These researchers studied a sample of 29 female schizophrenic out-patients (age range 21–65 years, median 38 years). All were receiving maintenance treatment with either oral or depot fluphenazine. Since starting antipsychotic drug treatment, a third (33 per cent) had noticed a change in the quality of orgasm, and 22 per cent complained of a decreased ability to achieve orgasm. Unlike the results in the male sample, reported above, there was no significant partial correlation coefficient (eliminating the effect of age) between log plasma prolactin and sexual dysfunction score.

Ghadirian *et al.* (1982) also reported that over 90 per cent of the women in the sample reported disturbance of menstruation since being administered antipsychotic drugs. Increased irregularity and change in quality of menstruation were both reported by 78 per cent of the sample. However, recent work by Prentice and Deakin (1992) challenges whether menstrual irregularities are necessarily a consequence of drug treatment. These investigators studied forty female schizophrenic patients who were premenopausal (age range 17–44 years, mean 34 years) and receiving regular depot medication. Eighteen patients (45 per cent) had menstrual irregularities: 12

with oligomenorrhoea and six with complete amenorrhoea. These patients had significantly higher scores on positive and negative symptoms than the 22 patients with regular menstrual cycles, and also significantly poorer scores for cognitive function. However, the two groups did not differ significantly on total dose of antipsychotic drug or serum prolactin concentrations. Prentice and Deakin concluded that menstrual irregularities in schizophrenic women may be largely a result of organic brain changes associated with the psychotic illness, rather than due to drug treatment alone.

Theoretical mechanisms Nestoros *et al.* (1980) suggested that antipsychotic drugs may mediate their detrimental effects on sexual function by antagonizing muscarinic cholinergic function and facilitating serotonergic function. In women, decreased sexual interest and orgasmic difficulties have been attributed to the anticholinergic effects of antipsychotic drugs. Degen (1982) reported on two women with delayed orgasm while receiving treatment with phenothiazine drugs, thioridazine, chlorpromazine and trifluoperazine. When the women were switched to loxapine and fluphenazine, drugs with less anticholinergic and anti-adrenergic activity, their sexual functioning returned to normal.

ANTIDEPRESSANT DRUGS

Antidepressant drugs are effective in the treatment of acute depressive illness of at least moderate severity, and are also useful in preventing recurrence of unipolar depression. This group of drugs consists of two main classes: heterocyclic antidepressants and monoamine oxidase inhibitors. Most of the heterocyclic antidepressants, which include the so-called tricyclic antidepressants and certain newer non-tricyclic compounds, are believed to act primarily by blocking the reuptake of monoamines from the synaptic cleft. They have a range of adverse effects, varying according to the compound, including sedation, postural hypotension, anticholinergic side-effects, and electrocardiographic changes. The newer serotonin reuptake inhibitors also act by monoamine reuptake inhibition, but this is selective for serotonin. Their chemical structures and hence side-effect profiles are different from those of the heterocyclic agents. Monoamine oxidase inhibitors (MAOIs) are most commonly used as second-line drugs for the treatment of depressive disorders. These drugs act by inhibiting the deamination of monoamines, specifically noradrenaline and serotonin.

Erectile problems
The majority of reports linking antidepressant drugs with erectile problems deal with small numbers of patients. There have been case reports of

impotence associated with heterocyclic antidepressants, including amitryptyline, imipramine, desipramine, nortriptyline, protriptyline, amoxapine, clomipramine, and maprotiline (Barnes 1984; Segraves 1988*a*, 1989). Case reports of erectile impotence also exist for MAOIs, including mebanazine, phenelzine, isocarboxazid, and tranylcypromine. In their review of antidepressant drug therapy and male sexual dysfunction, Mitchell and Popkin (1983) suggested that no single agent seems to be implicated more frequently than the other drugs. As Segraves (1989) highlighted, in those reports where the time of onset is clear, these side-effects usually appeared within one to two weeks of drug administration and often abated with drug discontinuation or dosage reduction. Nevertheless, the evidence for a direct causal relationship between erectile impotence and drug treatment is only suggestive.

Beaumont (1977) investigated the sexual side-effects of clomipramine administered to depressed patients in an uncontrolled study. The significance of the findings is somewhat limited by the retrospective nature of the data regarding sexual functioning prior to the depressive illness and the use of dosages at the lower end of the dose range, that is, 30 mg and 75 mg a day. He discussed the problems involved in differentiating between illness-related and drug-induced sexual dysfunctions. He found that 68 per cent of the males and 57 per cent of the females involved in the study showed some sexual symptoms before treatment which were attributable to their mood disorder. For example, impotence was present in 15 per cent of the males. Clomipramine affected the ability to obtain and maintain an erection in 20 per cent of the male patients (40 per cent if those patients reporting a doubtful effect are included). This was despite an overall improvement in sexual functioning following drug treatment, primarily due to recovery from the depressive illness.

Steiger (1988) reported a single-blind study of the effects of clomipramine on nocturnal penile tumescence in a normal young man receiving placebo medication initially, then increasing dosages of clomipramine and finally placebo again. Decreased amplitude and duration of nocturnal erections was confirmed at dosages of 20 mg to 75 mg a day of the drug and full erections were noted only after an increased latency. There were significant inverse correlations between plasma concentrations of clomipramine and the degree of nocturnal penile tumescence.

There are a limited number of controlled studies of the effects of antidepressant pharmacotherapy on erectile dysfunction. The findings are contradictory. For example, Kowalski *et al.* (1985) conducted a double-blind study of mianserin and amitriptyline in a non-psychiatric population. Both compounds at therapeutic doses significantly reduced the amplitude and duration of nocturnal erections. In contrast, two controlled studies of tricyclic antidepressants in patient populations reported no significant effect on erectile function. Harrison and colleagues (1986) investigated the effects of imipramine and phenelzine on sexual function in a double-blind study. They reported that neither treatment is associated with an increased frequency of erectile problems as assessed by self-report questionnaires. Further, in a double-blind, controlled study of the use of clomipramine in obsessive-compulsive disorder, Monteiro and co-workers (1987) found no change in erectile function while patients were taking the drug.

Theoretical mechanisms Erectile difficulties with tricyclics and related antidepressants may be related to their anticholinergic activity which could interfere with the parasympathetic control of erection. Alternatively, a central enhancement of noradrenergic activity might result in sexual impairment. The latter hypothesis is favoured by Kowalski *et al.* (1985) who concluded that the impairment of nocturnal erections by both amitriptyline and mianserin might result from an increased turnover of noradrenaline since mianserin has minimal anticholinergic effects and little effect on central serotonin reuptake. Since MAOIs also possess minimal affinity for muscarinic receptors, it seems likely that they exert their effects on sexual function via noradrenergic transmission.

Ejaculatory problems

It is increasingly evident that antidepressants influence ejaculatory function, especially orgasm attainment, although the incidence of such effects is still unknown. There are case reports of ejaculatory problems with antidepressants involving small numbers of patients. Heterocyclic antidepressants including amitriptyline, imipramine, desipramine, protriptyline, trimipramine, amoxapine, doxepin, and clomipramine are capable of producing retarded ejaculation and perhaps another problem described as 'inhibition' or 'absence' of ejaculation (Barnes 1984; Segraves 1989). In these latter cases, inadequate description often makes it difficult to decide whether ejaculation was so delayed that it never occurred or whether retrograde ejaculation should be suspected. Complete abolition of ejaculation may be a dose-related effect (Beaumont 1973). Rosenbaum and Pollack (1988) have reported ejaculation without orgasm in two patients starting treatment with desipramine. As with erectile difficulties, most reports indicate rapid reversal of ejaculatory dysfunction when the drugs are withdrawn.

In the study by Beaumont (1977) described previously, ejaculatory problems potentially attributable to clomipramine were reported in 20–40 per cent of the depressed male patients and achievement of orgasm was adversely affected in 26–42 per cent of these men. The case report by Steiger (1988) reported ejaculatory inhibition with 100 mg clomipramine.

In the controlled, double-blind study of clomipramine by Monteiro *et al.* (1987) already mentioned, 96 per cent of the sample that had been previously orgasmic became anorgasmic on a dosage of 200 mg taken orally while none of the four men on placebo became anorgasmic. Most patients noticed marked difficulty in achieving orgasm within the first few days, on doses of 25–50 mg a day. Depression scores in both the clomipramine and placebo groups were comparably low before and during treatment, so the anorgasmia after starting clomipramine is unlikely to be attributable to depressed mood. Harrison and colleagues (1986) showed that phenelzine (60–90 mg orally for six weeks) and imipramine (200–300 mg orally for six weeks) were associated with a number of adverse changes in sexual function in both sexes, although men reported more kinds of problems and a higher incidence. Significant anorgasmia during masturbation and significant difficulties with ejaculation occurred with both active treatments compared with placebo. However, for both these problems, impairment was more severe for patients treated with phenelzine than imipramine, and the same was true for level of sexual interest, enjoyment of sex, and the ability to achieve orgasm during intercourse.

Nurnberg and Levine (1987) commented that the current literature on MAOI-associated sexual dysfunction is sparse in view of its apparent frequency. Most authors agree that orgasmic and ejaculatory capacity is more often affected by MAOIs than erectile capacity (Remick and Froese 1990). In the study by Harrison *et al.* (1986), 40 per cent of the patients receiving phenelzine developed sexual problems, although figures were not presented for men and women independently. Rabkin *et al.* (1985) reported anorgasmia or impotence as the most prevalent side-effect in 22 per cent of moderately depressed patients treated with phenelzine. Spontaneous remission of phenelzine-induced anorgasmia has been reported in three patients, one of whom was male (Nurnberg and Levine 1987).

Case reports of impaired ejaculation with mebanazine, iproniazid, and isocarboxazid (Segraves 1988*a*, 1989) also exist. It has been suggested that the non-hydrazine MAOI, tranylcypromine, produces less sexual dysfunction than phenelzine (Remick and Froese 1990). L-Deprenyl, an MAOI that more selectively inhibits the B form of monoamine oxidase and therefore would be expected to cause less increase in serotonin, has not been reported to adversely affect sexual function (Quitkin *et al.* 1984). This could have implications for any theoretical explanations of the mechanisms by which MAOIs produce their effects on sexual function.

Theoretical mechanisms   For tricyclic antidepressants, the anticholinergic action may be responsible for retarded ejaculation by interfering with the cholinergic control of anterograde ejaculation. However, effects on the adrenergic system, either central potentiation or peripheral blockade, may be relevant. Since α_1-adrenergic receptors mediate ejaculation, the α-adrenergic antagonistic actions of certain antidepressants may be important. Segraves (1989) has suggested that, since muscarinic receptors are present in peripheral adrenergic nerve terminals, it is possible that the action of the parasympathomimetic, bethanecol, in reversing antidepressant-induced anorgasmia is secondary to muscarinic-agonist potentiation of adrenergic function.

It has also been suggested that serotonin may have a modulating effect on sexual behaviour, such that those antidepressants which increase serotonin levels in the brain thereby produce orgasmic inhibition. Some of the evidence for this mechanism includes case reports of the relief of anorgasmia by the substitution of an antidepressant with weaker effects on serotonin reuptake. Also the greater efficacy of cyproheptadine compared to diphenhydramine in alleviating anorgasmia associated with imipramine therapy is consistent with the hypothesis that the serotonergic action of imipramine is related to its inhibition of orgasm. Murphy (1987) has cited evidence that down-regulation of postsynaptic serotonin receptors is the best hypothesis for clomipramine-induced anorgasmia. The higher incidence of delayed ejaculation and anorgasmia with antidepressants selective for serotonergic neurotransmission lends further weight to the postulated role of serotonin.

It is not clear how MAOIs cause ejaculatory disturbances. They possess no anticholinergic properties but may have a sympatholytic action. A fall in peripheral sympathetic tone with chronic administration of these drugs has been attributed to the production of octopamine, a false adrenergic transmitter. Other recent theories postulate that the accumulation of monoamine neurotransmitters due to monoamine oxidase inhibition leads to either pre- or postsynaptic receptor changes.

Serotonin reuptake inhibitors

There is already evidence that this subgroup of antidepressants is associated with a higher incidence of adverse sexual effects, particularly delayed ejaculation and orgasmic difficulties, than standard heterocyclic antidepressants. For example, Herman *et al.* (1990) report that delayed orgasm or anorgasmia developed in five (8.3 per cent) of their initial 60 outpatients treated with fluoxetine and in only one case remitted with continued treatment. The patients were equally divided by sex, and most had a history of antidepressant-induced sexual dysfunction during treatment with other antidepressants. They were prescribed various doses of fluoxetine from 20 to 80 mg per day.

A similar proportion of patients with delayed orgasm or anorgasmia (7.8 per cent) was reported by Zajecka *et al.* (1991) in a series of 77 depressed out-patients. One man and five women were affected. However, the true incidence may be higher. Since the investigators had not systematically questioned the patients about adverse effects, this incidence figure represented only spontaneous complaints of orgasm dysfunction. Indeed, in a study of fluoxetine treatment of low-weight chronic bulimia nervosa in which side-effects were assessed using the 'Symptom and side-effect checklist', four out of ten women suffered from anorgasmia (Solyom *et al.* 1990).

Data on the newer serotonin reuptake inhibitors largely emanate from the multicentre comparison studies and concern male sexual dysfunction. Reimherr *et al*. (1990) found that male sexual dysfunction occurred with a statistically significantly higher frequency (21 per cent) in depressed outpatients treated with sertraline than in patients treated with either placebo or amitriptyline. The higher incidence of male sexual dysfunction in the sertraline group was largely a reflection of a greater frequency of delayed ejaculation, with occasional anorgasmia. The authors claimed that this disappeared with continued sertraline dosing in all but two cases. Cohn *et al*. (1990) reported male sexual dysfunction such as decreased libido, impotence, or ejaculation disturbance in 8.6 per cent of elderly depressed patients receiving sertraline compared with 4.7 per cent of amitriptyline patients.

Dechant and Clissold (1991) reviewed the data on the adverse effects of paroxetine from the manufacturer's report on the worldwide clinical experience with the drug. Among males receiving antidepressant therapy in short-term (less than six weeks) trials, abnormal ejaculation occurred with a frequency in excess of placebo in nine per cent of patients receiving paroxetine and three per cent of patients on active control. Curiously, this adverse effect did not appear in the side-effect profiles for long-term (greater than six weeks) administration. However, decreased libido was reported at an excess frequency of three per cent for paroxetine in both cases.

Priapism

Priapism has not been described with tricyclic antidepressants. In contrast, Banos *et al*. (1989) commented in their review that trazodone has frequently been described as being responsible for prolonged erections and priapism, following the first case report in 1983 (Scher *et al*. 1983). Priapism during trazodone treatment is most likely to appear in the first month of treatment and at a dosage of 150 mg or less. A case report of priapism as a side-effect of an MAOI, phenelzine, has also been published (Yeragani and Gershon 1987).

Theoretical mechanisms   The mechanism of these effects is unknown, but peripheral α-adrenergic blockade has been proposed (Abber *et al*. 1987). It is notable that trazodone, as compared with most antidepressants in current use, has substantial α_1-adrenergic receptor blocking activity and negligible anticholinergic activity.

Female sexual dysfunction

A number of case reports suggest that both heterocyclic antidepressants and MAOIs may cause anorgasmia. Imipramine, nortriptyline, amoxapine, clomipramine, phenelzine, isocarboxazid, and tranylcypromine have all been implicated (Barnes 1984; Segraves 1988*a*, *b*). It seems likely that monoamine oxidase inhibitors cause anorgasmia even more frequently than heterocyclic antidepressants. The case reports of delayed orgasm and anorgasmia in women receiving fluoxetine have already been mentioned (Herman *et al.* 1990; Solyom *et al.* 1990; Zajecka *et al.* 1991).

The controlled study by Harrison and colleagues (1986) already referred to indicated that both imipramine and phenelzine significantly impaired the ability of women to experience orgasm during masturbation. Only phenelzine significantly impaired the ability to experience coital orgasm. The adequacy of vaginal lubrication showed no significant treatment differences. Monteiro *et al.* (1987) in their placebo-controlled study of clomipramine noted that anorgasmia was equally likely to occur in females as in males. Among the female patients, six out of the seven who were previously orgasmic became anorgasmic on clomipramine whilst none of the women receiving placebo experienced this side-effect. The difference between the drug and placebo groups was highly significant.

In his uncontrolled study of the sexual side-effects of clomipramine, Beaumont (1977) described a dose-dependent effect on female orgasm. A low dose (30 mg daily) appeared to improve the ability of just over half of the patients (53 per cent) to achieve orgasm. However, detrimental effects on orgasm occurred in 11 per cent on low dose (26 per cent if doubtful cases were included) and 19 per cent (44 per cent) on the higher dose (75 mg daily). Overall, the drug proved beneficial concerning difficulties with orgasm in 31 per cent of patients and had definitely undesirable effects in 14 per cent, although this figure could be as high as 34 per cent taking doubtful cases into consideration. To date there is minimal evidence that any pharmacological agent facilitates orgasmic attainment beyond the improvement expected due to treatment of the depressive illness. Nevertheless, McLean and associates (1983) reported two cases where 75–100 mg of clomipramine had induced spontaneous orgasms with yawning. This effect occurred at a lower dosage than that causing anorgasmia, as reported in other studies.

There have been case reports of increased libido, to a greater level than premorbidly, in depressed women receiving trazodone (Gartrell 1986), coinciding with a remission of depressive symptoms. One controlled study by Crenshaw *et al.* (1987) suggests a similar effect for buproprion.

Theoretical mechanisms In his review of psychiatric drugs and inhibited female orgasm, Segraves (1988*a, b*) commented that the mechanism by which antidepressants induce anorgasmia is unclear. The same explanatory hypotheses postulated for male ejaculatory dysfunction (anticholinergic and serotonergic activity or α_1-blockade) have been entertained. Several lines of evidence argue against the anticholinergic hypothesis, including the failure to find effects of atropine or bethanecol on orgasm in human females. In addition, MAOIs, which apparently cause anorgasmia even more frequently than heterocyclic antidepressants, possess minimal affinity for muscarinic receptors. As described for male ejaculatory difficulties, the evidence for enhanced serotonergic neurotransmission is more compelling. The possibility that orgasmic inhibition is secondary to α_1 blockade is supported by a report from Riley and Riley (1983) suggesting that labetalol (a drug with both α- and β-adrenergic blocking activity) but not propranolol (a β-blocker) causes dose-related delay in orgasm attainment in females (Segraves 1988b).

CONCLUSIONS

The findings of the published surveys of patient samples receiving anti-depressant and antipsychotic drugs suggest that sexual dysfunctions occur commonly in such groups, and are commonly perceived as problems by the patients. While acknowledging the difficulties of teasing apart illness-related and drug-induced effects, a proportion of the dysfunctions un-doubtedly represent drug side-effects, and this must be taken into account by clinicians when weighing up the risks and benefits of such treatment, particularly with regard to long-term administration. Systematic enquiry is required to uncover these problems, which otherwise tend to remain covert, despite the personal distress and damage to intimate relationships they can cause.

REFERENCES

Abber, J.C., Lue, T.F., Luo, J., Juenemann, K., and Tanagho, E.A. (1987). Priapism induced by chlorpromazine and trazodone: mechanism of action. *Journal of Urology*, **137**, 1039–42.

Arato, M., Erdos, A., and Polgar, M. (1979). Endocrinological changes in patients with sexual dysfunction under long-term neuroleptic treatment. *Pharmako-psychiat*, **12**, 426–31.

Banos, J.E., Bosch, F., and Farre, M. (1989). Drug-induced priapism. Its aetiology, incidence and treatment. *Medical Toxicology*, **4**, 46–58.

Barnes, T.R.E. (1984). Drugs and sexual dysfunction. In *Current themes in psychiatry* (Vol. 3), (ed. R.N. Gaind, F.L. Fawzy, B.L. Hudson, and R.O. Pasnau), pp. 51–92. Spectrum, New York.

Beaumont, G. (1973). Sexual side-effects of clomipramine (Anafranil), *Journal of International Medical Research*, **1**, 469–72.

Beaumont, G. (1977). Sexual side-effects of clomipramine (Anafranil). *Journal of International Medical Research*, **5** (Suppl. 1), 37–44.

Becker, L.E. and Mitchell, A.D. (1965). Priapism. *Surgical Clinics of North America*, **45**, 1523–34.

Blair, J.H. and Simpson, G.M. (1966). Effect of antipsychotic drugs on reproductive functions. *Diseases of the Nervous System*, **27**, 645–7.

Brambilla, F., Guerrini, A., Guastalla, A., Rovere, C., and Riggi, F. (1974). Neuro-endocrine effects of haloperidol therapy in chronic schizophrenia. *Psychopharmacology*, **44**, 17–22.

Brindley, G.S. (1983). Cavernosal alpha-blockade: a new technique for investigating and treating erectile impotence. *British Journal of Psychiatry*, **143**, 332–7.

Brindley, G.S. (1984). New treatment for priapism. *Lancet*, **i**, 220–1.

Buddeberg, C., Furrer, H., and Limacher, B. (1988). Sexualle Schwierigkeiten ambulant behandelter Schizophrener. *Psychiat Prax*, **15**, 187–91.

Buvat, J., Lemaire, A., Buvat-Herbaut, J.C., Fourlinnie, J.C., Racadot, A., and Fossati, P. (1985). Hyperprolactinaemia and sexual function in men. *Hormone Research*, **22**, 196–203.

Carter, J.N., Tyson, J.E., Tolis, G., Van Vliet, S., Faiman, C., and Friesen, H.G. (1978). Prolactin-secreting tumors and hypogonadism in 22 men. *New England Journal of Medicine*, **299**, 845–52.

Cohn, C.K., Shrivastava, R., Mendels, J., Cohn, J.B., Fabre, L.F., Claghorn, J.L, Dessain, E.C., Itil, T.M., and Lautin, A. (1990). *Journal of Clinical Psychiatry*, **51** (Suppl. B), 28–33.

Crenshaw, T.L., Goldberg, J.P., and Stern, W.C. (1987). Pharmacological modification of psychosexual dysfunction. *Journal of Sex and Marital Therapy*, **13**, 239–52.

Cunningham, G.R., Karacan, I., Ware, J.C., Lantz, G.D., and Thornby, J.I. (1982). The relationship between serum testosterone and prolactin levels and nocturnal penile tumescence (NPT) in impotent men. *Journal of Andrology*, **3**, 241–7.

Dechant, K.L. and Clissold, S.P. (1991). Paroxetine. A review of its pharmaco-dynamic and pharmacokinetic properties, and therapeutic potential in depressive illness. *Drugs*, **41**, 225–53.

Degen, K. (1982). Sexual dysfunction in women using major tranquilizers. *Psychosomatics*, **23**, 959–61.

El-Beheiry, A., Souka, A., El-Kamshoushi, A., Hussein, S., and El-Sabah, K. (1988). Hyperprolactinaemia and impotence. *Archives of Andrology*, **21**, 211–14.

Erlenmeyer-Kimling, L., Nicol, S., Rainer, J.D., and Deming, W.E. (1969). Changes in fertility rates of schizophrenic patients in New York State. *American Journal of Psychiatry*, **125**, 916–27.

Essen-Moller, E. (1935). Untersuchungen uber die Fruchtbarkeit gewisser Gruupen von Geisteskranken. *Acta Psychiatrica Neurologica Scandinavica* (Suppl. 8).

Everett, G.M. (1975). Role of biogenic amines in the modulation of aggressive and sexual behavior in animals and man. In *Sexual behavior: pharmacology and biochemistry* (ed. M. Sandler and G.L. Gessa). Raven, New York.

Fishbain, D.A. (1985). Priapism resulting from fluphenazine hydrochloride treatment reversed by diphenhydramine. *Annals of Emergency Medicine*, **14**, 600–2.

Friedman, S. and Harrison, G. (1984). Sexual histories, attitudes, and behavior of schizophrenic and 'normal' women. *Archives of Sexual Behavior*, **13**, 555–67.

Gartrell, N. (1986). Increased libido in women receiving trazodone. *American Journal of Psychiatry*, **143**, 781–2.

Gessa, G.L. and Tagliamonte, A. (1974). Possible role of brain serotonin and dopamine in controlling male sexual behavior. *Advances in Biochemical Psychopharmacology*, **11**, 217–28.

Ghadirian, A.M., Chouinard, G., and Annable, L. (1982). Sexual dysfunction and plasma prolactin levels in neuroleptic-treated schizophrenic outpatients. *Journal of Nervous and Mental Disease*, **170**, 463–7.

Gould, R.J., Murphy, K.M.M., Reynolds, I.J., and Snyder, S.H. (1984). Calcium channel blockers: a possible explanation for thioridazine's peripheral side-effects. *American Journal of Psychiatry*, **141**, 352–7.

Griffith, S.R. and Zil, J.S. (1984). Priapism in a patient receiving antipsychotic therapy. *Psychosomatics*, **25**, 629–31.

Harrison, W.M., Rabkin, J.G., Ehrhardt, A.A., Stewart, J.W., McGrath, P.J., Ross, D., *et al.* (1986). Effects of antidepressant medication on sexual function: a controlled study. *Journal of Clinical Psychopharmacology*, **6**, 144–9.

Herman, J.B., Brotman, A.W., Pollack, M.H., Falk, W.E., Biederman, J., and Rosenbaum, J.F. (1990). Fluoxetine-induced sexual dysfunction. *Journal of Clinical Psychiatry*, **51**, 25–7.

Hughes, J.M. (1964). Failure to ejaculate with chlordiazepoxide. *American Journal of Psychiatry*, **121**, 610–11.

Hugues, F.C. (1989). Effets indesirables psychosexuels des medicaments. *Annales de Psychiatrie*, **4**, 335–8.

Kedia, K. and Markland, C. (1975). The effect of pharmacological agents on ejaculation. *Journal of Urology*, **114**, 569–72.

Kogeorgos, J. and de Alwis, C. (1986). Priapism and psychotropic medication. *British Journal of Psychiatry*, **149**, 241–3.

Kotin, J., Wilbert, D.E., Verburg, D., and Soldinger, S.M. (1976). Thioridazine and sexual dysfunction. *American Journal of Psychiatry*, **133**, 82–5.

Kowalski, A., Stanley, R.O., Dennerstein, L., Burrows, G., and Maguire, K.P. (1985). The sexual side-effects of antidepressant medication: a double-blind comparison of two antidepressants in a non-psychiatric population. *British Journal of Psychiatry*, **147**, 413–18.

Leconte, M., Halpern, B., and Arnulf, G. (1960). What can be learned from the total suppression of neuroleptics in a closed ward of restless patients. *Semaine des Hôpitaux Therapeutique*, **36**, 154–7.

McLean, J.D., Forsythe, R.G., Kapkin, I.A. (1983). Unusual side-effects of clomipramine associated with yawning. *Canadian Journal of Psychiatry*, **28**, 569–70.

McWaine, D.E. and Procci, W.R. (1988). Sexuality in the elderly. *Seminars on Urology*, **5**, 141–5.

Martin-du-Pan, R., Baumann, P., Magrini, G., and Felber, J.P. (1979). Neuroendocrine effects of chronic neuroleptic therapy in male psychiatric patients. *Psychoneuroendocrinology*, **3**, 245–52.

Meco, G., Falaschi, P., Casacchia, A., Rocco, A., Petrini, P., Rosa, M., and Agnoli, A. (1985). Neuroendocrine effects of haloperidol decanoate in patients with chronic schizophrenia. In *Chronic treatments in neuropsychiatry* (ed. D. Kemali and G. Racagni), pp. 89–93. Raven, New York.

Mitchell, J.E. and Popkin, M.K. (1982). Antipsychotic drug therapy and sexual dysfunction in men. *American Journal of Psychiatry*, **139**, 633–7.

Mitchell, J.E. and Popkin, M.K. (1983). Antidepressant drug therapy and sexual dysfunction in men: a review. *Journal of Clinical Psychopharmacology*, **3**, 76–9.

Monteiro, W.O., Noshirvani, H.F., Marks, I.M., and Lelliott, P.T. (1987). Anorgasmia from clomipramine in obsessive–compulsive disorder. A controlled trial. *British Journal of Psychiatry*, **151**, 107–12.

Morley, J.E. (1986). Impotence. *American Journal of Medicine*, **80**, 897–905.

Murphy, M. (1987). Down-regulation of post-synaptic serotonin receptors as a mechanism for clomipramine-induced anorgasmia. *British Journal of Psychiatry*, **151**, 704.

Nestoros, J.N., Lehmann, H.E., and Ban, T.A. (1980). Neuroleptic drugs and sexual function in schizophrenia. *Modern Problems in Pharmacopsychiatry*, **15**, 111–30.

Nininger, J.E. (1979). Inhibition of ejaculation by amitriptyline. *American Journal of Psychiatry*, **135**, 750–1.

Nurnberg, H.G. and Levine, P.E. (1987). Spontaneous remission of MAOI-induced anorgasmia. *American Journal of Psychiatry*, **144**, 805–7.

Opler, L.A. and Feinberg, S.S. (1991). The role of pimozide in clinical psychiatry: a review. *Journal of Clinical Psychiatry*, **52**, 221–33.

Osborne, M.P. (1974). Penile parkinsonism. *Postgraduate Medical Journal*, **50**, 523–4.

Pomme, B., Girard, J., and Debost, M. (1965). Troubles de la sexualite et medications psychotropes. *Annales de Medico-psychologique*, **123**, 551–62.

Prentice, D.S. and Deakin, J.F.W. (1992). Role of neuroleptic drugs and organic mechanisms in the aetiology of menstrual irregularities in schizophrenic women. *Schizophrenia Research*, **6**, 114.

Quitkin, F.M., Liebowitz, M.R., Stewart, J.W., McGrath, P.J., Harrison, W., Rabkin, J.G. *et al.* (1984). L-deprenyl in atypical depressives. *Archives of General Psychiatry*, **41**, 777–81.

Rabkin, J., Quitkin, F., McGrath, P., Harrison, W., and Tricamo, E. (1985). Adverse effects to monoamine oxidase inhibitors: part II: treatment correlates and clinical management. *Journal of Clinical Psychopharmacology*, **5**, 2–9.

Reimherr, F.W., Chouinard, G., Cohn, C.K., Cole, J.O., Itil, T.M., LaPierre, Y.D., Masco, H.L., and Mendels, J. (1990). Antidepressant efficacy of sertraline: a double-blind, placebo- and amitriptyline-controlled, multicenter comparison study in outpatients with major depression. *Journal of Clinical Psychiatry*, **51** (Suppl. B), 18–27.

Remick, R.A. and Froese, C. (1990). Monoamine oxidase inhibitors: clinical review. *Canadian Family Physician*, **36**, 1151–5.

Riley, A.J. and Riley, E.J. (1983). Cholinergic and adrenergic control of human sexual responses. In *Psychopharmacology and sexual disorders* (ed. D. Wheatley). Oxford University Press.

Rosenbaum, J.F. and Pollack, M.H. (1988). Anhedonic ejaculation with desipramine. *International Journal of Psychiatry in Medicine*, **18**, 85–8.

Scher, M., Krieger, J., and Juergens, S. (1983). Trazodone in priapism. *American Journal of Psychiatry*, **140**, 1362–3.

Schwartz, M.F., Bauman, J.E., and Masters, W.H. (1982). Hyperprolactinemia and sexual disorders in men. *Biological Psychiatry*, **17**, 861–76.

Segraves, R.T. (1988a). Sexual side-effects of psychiatric drugs. *International Journal of Psychiatry in Medicine*, **18**, 243–52.

Segraves, R.T. (1988b). Psychiatric drugs and inhibited female orgasm. *Journal of Sex and Marital Therapy*, **14**, 202–7.

Segraves, R.T. (1989). Effects of psychotropic drugs on human erection and ejaculation. *Archives of General Psychiatry*, **46**, 275–94.

Shen, W.W. and Park, S. (1982). Thioridazine-induced inhibition of female orgasm. *Psychiatric Journal of the University of Ottawa*, **7**, 249–51.

Slater, E., Hare, E.H., and Price, J.S. (1971). Marriage and fertility of psychiatric patients compared with national data. *Social Biology*, **18** (Suppl.), 60–73.

Smith, P.J. and Talbert, R.L. (1986). Sexual dysfunction with antihypertensive and antipsychotic agents. *Clinical Pharmacy*, **5**, 373–83.

Solyom, L., Solyom, C., and Ledwidge, B. (1990). The fluoxetine treatment of low-weight, chronic bulimia nervosa. *Journal of Clinical Psychopharmacology*, **10**, 421–5.

Steiger, A. (1988). Effects of clomipramine on sleep EEG and nocturnal penile tumescence: a long-term study in a healthy man. *Journal of Clinical Psychopharmacology*, **8**, 349–54.

Vanelle, J.M. and Poirier, M.F. (1989). La prise en compte des effets des medicaments psychotropes sur le comportement sexual. *Annales Psychiatriques*, **4**, 339–42.

Verhulst, J. and Schneidman, B. (1981). Schizophrenia and sexual functioning. *Hospital and Community Psychiatry*, **32**, 259–62.

Wein, A.J. and Van Arsdalen, K.N. (1988). Drug-induced male sexual dysfunction. *Urologic Clinics of North America*, **15**, 23–31.

Winter, C.C. (1981). Priapism. *Journal of Urology*, **125**, 212.

Yeragani, V.K. and Gershon, S. (1987). Priapism related to phenelzine therapy. *New England Journal of Medicine*, **317**, 117–18.

Zajecka, J., Fawcett, J., Schaff, M., Jeffriess, H., and Guy, C. (1991). The role of serotonin in sexual dysfunction: fluoxetine-associated orgasm dysfunction. *Journal of Clinical Psychiatry*, **52**, 66–8.

10
Recreational drugs and sexuality
Rhodri Huws and Gwyneth Sampson

INTRODUCTION

For centuries people of most cultures have used drugs for recreation. The sought-for effect is either a change in consciousness, altered interactions with other people, or in some cases improved sexual performance. In Old Testament days, Rachael exchanged her marital rights for her sister Leah's mandrakes, which were presumed to be an aphrodisiac (Genesis 30, 14–17).

Interestingly, the debate about a relationship between drug misuse and sexual morality has continued, and is often a media topic. The tone of the debate reflects the differing moral codes applied to recreational drug use, and this varies within cultures and with time. This interrelationship between drug use and sexuality can be viewed from a number of perspectives.

1. Psychoanalytic hypotheses propose that addicts are regressed to the oral level of sexual development. Injecting heroin gives a sudden feeling of excitement followed by a feeling of satisfaction that has been described as the 'pharmacogenic orgasm' (Chessick 1960). Tenhouten (1982) studied 1684 addicts. Those with high 'strength of addiction' found erotic stimulation in an injection-induced 'orgasm', while those with a low 'strength of addiction' found a genital orgasm more pleasurable. She concluded that for some people opiate injection becomes a symbolic sexual substitute for genital sex (for example, the needle representing the erect penis). Whilst this formulation may be helpful when viewing heroin addiction within a psycho-analytic paradigm it is simplistic when reviewing the majority of drug users.

2. Psychological factors are important, often in relation to childhood and adolescent experiences. Shedler and Block (1990) showed that the pattern of drug use at 18 years had a psychological basis which could be related to early upbringing and it is accepted that early disturbances can be involved in the genesis of both relationship and sexual difficulties.

3. Sociological research finds factors common to both sexuality and drug abuse. Numerous studies have looked at drug use and sexual activity among students. Goode (1972) surveyed 564 undergraduates. Those who had used

drugs (usually cannabis) were more likely to be sexually experienced, to have commenced sexual activity earlier in life, and to have had a greater number of partners. An increased cannabis 'dose' was associated with increased sexual activity. If the student was sexually active prior to entering college then he or she was more likely to participate in the use of drugs. This demonstrates a connection between drug use and sex but does not allow any inferences about causality to be made. Pope *et al.* (1981) surveyed 710 college students, looking at social and psychological factors, drug use, and sexual activity: 44 per cent used alcohol once a week and 26 per cent used cannabis once a week. Other drugs were used infrequently with cocaine being used weekly by 1.6 per cent. Drug users and non-users were indistinguishable on a range of variables including standard of work, social activities, career plans, or feelings of subjective alienation. Male users were more likely to have visited a psychiatrist but few felt that their visits were related to their use of drugs. Users were far more likely than non-users to have been sexually active with more than one partner. A study of 335 young adults in Scotland found similar results, the strongest correlation being between alcohol use and age of first intercourse (Robertson and Plant 1988).

Surveys demonstrate that whilst use of drugs including cannabis was limited to a small group of students and young people in the 1960s, during the past twenty years drug use has increased and is now common. It seems that those people with a younger age of first intercourse and who have more sexual partners are also more likely to use alcohol and/or cannabis. This could include at least a quarter of the population under 25.

Historically, literature and the media have painted stereotypes such as the 'male, heavy drinker', 'cannabis-using student', and 'drug addict', and have indicated that these groups have different views and attitudes towards sexuality. However, with such a high percentage of the population using alcohol and/or cannabis it is difficult to produce one stereotype of drug user.

4. The physical and physiological effects of drug use on sexual function are important. The human sexual response involves the cardiovascular, genitourinary, and nervous systems. The musculoskeletal system is involved in sexual performance, and disturbances in the gastrointestinal tract or respiratory system often interfere with sexual activity. Drug use can affect all these body systems either immediately or with longer term damage.

Alcohol is the recreational drug which has been most investigated in terms of its relationship with human sexuality. Research which is directed at preventing HIV transmission has produced further information on human sexual behaviour in general and the sexual behaviour of heroin users. The research on other recreational drugs and sexuality is limited, with much of the information derived from case reports and uncontrolled surveys.

ALCOHOL

Alcohol was one of the first drugs to be used recreationally and the problems associated with its use were known in 1700 BC when the Laws of Hammurabi regulated the sale of wine and prohibited drunkenness on the wine-seller's premises. The relationship between alcohol and sex is perhaps best summarized by Shakespeare in Macbeth (Act II, Scene 3):

Macduff: What three things does drink especially provoke?
Porter: Marry, sir, nose painting, sleep and urine. Lechery, sir, it provokes and unprovokes. It provokes the desire but takes away the performance.

In the survey of Athanasiou *et al.* (1970) 45 per cent of men and 68 per cent of women felt that alcohol enhanced sexual enjoyment; 42 per cent of men and 21 per cent of women felt that enjoyment was decreased. Rubin and Henson (1976) recruited 16 males aged 21 to 29 who were given either alcohol or placebo and their sexual responses to erotic videos were measured. High-dose alcohol inhibited all parameters of sexual functioning but low-dose alcohol had no overall effect (there was a small but significant reduction in mean sexual arousal). A dose-related reduction in arousal was found in a similar study of 48 male undergraduates (Briddell *et al.* 1976) and in chronic alcoholics (Wilson *et al.* 1978). The effect of alcohol on orgasm and ejaculation in males also shows impairment with increasing doses (Malatesta *et al.* 1979). In women, Wilson and Lawson (1976*a*) measured the effects of alcohol and placebo on vaginal responses in 16 college attenders and found a dose-related reduction in sexual response following alcohol ingestion. A later study of 18 female college attenders found longer orgasmic latencies and decreased intensity of orgasm with increasing amounts of alcohol, but the women reported greater arousal and orgasmic pleasurability with increasing levels of alcohol (Malatesta *et al.* 1982). This study was not placebo controlled so the results may have been influenced by expectation.

As Shakespeare indicated, people have expectations of the effect of alcohol upon sexuality. In a controlled study of 40 males, those who thought that they had drunk alcohol experienced an increased sexual response to erotic videos whilst those who thought that they had not imbibed alcohol exhibited no response. This effect was independent of whether alcohol had in fact been drunk (Wilson and Lawson 1976*b*).

It has been shown that alcohol does not affect man's ability to control sexual arousal (Rubin and Henson 1976), supporting Wilson's (1977) suggestion that the so-called pharmacological disinhibiting effect of alcohol may be used to justify otherwise unacceptable behaviour. In both men and women, beliefs about the effect of alcohol and sexuality can lead to increased drinking and can influence sexual activity whilst intoxicated (Leigh 1990).

A failure to obtain an erection for pharmacological reasons can generate performance anxiety during further attempts at intercourse, leading to secondary psychological impotence. Tan *et al.* (1984) investigated 13 alcoholics who complained of impotence and found that in seven the impotence was psychological in origin.

The acute effect of alcohol on arousal is probably mediated via the spinal reflexes and, at a certain level, will cause impotence. The direct pharmacological effect on alcohol and sexual performance seems to occur at blood levels above 40 mg l^{-1} (Bancroft 1989). Acute intoxication with alcohol causes a transient decrease in plasma testosterone (Ylikahri *et al.* 1974; Mendelson *et al.* 1977). This is probably a direct toxic effect (of either alcohol or acetaldehyde, its metabolite) on the testes but it is not known if this has any effect on sexuality. Alcohol does not appear to acutely affect the pituitary–gonadal hormones in women (McNamee *et al.* 1979).

Long-term alcohol abuse affects the body in a variety of ways. The main nervous system abnormality seen is peripheral neuropathy which can affect sexual functioning directly by impairing sensory input. It can also cause damage to the autonomic nerves with resultant damage to the mechanism of erection and ejaculation. Alcohol also affects the endocrine system with a decrease in testosterone level in men which is independent of weight loss or liver damage (Gordon *et al.* 1976). Lowered testosterone, raised sex-hormone-binding globulin, and raised oestrogen is occasionally found with gynaecomastia and loss of sexual interest. This is probably mediated via the hypothalamo–pituitary–gonadal system rather than via alcohol-induced liver damage. Prolonged abuse can also cause ovarian atrophy in women and testicular atrophy in men (Van Thiel and Lester 1979). Of 60 chronic alcoholics with sexual dysfunction, 38 had testicular atrophy and 22 did not. After six months of abstinence from alcohol the sexual dysfunction improved in 15 of the non-atrophied group (68 per cent) compared with seven out of the 38 with atrophy (18 per cent). Hormonal treatment did not help those who remained dysfunctional (Van Thiel *et al.* 1982).

It is often presumed that chronic alcoholics have sexual difficulties. Uncontrolled studies of alcoholics report rates of impotence of 44–59 per cent (Jensen 1979; Mandell and Miller 1983). A controlled study of 50 male alcoholics found that the alcoholic group had a significantly higher rate of impotence than the controls (54 per cent vs 28 per cent) and also reported less sexual satisfaction (Whalley 1978). A survey of 917 women showed that heavy drinkers had a high rate of sexual dysfunction, especially lack of interest and anorgasmia. Moderate drinkers, however, had lower levels of sexual dysfunction than both heavy drinkers and light or abstinent drinkers (Klassen and Wilsnack 1986).

As with all recreational drugs there is a complex interrelationship between chronic alcohol misuse and sexual and relationship dysfunction. Both may have similar aetiological or precipitating factors. In a study comparing

female alcoholics with controls, the alcohol abusers were more likely to
have been sexually abused as children but were also more likely to have
developed sexual dysfunction prior to developing problems with alcohol
(Covington and Kohen 1984). Alcohol may be used as a tranquillizer to
blunt the emotional pain of relationship or sexual problems; becoming
intoxicated may be a way of avoiding intercourse with a partner you dislike.
Relationship difficulties that are secondary to alcoholism may lead to an increase in drinking, leading into a spiral of increasing abuse and dysfunction.

Alcohol produces short-term psychological effects of expectation and
short-term pharmacological effects on sexual performance. Its disinhibiting
and sedative effects also impair relationships and sexual performance. Its
long-term effects may permanently damage relationships and sexuality.

HEROIN

Opiates were used medically by the Sumerians 6000 years ago and later by
the Greeks and Romans. They were used recreationally by the Chinese in
the seventeenth century. Heroin is made from opium and its abuse is an
increasing problem. The drug is either injected or smoked. The sharing of
needles has led to the spread of HIV infection amongst heroin users.

The heroin addict is likely to be taking drugs other than heroin such as
opiates, hypnotics, alcohol, nicotine, and cannabis. Heroin addiction
causes major social and interpersonal problems with many addicts having
disturbed personalities prior to drug use.

Heroin use is associated with a variety of sexual problems with decreased
libido, retarded ejaculation, and impotence being reported (Mintz *et al.*
1974; Parr 1976). Cushman (1972) found significant sexual dysfunction

Table 10.1 Impairment of sexual behaviour in heroin addiction and
methadone maintenance (Cushman 1972)

Group	Number	Loss of libido (arousal by appropriate stimuli)	Impotence (ability to conclude coital act)	Delayed ejaculation (normal 4–25 minutes)
Heroin addicts	13	61%	39%	70%
Methadone users	27	25%	32%	22%
Abstinent	13	0%	0%	0%
Control	14	0%	7%	0%

(loss of libido, impotence, delayed ejaculation) in heroin addicts and methadone users (see Table 10.1).

Cicero *et al.* (1975) found heroin and methadone users had delayed ejaculation and impotence, and in 95 per cent of both groups there was a reduction in libido. Abnormal hormonal status has been reported in opiate users. Menstrual abnormalities are common, with 50 per cent of heroin addicts being amenorrhoeic (Gaulden *et al.* 1964; Bai *et al.* 1974). Testosterone levels have been found to be normal or low in heroin addicts and consistently low on methadone maintenance. There is not a clear correlation between low testosterone and the degree of dysfunction (Cicero *et al.* 1975). Luteinizing hormone (LH) and follicle-stimulating hormone (FSH) have usually been found to be normal (Azizi *et al.* 1973). Acute opiate use causes a large increase in prolactin levels and a few studies have shown a high level of prolactin in chronic use. The mid-cycle peak in gonadotrophins and the luteal peak in progesterone does not occur.

Many addicts develop chronic illnesses which further affect their sexual functioning. Heroin addicts gave two main reasons for their sexual problems, one being lack of time due to drug-seeking behaviour and the second that sex reduced the effect of the drug. Methadone users said that they had an inability to obtain and maintain an erection and that a reduction in sensation made sex less desirable (Cicero *et al.* 1975).

Heroin addicts are seen as a high-risk group in relation to HIV infection and its transmission through sexual contact. This could influence the sexuality of the addict and their partners. In those who have become HIV positive there is a clear relationship between recreational drugs and sexuality. It could be expected that heroin addicts have relationship and sexual problems, the sexual problems having a direct physical as well as psychological aetiology.

Abstinent addicts often describe a stable sexual relationship with a drug-free partner as being a major reason for abstinence. Such people may present with sexual dysfunction which will require physical investigation as well as psychosexual assessment.

CANNABIS

The use of cannabis is now common in all strata of British and American society. It is usually smoked mixed with tobacco but can be eaten. Alcohol is often consumed at the same time.

There are many reports of cannabis enhancing sexual pleasure (Athanasiou *et al.* 1970; Gay and Sheppard 1972; Gay *et al.* 1982). In a study of 100 users by Halikas *et al.* (1982) 72 per cent felt that it had an aphrodisiac effect, but only nine per cent felt that this effect was strong. The issue is complicated by the placebo effect. The effects reported by 11 subjects given cannabis or a placebo were similar and none reported any enhancement of sexual feelings (Jones 1971). Kolodny *et al.* (1979) reported that 83 per cent of male and 81 per cent of female users reported enhanced sexual feelings due to an increased sense of touch as well as relaxation rather than any specific improvement in sexual performance. Interestingly he found that if the partner was not also intoxicated, this effect was not seen. Gay *et al.* (1975) also felt that the enhancement of sexual feelings was due to an enhancement of sensory experience. Dawley *et al.* (1979) found that heavy users with an expectation of sexual enhancement reported that it occurred but infrequent users with no expectations did not. Users have also reported that cannabis can lead to delayed ejaculation and thus increase sexual satisfaction but this has not been investigated.

The Indian Hemp Drugs Commission of 1894 (Taberner 1985) reported that cannabis preparations 'have no aphrodisiac power whatsoever: and as a matter of fact, they are used by ascetics in this country [India] with the ostensible object of destroying sexual appetite'. More recent research has equally failed to demonstrate any clear evidence that cannabis directly affects sexual performance.

Reports of cannabis causing dysfunction are equally difficult to interpret but many reports suggest decreased sexual function with heavy use (Chopra 1969). Although one study (Kolodny *et al.* 1974) reported lower plasma testosterone and sperm count in cannabis users, others (Mendelson *et al.* 1974; Cushman 1975) failed to replicate the findings.

AMPHETAMINES

Amphetamines are used for their euphoric effect and for the fact that they reduce the desire to sleep. They are taken orally or snorted (intranasally) but rarely injected. When taken by injection they produce a 'rush' similar to that obtained with opiates, which again prompts speculation about a 'pharmacogenic orgasm'. Small studies (Bell and Trethowan 1961; Gay and Sheppard 1972; Angrist and Gershon 1976) describe addicts who reported improvements in sexual behaviour and others who developed delayed ejaculation. Gossop *et al.* (1974) found that oral amphetamine users had fewer sexual difficulties than intravenous heroin users.

There is insufficient data, especially in comparison with a control group, to be clear about sexual dysfunction or improvement in relation to amphetamine use.

COCAINE

Cocaine is obtained from the coca leaf cultivated in South America. The leaf has been used locally for centuries as a mild euphoriant and the purified form is used for this effect in America and Europe. Freud promoted its use, taking it himself to ward off depression, with apparent success. It is usually taken intranasally and a more purified form, 'crack', can be smoked. Crack was initially regarded in America as a 'clean' drug. It was pure, did not need injecting, and could be smoked without tobacco. The euphoriant effect occurs quickly, especially when smoked—again with connotations of orgasm. The drug is very expensive and until recently has not been widely available in Britain. It is not physically addictive but a psychological dependence can occur and chronic use leads to personal and psychological problems. Wesson (1982) studied cocaine use in massage parlours. Male clients felt that cocaine improved their desire but it made obtaining an erection and ejaculating more difficult. The female prostitutes found that the main effect was to keep them awake and to help them suppress negative emotions. Cocaine is also used as a local anaesthetic to the head of the penis or the clitoris, which delays ejaculation and orgasm and can therefore prolong intercourse (Gay *et al.* 1982). It has also been used anally and can allow violent sexual behaviour to take place. Reports of cocaine causing sexual dysfunction, mainly impotence, are more common (Siegel 1982; Cocores *et al.* 1986) but again these are all uncontrolled studies. They do, however, confirm the view expressed in 1903 by the American Journal of Pharmacy (Taberner 1985) who reported on a positive note 'One redeeming feature there is, the habit of cocaine seems to lessen both sexual desire and ability, so there is less danger of its transmission by heredity'. Claims that cocaine is the champagne of sexual drugs appear unjustified (Taberner 1985).

AMYL NITRITE

Amyl nitrite is widely used in the male homosexual population and can be bought, from sex shops, in a small glass ampoule which is broken open and the contents inhaled. Israelstam *et al.* (1978) interviewed 70 male homosexuals and found that 63 used the drug. It relaxes the anal sphincter and can therefore facilitate anal intercourse and also delays ejaculation. It also gives a tachycardia and users report a loosening of inhibitions and euphoria. Some users reported that when taking amyl nitrite the choice of partner became less important. The effect lasts for about two minutes. The only side-effect that they reported was headache. Other papers confirmed the relative safety of the drug (Sigell *et al.* 1978; Lowry 1982). When taken to facilitate intercourse it is inhaled just prior to penetration as it can otherwise cause a loss of erection (Welti and Brodski 1980). Studies in the early 1980s suggested an association between amyl nitrite use and Kaposi's sarcoma, which often occurs in people with AIDS (Goedert *et al.* 1982). It now appears that Kaposi's sarcoma is more common when AIDS had been acquired by sexual contact rather than parenterally (Beral *et al.* 1990) which is the likely explanation for the earlier suggestions.

ECSTASY AND LSD

Lysergic acid diethylamide (LSD) is an hallucinogenic drug which gained some notoriety amongst the intelligentsia in the early 1970s but is now used mainly by teenagers. It is relatively easy to manufacture, and a dose lasts for about 12 hours. 'Ecstasy', 3,4-methylenedioxymethamphetamine, is chemically related to both hallucinogens and amphetamines and is reported to induce a unique state of euphoria and self-awareness without hallucinatory symptoms.

Kolodny *et al.* (1979) found that out of 140 regular LSD users less than 15 per cent reported any sexually enhancing effect. LSD dramatically changes the perception of external stimuli so it would be expected that the experience of sex would also be changed. Ecstasy has been widely reported in the press as being a 'love drug' and that users become sexually disinhibited. There appears to be little evidence for this. Ninety out of 100 users describe a sense of 'closeness' with other people but sexual effects were not mentioned (Peroutka 1988). Our knowledge of the sexual effects of these drugs remains minimal.

ANABOLIC STEROIDS

The use of anabolic steroids among athletes and body builders to gain strength and increase muscle mass is increasing, in spite of their illegality and known physical and psychological complications. Doses of 10 to 100 times the recommended medical dose are taken in cycles of 4 to 12 weeks in association with training (Pope and Katz 1988).

Studies have shown an increase in aggression, mood disturbances, and both increased and decreased libido; however, such studies are small, largely uncontrolled and may well not be representative of the steroid-using athlete population (Bahrke *et al.* 1990). There are no studies specifically looking at sexuality and sexual dysfunction among users.

NICOTINE

Nicotine is the active ingredient in tobacco leaves. It was introduced to Europe in the sixteenth century at the same time as coca leaves and quickly became a recreational drug whilst the use of coca leaves did not. In the past, tobacco companies have tried to persuade the public that smoking is sexually attractive and socially acceptable (Taberner 1985) but now with increasing recognition of the physical dangers of smoking, this is becoming less so.

'Smoking' is seen as a 'high-risk' factor in relation to organic erectile failure (Virag *et al.* 1985). Its detrimental effect is presumably via the cardiovascular system, and less frequently the respiratory system.

Impotence can improve after cessation of smoking but with severe cardiovascular damage, the erectile failure is permanent (Forsberg *et al.* 1979).

BENZODIAZEPINES

Benzodiazepines were introduced in the 1970s as non-addictive alternatives to barbiturate hypnotics. Now it is known that they have considerable addictive potential and their medical use is diminishing. They are widely used as drugs of abuse by heroin users who use them as a supplement to heroin. They are often taken in doses far in excess of their recommended medical dose. In large doses their effect will be as a sedative and they are, therefore, likely to diminish sexual feelings; at lower doses they act as anxiolytics and this may lead to improved sexuality. In a study looking at the effect of testosterone and using diazepam as a control, there was no effect on sexuality when comparing pre- and post-treatment with benzodiazepine use, even in patients with high anxiety (Carney *et al.* 1978). A double-blind placebo study of pharmacological doses of diazepam showed a dose-related reduction in female sexual response (Riley and Riley 1986). There have been case reports of impotence (Usdin 1960) and failure to ejaculate (Hughes 1964) but in view of the few reports and the widespread use of these drugs it is likely that this is a rare occurrence. There have been no studies on the effect of high-dose benzodiazepines on sexuality.

SOLVENTS

Volatile solvents are used mainly by young teenage boys for their euphoriant and hallucinogenic effects. Interestingly, when chloroform was first used in the mid-nineteenth century cases were reported of women behaving obscenely whilst under its effect. Ether was also reported to have caused sexual dreams in a prostitute, prompting some surgeons to withdraw its use as an anaesthetic in women. There is no current work on their effect on sexuality when used as drugs of abuse.

CONCLUSION

It is evident that the relationship between recreational drugs and sexuality is a complex one.

Many people use recreational drugs, especially nicotine and alcohol. Alcohol is associated with changes in expectation and short- and long-term physical changes, both of which can produce sexual dysfunction. Long-term nicotine use significantly increases the risk of organic sexual difficulties. Cannabis is commonly used, often in combination with alcohol and nicotine—it appears to be 'safer' than either alcohol or nicotine in its effects upon sexual behaviour. Heroin clearly produces sexual dysfunction.

There is a correlation between increasing levels of substance abuse and the adoption of high-risk behaviour and attitudes (Klee *et al.* 1990; Rolf *et al.* 1991). Addicts often engage in high-risk sexual behaviour, exposing themselves and others to HIV infection—such behaviour impairs relationships, producing further psychosexual problems.

There is insufficient data to be sure of the sexual consequences of amphetamines, cocaine, LSD, amyl nitrite, anabolic steroids, and solvent misuse.

REFERENCES

Angrist, B. and Gershon, S. (1976). Clinical effects of amphetamine and L-dopa on sexuality and aggression. *Comprehensive Psychiatry*, **17**, 715–27.

Athanasiou, R., Shaver, P., and Tavris, C. (1970). Sex. *Psychology Today*, **4**, 39–52.

Azizi, F., Vagenais, A., Longscope, C., Ingbar, S., and Braverman, L. (1973). Decreased serum testosterone in male heroin and methadone addicts. *Steroids*, **22**, 467–72.

Bahrke, M.S., Yesalis, C.E., and Wright, J.E. (1990). Psychological and behavioural effects of endogenous testosterone levels and anabolic-androgenic steroids among males. *Sports Medicine*, **10**, 303–37.

Bai, J., Greenwald, E., Caterini, H., and Kaminetsky, H.A. (1974). Drug related menstrual abnormalities. *Obstetrics and Gynaecology*, **44**, 713–18.

Bancroft, J. (1989). *Human sexuality and its problems*. Churchill Livingstone, Edinburgh.

Bell, D.S. and Trethowan, W.A. (1961). Amphetamine addiction and disturbed sexuality. *Archives of General Psychiatry*, **4**, 74–8.

Beral, V., Peterman, T.A., Berkelman, R.L., and Jaffe, H.W. (1990). Kaposi's sarcoma among persons with AIDS: a sexually transmitted infection? *Lancet*, **335**, 123–8.

Briddell, D.W. and Wilson, C.T. (1976). Effect of alcohol and expectancy set on male sexual arousal. *Journal of Abnormal Psychology*, **85**, 225–34.

Carney, A., Bancroft, J., and Mathews, A. (1978). Combination of hormonal and psychological treatment for female sexual unresponsiveness: a comparative study. *British Journal of Psychiatry*, **132**, 339–46.

Chessick, R.D. (1960). The 'Pharmacogenic orgasm' in the drug addict. *Archives of General Psychiatry*, **3**, 545–6.

Chopra, G.S. (1969). Man and marijuana. *The International Journal of the Addictions*, **4**, 215–47.

Cicero, T.J., Bell, R.D., Wieat, W.G., Allison, J.H., Polakoski, K., and Robins, E. (1975). Function of the male sex organs in heroin and methadone users. *New England Journal of Medicine*, **292**, 882–7.

Cocores, J.A., Dackis, C.A., and Gold, M.S. (1986). Sexual dysfunction secondary to cocaine abuse in two patients. *Journal of Clinical Psychiatry*, **47**, 384–5.

Covington, S.S. and Kohen, J. (1984). Women, alcohol and sexuality. In *Cultural and sociological aspects of alcoholism and substance abuse*, pp. 41–56. Howarth Press.

Cushman, P. (1972). Sexual behaviour in heroin addiction and methadone maintenance. *New York State Journal of Medicine*, **72**, 1261–5.

Cushman, P. (1975). Plasma testosterone levels in healthy male marijuana smokers. *American Journal of Drug and Alcohol Abuse*, **2**, 269–75.

Dawley, H.H., Winstead, D.K., Baxter, A.S., and Gay, J.R. (1979). An attitude survey of the effects of marijuana on sexual enjoyment. *Journal of Clinical Psychology*, **35**, 212–17.

Forsberg, L., Gustavee, B., Hojerback, T., and Olsson, A.M. (1979). Impotence, smoking and beta-blocking drugs. *Fertility and Sterility*, **31**, 589–91.

Gaulden, E.C., Littlefield, D.C., Putoff, O.E., and Selvert, A.L. (1964). Menstrual abnormalities associated with heroin addiction. *American Journal of Obstetrics and Gynaecology*, **90**, 155–60.

Gay, G.R. and Sheppard, C. (1972). Sex in the 'Drug culture'. *Medical Aspects of Human Sexuality*, **6**, 28–50.

Gay, G.R., Newmeyer, J.A., Ellon, R.A., and Wieder, S. (1975). Drug–sex practice in the Haight–Ashbury or 'The sensuous hippie'. In *Sexual behaviour: pharmacology and biochemistry* (ed. M. Sandler and G.L. Gessa), pp. 63–79, Raven, New York.

Gay, G.R., Newmeyer, J.A., Perry, M., Johnson, G., and Kurland, M. (1982). Love and Haight: the sensuous hippie revisited. Drug/sex practices in San Francisco 1980–81. *Journal of Psychoactive Drugs*, **14**, 111–24.

Goedert, J.J., Wallen, W.C., Mann, D.L., Strong, D.M., Neuland, C.Y., Greene, M.H., Murray, C., Fraument, J.F., and Blattner, W.A. (1982). Amyl nitrate may alter T-lymphocytes in homosexual men. *Lancet*, **i**, 412–15.

Goode, E. (1972). Drug use and sexual activity on a college campus. *American Journal of Psychiatry*, **128**, 1272–6.

Gordon, G.G., Altman, K., Southern, L., Rubin, E., and Leber, C.S. (1976). Effect of ethanol administration on sex hormone metabolism in normal men. *New England Journal of Medicine*, **295**, 793–7.

Gossop, M.R., Stern, R., and Connell, P.H. (1974). Drug dependence and sexual dysfunction: a comparison of intravenous users of narcotics and oral users of amphetamines. *British Journal of Psychiatry*, **124**, 431–4.

Halikas, J., Weller, R., and Morse, C. (1982). Effect of regular marijuana use on sexual performance. *Journal of Psychoactive Drugs*, **14**, 59–70.

Hughes, J.M. (1964). Failure to ejaculate with chlordiazepoxide. *American Journal of Psychiatry*, **121**, 610–11.

Israelstram, S., Lambert, S., and Oki, G. (1978). Poppers, a new recreational drug craze. *Canadian Psychiatric Association Journal*, **23**, 493–5.

Jensen, S.B. (1979). Sexual customs and dysfunction in alcoholics: part I. *British Journal of Sexual Medicine*, **6**, 29–32.

Jones, R.T. (1971). Marijuana-induced 'high': influence of expectation, setting and previous drug experience. *Pharmacology Reviews*, **23**, 359–69.

Klassen, A.D. and Wilsnack, S.C. (1986). Sexual experience and drinking among women in a US national survey. *Archives of Sexual Behaviour*, **15**, 363–92.

Klee, H., Faugier, J., Hayes, C., Boulton, T., and Morris, J. (1990). Factors associated with risk behaviour among injecting drug users. *AIDS*, **2**, 133–45.

Kolodny, R.C., Masters, W.H., Kolodner, R.M., and Toro, G. (1974). Depression of plasma testosterone levels after chronic intensive marijuana use. *New England Journal of Medicine*, **290**, 872–4.

Kolodny, R.C., Masters, W.H., and Johnson, V.E. (1979). *Textbook of sexual medicine*. Little Brown, Boston.

Leigh, B.C. (1990). The relationship of sex-related alcohol expectancies to alcohol consumption and sexual behaviour. *British Journal of Addiction*, **85**, 919–28.

Lowry, T.P. (1982). Psychosexual effects of volatile nitrites. *Journal of Psychoactive Drugs*, **14**, 77–80.

McNamee, B., Ratcliffe, J., Ratcliffe, W., and Oliver, J. (1979). Lack of effect of alcohol on pituitary–gonadal hormones in women. *British Journal of Addiction*, **74**, 316–17.

Malatesta, V.J., Pollack, R.H., Wilbanks, W.A., and Adams, H.E. (1979). Alcohol effects on the orgasmic ejaculatory response in human males. *Journal of Sex Research*, **15**, 101–7.

Malatesta, V.J., Pollack, R.H., Crotty, T.D., and Peacock, L.J. (1982). Acute alcohol intoxication and female orgasmic response. *Journal of Sex Research*, **18**, 1–17.

Mandell, W. and Miller, C.M. (1983). Male sexual dysfunction as related to alcohol consumption: a pilot study. *Alcoholism: Clinical and Experimental Research*, **7**, 65–9.

Mendelson, J.H., Kuehnle, J., Ellingbore, J., and Babor, T.F. (1974). Plasma testosterone levels before, during and after chronic marijuana smoking. *New England Journal of Medicine*, **290**, 1051–5.

Mendelson, J.H., Mello, N.K., and Ellingboe, J. (1977). Effect of acute alcohol intake in pituitary–gonadal hormones in normal human males. *Journal of Pharmacology and Experimental Therapeutics*, **202**, 676–82.

Mintz, J., O'Hare, K., O'Brien, C.P., and Goldschmidt, J. (1974). Sexual problems of heroin addicts. *Archives of General Psychiatry*, **31**, 700–3.

Parr, D. (1976). Sexual aspects of drug abuse in narcotic addicts. *British Journal of Addiction*, **71**, 261–8.

Peroutka, S.J., Newman, H., and Harris, H. (1988). Subjective effects of 3,4-methylenedioxymethampetamine in recreational users. *Neuropsychopharmacology*, **1**, 273–7.

Pope, H.G. and Katz, D.L. (1988). Affective and psychotic symptoms associated with anabolic steroid use. *American Journal of Psychiatry*, **145**, 487–90.

Pope, H.G., Ionescu-Pioggia, M., and Cole, J.O. (1981). Drug use and life-style among college undergraduates. *Archives of General Psychiatry*, **38**, 588–91.

Riley, A.J. and Riley, E.J. (1986). The effect of single dose diazepam on female sexual response induced by masturbation. *Sexual and Marital Therapy*, **1**, 49–53.

Robertson, J.A. and Plant, M.A. (1988). Alcohol, sex and risk of HIV infection. *Drug and Alcohol Dependence*, **22**, 75–8.

Rolf, J., Nanda, J., Baldwin, J., Chandra, A., and Thompson, L. (1991). Substance misuse and HIV/AIDS risk among delinquents: a prevention challenge. *The International Journal of the Addictions*, **25**, 533–59.

Rubin, H.B. and Henson, D.E. (1976). Effect of alcohol on male sexual responding. *Psychopharmacology*, **47**, 123–34.

Shedler, J. and Block, J. (1990). Adolescent drug use and psychological health. *American Psychologist*, **45**, 612–30.

Siegel, R.K. (1982). Cocaine and sexual dysfunction: the curse of mama coca. *Journal of Psychoactive Drugs*, **14**, 71–4.

Sigell, L.T., Kapp, F.T., Fusaro, G.A., Nelson, E.D., and Falck, R.S. (1978). Popping and snorting volatile nitrites: a current fad for getting high. *American Journal of Psychiatry*, **135**, 1216–18.

Taberner, P.V. (1985). *Aphrodisiacs. The science and the myth*. Croom Helm, London.

Tan, E.T.H., Johnson, R.H., Lambie, D., Vijayason, M.E., and Whiteside, E.A. (1984). Erectile impotence in chronic alcoholics. *Alcoholism: Clinical and Experimental Research*, **8**, 297–301.

Tenhouten, S. (1982). Sexual dynamics and strength of heroin addiction. *Journal of Psychoactive Drugs*, **14**, 101–9.

Usdin, G.L. (1960). Preliminary report on librium. *Journal of Louisiana State Medical Society*, **112**, 142–7.

Van Thiel, D.H. and Lester, R. (1979). The effect of chronic alcohol abuse on sexual function. *Clinics in Endocrinology and Metabolism*, **8**, 499–510.

Van Thiel, D.H., Gavaler, J.S., and Sanghvi, A. (1982). Recovery of sexual function in abstinent alcoholic men. *Gastroenterology*, **84**, 677–82.

Virag, R., Bouilly, P., and Frydman, D. (1985). Is impotence an arterial disorder? *Lancet*, **i**, 181–4.

Welti, R.S. and Brodski, J.B. (1980). Treatment of intraoperative penile tumescence. *Journal of Urology*, **124**, 925–6.

Wesson, P.R. (1982). Cocaine use by masseuses. *Journal of Psychoactive Drugs*, **14**, 75–6.

Whalley, L.J. (1978). Sexual adjustments of male alcoholics. *Acta Psychiatrica Scandinavia*, **58**, 281–98.

Wilson, G.T. (1977). Alcohol and human sexual behaviour. *Behaviour Research and Therapy*, **15**, 239–52.

Wilson, G.T. and Lawson, D.M. (1976*a*). Effects of alcohol on sexual arousal in women. *Journal of Abnormal Psychology*, **85**, 489–97.

Wilson, G.T. and Lawson, D.M. (1976*b*). Expectancies, alcohol and sexual arousal in male social drinkers. *Journal of Abnormal Psychology*, **85**, 587–94.

Wilson, G.T., Lawson, D.M., and Abrahams, D.B. (1978). Effects of alcohol on sexual arousal in male alcoholics. *Journal of Abnormal Psychology*, **87**, 609–16.

Ylikahri, R., Huttunen, M., Harkonen, M., Seuderling, U., Onikki, S., Karonen, S.L., and Adleurcreutz, H. (1974). Low plasma testosterone values in men during hangover. *Journal of Steroid Biochemistry*, **5**, 655–8.

11

Pharmacotherapy for sexual dysfunction: current status

Alan J. Riley and Elizabeth J. Riley

INTRODUCTION

Throughout the ages, man of all cultures has sought drugs to modify his sexual performance and an enormous number of preparations of vegetable, animal, and mineral origin have been extolled to have aphrodisiac properties. Even today, vast sums of money are spent on alleged aphrodisiacs, the majority of which are at best ineffective and at worse toxic. In the past there has been very little research effort directed at finding drugs to treat sexual dysfunction and, with few exceptions, most of the drugs that are now used for this purpose were originally developed for other indications. Indeed in the United Kingdom today no drug has been licensed by the Department of Health specifically for the treatment of sexual dysfunction although the butyrophenone, benperidol, is registered for the control of deviant and antisocial behaviour and the anti-androgen, cyproterone acetate, is licensed for severe hypersexuality and sexual deviance in the male.

During the coming years pharmacotherapy will play an increasingly important role in the management of sexual dysfunction. Sexual indications for established drugs will be evaluated and novel drugs will be developed specifically to treat sexual dysfunction. In this chapter the current state of pharmacotherapy for sexual dysfunction is reviewed.

ERECTILE DYSFUNCTION

There is considerable interest in pharmacotherapy for erectile dysfunction. In part this is because erectile dysfunction affects a large number of men and other management approaches are either inconvenient or not very effective. Erectile dysfunction is a symptom with a multifactorial aetiology and it is therefore unrealistic that there will ever be a treatment which is effective in all cases. Few pharmacological approaches to this problem have been evaluated by means of adequately controlled trials. Nevertheless, drugs that have been reported to benefit a few patients in uncontrolled case studies are sometimes worth trying and may, in the light of further experience, be found to be more generally useful.

The most extensively studied pharmacotherapeutic approach to the management of erectile dysfunction is intracorporeal administration of vasoactive drugs. Of oral approaches, yohimbine hydrochloride is receiving increasing attention, while early studies of the use of opioid antagonists, pentoxifylline and nitrites, in this indication have produced some interesting results. These preparations deserve further investigation. The dopamine-uptake inhibitor, bupropion, has been evaluated in a series of 30 patients with psychogenic erectile dysfunction but was found to be no better than placebo, although the power of the study was low (Goldberg and Crenshaw 1992).

Intracorporeal treatment

Although Michal et al. (1977) were the first to demonstrate the erection-inducing effect of papaverine when they accidentally injected the drug into the penile circulation during a revascularization operation, it was Virag who first utilized this property of papaverine therapeutically (Virag 1982). He injected the drug directly into the corpus cavernosum (intracorporeal or intracavernosal injection). In the following year Brindley personally demonstrated erection following phenoxybenzamine administered by the same route (Brindley 1983). Following these observations, Brindley investigated the possible erection-inducing properties of a number of drugs administered intracorporeally (Brindley 1986). He found that phentolamine, thymoxamine, imipramine, verapamil, and naftidrofuryl possessed this property. Intracorporeal injection of vasoactive intestinal polypeptide (VIP) (Ottesen et al. 1984) and prostaglandin E_1 (PGE_1) (Virag and Adaikan 1987; Stackl et al. 1988) also induce erection.

That the erection following the administration of vasoactive drugs is pharmacological rather than psychological or mechanical has been confirmed in double-blind placebo-controlled studies. Kiely et al. (1987) reported that a combination of papaverine (30 mg) and phentolamine (1 mg) induced erection in men complaining of erectile failure whereas the injection of a similar quantity of saline had no effect. Szasz et al. (1987) reported a positive erectile response in all of 11 erectile dysfunctional men to either phenoxybenzamine (5 mg) or papaverine (30 mg) plus phentolamine (1 mg) but not to intracorporeal saline injections. Furthermore, dose-related responses have been demonstrated (Schramek and Waldhauser 1989).

Intracorporeal injection of vasoactive drugs has become an established procedure used in the investigation of erectile dysfunction (Lue and Tanagho 1987). Failure to attain a sustained rigid erection following an adequate intracorporeally administered dose of a vasoactive drug raises the probability of a vasculogenic aetiology. However, up to 15 per cent of non-responders may show predominance of psychological factors, the failure to attain erection probably resulting from anxiety-induced excessive nor-adrenergic tone constricting the penile vasculature (Buvat *et al.* 1986). Papaverine or PGE_1 are the drugs most frequently used for this diagnostic test. There are suggestions that PGE_1 may be more effective than papaverine. Kattan *et al.* (1991) reported a double-blind crossover study in 54 men with vasculogenic erectile dysfunction in which they compared the two drugs. Satisfactory erection occurred in 46 per cent of the men with PGE_1 (20 mcg) and in 14 per cent with papaverine (60 mg).

For some patients with predominantly psychogenic erectile dysfunction, the reassurance that erection is still possible, which follows pharmacologically induced erection in the consulting room, is sufficient to resolve their erectile dysfunction, especially if they are able to use the induced erection for intercourse. In a series of 250 consecutive unselected erectile dysfunctional patients, 109 completed a within-office programme of papaverine injections for diagnostic purposes and of these, 34 per cent regained normal erectile function without any further therapy (Puppo *et al.* 1988).

Patients who do not respond favourably in this way and who do not have severe arteriogenic erectile dysfunction can be taught to self-inject the drug (Brindley 1983; Zorgniotti and Lefleur 1985; Williams *et al.* 1987). Not all men readily accept this management approach. Gilbert and Gingell (1991) found that 49.9 per cent of their patients declined to use self-injection despite satisfactory responses obtained in 65.3 per cent of these men. Other workers have reported higher uptake rates for this treatment (Sidi *et al.* 1986). A significant number (5–41 per cent) of men drop out of self-injection programmes for a variety of reasons. One reason for non-compliance is the fear of needles and the inconvenience of administering the drug (Sidi and Chen 1987). To improve compliance, insulin injection pens modified for intracorporeal self-injection have been used with success (Kromann-Andersen and Nielsen 1989) and attempts to develop implantable drug reservoirs are being made (Helmy 1991). In a series of 194 patients, 80 (41.2 per cent) benefited from self-injection and 21 (10.8 per cent) of these enjoyed the return of spontaneous erections after the use of one to eight (mean 6.2) injections (Gilbert and Gingell 1991). Other workers have also reported recovery of spontaneous erections following short courses of self-injection (Virag 1982; Crowe and Qureshi 1991).

A clinically significant risk associated with intracorporeal injection of vasoactive drugs is prolonged erection. Patients are usually advised to seek medical advice if their erection persists for longer than four hours (Crowe and Qureshi 1991) or six hours (Gilbert and Gingell 1991), when active treatment to induced detumescence may be required. The risk of prolonged erection can be minimized by careful selection of the dose of the agents used; this requires dose titration to a level which induces an erection which lasts for 30 to 120 minutes. Particular caution must be exercised in patients whose erectile dysfunction has a neurological aetiology because the erectile mechanism of such patients is frequently extremely sensitive to vasoactive agents, so they require lower doses. Starting doses of papaverine range from 8 to 15 mg, in patients in whom neuropathy is suspected, to 60 mg in cases of suspected arterial inadequacy. There is no uniform incremental dosing schedule, each worker having evolved his own. The maximum dose of papaverine is 120 mg, though usually, if 80 mg fails to induce an erection, 120 mg is also ineffective (Crowe and Qureshi 1991). Phentolamine can be added if a satisfactory response is not provided by papaverine alone (Keogh et al. 1989). Older patients generally require larger doses of papaverine than younger men (Crowe and Qureshi 1991). Even in studies where the dose of papaverine has been carefully selected, prolonged erections can occur and may reflect changes in sensitivity of the patient to the agent or alteration in its metabolic clearance due to factors yet to be defined, although anecdotally, alcohol consumption appears to reduce the erectile response to papaverine (Crowe and Qureshi 1991). In a series of patients who experienced 838 injections over a 12 month period, the incidence of prolonged erection was 2.6 per cent (Gilbert and Gingell 1991). The risk of prolonged erections may be lower with PGE_1 (Stackl et al. 1988). The dose of PGE_1 required to induce erection ranges from 5 mcg to 20 mcg (Waldhauser and Schramek 1988; Schramek and Waldhauser 1989).

Prolonged erection, if not treated within 24 h, may progress to priapism with intracavernosal thrombosis and fibrosis of the corpora cavernosa resulting in irreversible loss of erectile function. This has occurred in patients using self-injection programmes (Sidi et al. 1986; Hashmat and Abraham 1987; Crowe and Qureshi 1991). Repeated intracavernosal injections of phentolamine and papaverine over a nine-month period induce penile fibrosis in monkeys (Larsen et al. 1987) and corporal fibrosis has been reported in men following self-injection programmes (Corriere et al. 1988). Results from animal studies suggest that PGE_1 is less likely than papaverine to cause penile fibrosis (Aboseif et al. 1989). However, a possible disadvantage of PGE_1 compared with papaverine is that in some studies its administration has been associated with pain more frequently (Schramek and Waldhauser 1989) although in other studies the side-effect profile of PGE_1 and papaverine are similar (Kattan et al. 1991).

Other drugs administered intracorporeally are being evaluated in the management of erectile dysfunction. Buvat et al. (1989) showed that thymoxamine (moxisylyte) was less active than papaverine and in their series of 170 patients, only two had prolonged erections. Intracorporeal injection of vasoactive intestinal polypeptide (VIP) can induce erection (Ottesen et al. 1984) although Wagner and Gerstenberg (1988) failed to induce erection with high doses (60 mcg) of VIP but that the treatment facilitated normal erection when used in conjunction with erotic visual or vibratory stimulation. VIP has been used to potentiate the erection-inducing property of papaverine (Kiely *et al.* 1989). There are preliminary reports of the erectogenic property of intracorporeally administered calcitonin gene-related peptide (CGRP) and the enhancement by this peptide of PGE_1, (Stief *et al.* 1991) but data to date are limited.

Self-injection programmes for the management of erectile dysfunction have become commonplace but, regrettably, are being overused and even abused in some clinics. It is often less time consuming to teach self-administration than to explore possible psychogenic factors and manage the problem by behavioural or other psychological approaches. An important cause for non-acceptance of this approach by patients is the adverse reaction it engenders in the partners. This can be reduced by proper pre-treatment counselling and involving the partner in the injection programme. It is important that patients and their partners understand that intracorporeal administration of vasoactive drugs produces an erection but does not induce sexual arousal or sexual drive, except where these were reduced as a result of the erectile dysfunction. In fact, as Gilbert *et al.* (1990) have demonstrated, while intracorporeal papaverine will induce erection in androgen-deprived men (e.g. as a result of hormonal manipulation for the treatment of prostatic cancer), few will use it as a treatment for their erectile dysfunction due to their lack of libido. Those few who do continue to use this treatment are motivated to do so by their partners.

Yohimbine

Yohimbine, an indole alkaloid obtained from the bark of the yohimbine tree, *Pausinystalia yohimbe*, was being used as a treatment for sexual difficulties in both men and women more than seventy years ago (Hunner 1926). It has recently had a revival. There is now increasing evidence from clinical trials and clinical experience that yohimbine is effective in restoring erectile function in some men with either organic or psychogenic erectile dysfunction. Interesting trials of yohimbine have been undertaken by Morales and his colleagues working in Canada. In a pilot study involving 23 men with organic erectile dysfunction, yohimbine treatment resulted in 'full and sustained erections and resumption of satisfactory sexual performance' in six men and 'partial improvement' in four additional men (Morales *et al.* 1982). The same workers followed this pilot study with a placebo-controlled double-blind study of yohimbine in 62 men with erectile dysfunction conclusively diagnosed as having an organic aetiology (Morales *et al.* 1987). Twice as many men experienced complete return of erectile function on yohimbine (38 per cent) than on placebo (18.7 per cent), a statistically significant difference. This group of workers also studied yohimbine in 48 men with psychogenic erectile dysfunction (Reid *et al.* 1987). After ten weeks treatment with yohimbine, 62 per cent of men reported improvement in erectile function compared with only 16 per cent of men receiving placebo.

When placebo was changed to yohimbine in the men who had not responded, 21 per cent noticed some improvement.

In an English multicentre trial involving 61 men with erectile dysfunction of mixed aetiology, 36.7 per cent of men reported good stimulated erections after eight weeks treatment with yohimbine compared with only 12.9 per cent after placebo (Riley *et al.* 1989). When placebo was replaced by yohimbine, the percentage of men reporting good stimulated erections increased to 41.9 per cent. In this study yohimbine had no effect on morning erections, ejaculation, sexual interest, or sexual thoughts.

The dose of yohimbine used in the above mentioned trials was either 6 mg tds or 5.4 mg tds. The latter dose (5.4 mg tds) was also employed in a double-blind crossover study, undertaken in America, in patients with probable organic erectile dysfunction (Sonda *et al.* 1990). Of the 40 patients who were recruited, 33 completed the study and 33 per cent of these men had improved sexual function during the four weeks treatment with yohimbine. Fifteen per cent of men responded in both the yohimbine and placebo treatment periods while another 15 per cent responded to placebo alone. The remaining 36 per cent failed to respond to both yohimbine and placebo. These authors also reviewed 215 of their patients, with probable organic impotence, who had been treated with yohimbine. Partial and complete subjective improvement had occurred in 33 per cent and 5 per cent respectively. This series of patients included a large proportion of diabetics (60 per cent), hypertensives (33 per cent) and men with a history of alcoholism (25 per cent).

Higher doses of yohimbine have been evaluated. Daily doses up to 42 mg for one month were used in a placebo-controlled double-blind partial cross-over study in 82 patients (Susset *et al.* 1989). At the end of the yohimbine treatment period, 14 per cent of men reported the return of full and sustained erections, 20 per cent experienced partial improvement (with occasional penile rigidity sufficient to enable penetration), while 65 per cent failed to respond. Only three patients reported a positive placebo response. The authors considered this to be an encouraging outcome in view of the high incidence of diabetes and vascular pathologies in their study population. Of the 25 patients who reported either total or partial improvement, 15 considered that the maximum dose (42 mg daily) produced the greatest improvement, eight reported 32.4 mg to be the optimal daily dose, while the remaining two patients reported good results with a daily dose of 21.6 mg yohimbine.

In all the trials published to date, yohimbine has been administered on a regular basis over the course of four to ten weeks. Yohimbine is generally well tolerated. Reported side-effects include hypertension, anxiety, manic symptoms, restlessness, agitation, skin rash, and diarrhoea. Although some authors state that there is a delay in therapeutic effect of some two to three weeks after starting yohimbine (Morales *et al.* 1987; Susset *et al.*

1989), clinical experience suggests that some men gain benefit from using yohimbine on an 'as required basis' with the treatment being taken within an hour of anticipated intercourse. This approach to dosing requires careful evaluation.

Animal studies have confirmed a positive effect of yohimbine on sexual arousal and sexual motivation which is mediated through central mechanisms (Clark *et al.* 1985). Yohimbine has a number of pharmacological properties (Goldberg and Robertson 1983) the majority of which are only evident at high concentrations. The best established property of yohimbine at concentrations attained during treatment is α_2-adrenoceptor antagonism and it is probably by this mechanism that yohimbine improves erectile function. Other α_2-adrenoceptor antagonists have been (e.g. idoxazan) or are being (e.g. fluparoxan) evaluated in the management of erectile dysfunction. Idoxazan was marginally better than placebo but its use was associated with adverse effects (Haslam 1992).

Although most of the studies of yohimbine so far reported can be criticized on methodological grounds, there is now accumulating data to confirm that yohimbine is effective in the management of erectile dysfunction. The therapeutic effect of yohimbine in terms of numbers of patients responding favourably may not be very great, but this is to be expected in view of the multifactorial aetiology of impotence. Even considering the small therapeutic benefit that may be gained, yohimbine may be worth considering as a first-line treatment while the patient is waiting for specialist advice.

Opioid antagonists

Stress and anxiety induce a central release of endogenous opioids (Madden *et al.* 1977). The effect of endogenous opioids on sexual function of animals is complicated and may involve both stimulating and inhibiting effects depending on their site of action (see Chapter 1). They can inhibit initiation of copulatory behaviour and suppress penile reflexes. Erectile dysfunction can be an extremely stressful experience for men. The hypothesis that increased endogenous opioid release, resulting from such stress, may contribute to the development or maintenance of erectile dysfunction has been advanced and investigated by the use of opioid antagonists in erectile dysfunctional men. In an open study, Goldstein (1986) found that naltrexone (25–50 mg per day) produced full return of erectile function, including nocturnal penile tumescence in six patients suffering erectile dysfunction. In a single-blind placebo-controlled study, naltrexone (50 mg per day) significantly increased the frequency of morning and spontaneous full penile erections in a series of 30 patients with idiopathic erectile dysfunction (Fabbri *et al.* 1989). In addition, naltrexone treatment significantly increased the number of successful coitus compared to placebo. These observations are interesting and must be confirmed by further investigation.

Nitrites and nitrates

In vitro, nitroglycerine (propane-1,2,3-triyl trinitrate) and isorbide nitrate relax strips of human corpus cavernosum (Heaton 1989) and studies have shown that glyceryl trinitrate applied transdermally to the penis induce marked dilatation of the cavernosal arteries (Heaton *et al.* 1990). Mudd (1977) described an impotent man, who also suffered intermittent claudication, who began to experience erections, sufficient for intercourse, when he used sublingual glyceryl trinitrate or oral pentaerythritol tetranitrate. Ahmad (1990) reported the case of an impotent man with scleroderma who experienced the return of erection, sufficient for sexual intercourse, when he applied a nitroglycerine patch to the shaft of his penis. The effect of nitroglycerine applied as an ointment to the penis has been evaluated in erectile dysfunctional men by means of a double-blind placebo-controlled trial (Owen *et al.* 1989). Nitroglycerine increased penile circumference significantly in 18 out of 26 men studied. In another controlled trial, nitroglycerine patches applied to the penis induced a complete erection in 12 out of 26 impotent men and an additional nine patients had a partial response with this treatment (Claes and Baert 1989).

Pentoxifylline

Pentoxifylline is a methylxanthine marketed for the treatment of intermittent claudication caused by chronic occlusive arterial disease. In a double-blind placebo-controlled study, three of five patients with the diagnosis of vasculogenic erectile dysfunction reported improved erectile function while taking pentoxifylline (Korenman *et al.* 1988). In the same publication, Korenman *et al.* reported that, in an uncontrolled trial, five or seven men with the same diagnosis also improved with this treatment. More recently, Allenby *et al.* (1991) presented three cases of erectile dysfunction associated with occlusive vascular disease in which pentoxifylline also improved erectile function.

PREMATURE EJACULATION

The first choice of therapeutic approach to premature ejaculation is behavioural and pharmacotherapy is best reserved for those cases where this approach has failed or where there are factors that make it difficult or undesirable to use behavioural therapy.

Local anaesthetics

Over the years, various local anaesthetic agents have been used in an attempt to delay ejaculation by reducing penile sensory input. These have become known as genital desensitizers and included dibucaine (Aycock 1942), benzocaine (Damrau 1963) and nupercaine (Schapiro 1943). An 'over the counter' preparation of 10 per cent lidocaine, formulated as a spray (Studd 100®, Studd Holdings) is available as an aid to the management of premature ejaculation. The Food and Drug Advisory Review Panel has considered this product to be safe and effective for use as a male genital desensitizer (Federal Register 1982). Many men will have tried one of these proprietary products before seeking professional advice.

Psychotropic agents

A variety of psychotropic agents have been used in the management of premature ejaculation, including monoamine oxidase inhibitors (Bennett 1961), thioridazine (Mellgren 1967), and more recently clomipramine (Eaton 1973). While there is no doubt that these drugs are effective in delaying ejaculation, their effectiveness in treating premature ejaculation has not been evaluated in adequately controlled trials. A combination of amitriptyline and perphenazine (Triptafen DA®, Allen and Hanbury's), used as an adjunct to the 'Squeeze technique' in the management of premature ejaculation was evaluated by means of a double-blind placebo-controlled trial (Riley and Riley 1979). The active medication promoted the attainment of ejaculatory control early in the treatment programme but did not influence the overall results at twelve weeks. While adverse effects of this treatment were not a problem, subsequent use of an amitriptyline–perphenazine combination outside the clinical trial situation has been associated with a high incidence of side-effects which has lead frequently to non-compliance (Riley, personal observation).

Other drugs

Other classes of drugs have been used in the management of premature ejaculation. Propranolol (120 mg per day) was found to be no better than placebo (Cooper and Magnus 1984) and the combined α- and β-adrenoceptor antagonist, labetalol, has not been found to be effective (Riley, personal observation) even though this drug delayed ejaculation in a dose-related manner in healthy volunteers (Riley *et al.* 1982). Good results from the use of orally administered phenoxybenzamine in the treatment of premature ejaculation have been claimed by Shilon *et al.* (1984) on the basis of an uncontrolled trial; failure of ejaculation was a noted side-effect.

At the present time, clomipramine appears to be the most useful pharmacological agent for the management of premature ejaculation. There is no generally accepted dosing schedule but best results are attained if the dose is gradually titrated against response, starting with 10 mg daily (Goodman 1986). Clomipramine and other antidepressant drugs probably delay ejaculation by increasing 5-hydroxytryptaminergic activity because anorgasmia induced by such agents can be reversed by the concurrent administration of the 5-hydroxytryptamine (5-HT) antagonist, cyproheptadine (see p. 221). However, Colpi *et al.* (1991) using neurophysiological tests found that clomipramine increased the sensory threshold of the penis without affecting latency times or amplitudes of sacral-evoked response or dorsal nerve somatosensory cortical-evoked potential in premature ejaculators. The new class of selective 5-HT agonists and uptake inhibitors may prove to be useful for the management of premature ejaculation.

RETROGRADE EJACULATION AND FAILURE OF EMISSION

The ejaculatory process comprises three distinct but related events. The first event is emission, during which semen is deposited in the posterior urethra by contractile activity of the internal duct system. The second event is closure of the internal urethral sphincter of the bladder which prevents retrograde passage of semen into the bladder. The final event is ejaculation during which the bolus of semen is antegradely projected through the urethra to be forcibly emitted from the urethral meatus. The first two events are under the control of the sympathetic nervous system with α-adrenoceptor activation stimulating both the contractions of the internal ducts and closure of the internal urethral sphincter. Other neurotransmitters, such as oxytocin, may also be involved in these mechanisms.

Impairment of closure of the sphincter gives rise to retrograde ejaculation in which the patient generally has normal orgasmic sensation but no ejaculation of semen from the external urethral meatus. Instead, semen may be detected in urine voided after the event. Failure of emission and/or retrograde ejaculation can result from impairment of the nerve supply by either disease or surgical trauma or can be associated with the administration of drugs that block α adrenoceptors. There are anecdotal reports of beneficial effects of sympathomimetic agents in the management of these conditions. Ephedrine taken one or two hours before intercourse has been successful in the treatment of retrograde ejaculation (Stewart and Bergant 1974) and good results have also been claimed with phenylpropanolamine (Sandler 1979). Midodrine, a more potent orally active α-adrenoceptor agonist, has been found useful in the treatment of retrograde ejaculation (Jonas *et al.* 1979; Schwale *et al.* 1980). Pharmacotherapy is unlikely to be helpful where

retrograde ejaculation results from extensive surgical damage of the sphincter mechanism. However, Jonas *et al.* (1979) reported that normal ejaculation could be restored with midodrine in patients with anejaculation
resulting from extensive damage to the nerve supply of the internal genital
organs following abdominal surgery. Midodrine has also been found to be
helpful in the treatment of partial ejaculatory incompetence in some
patients (Riley and Riley 1982). Partial ejaculatory incompetence is characterized by reduced ejaculatory sensation and dribbling of the semen from
the urethra instead of it being forcibly ejected.

MIXED SEXUAL DYSFUNCTION

Bupropion hydrochloride, a non-tricyclic antidepressant, was evaluated by
means of a placebo-controlled study in a series of 60 men and women complaining of sexual aversion/inhibited sexual desire, inhibited sexual excitement, and/or inhibited orgasm (Crenshaw *et al.* 1987). Initial placebo
responders were eliminated during an eight week single-blind placebo phase
which was accompanied by sex education for the patients and their partners.
Non-responders were then treated with either placebo or bupropion for
12 weeks. At the end of the 12 week treatment period, 63 per cent of the
bupropion-treated patients reported themselves much or very much improved in terms of sexual desire and global assessment of sexual functioning, compared with three per cent for the placebo group. Sex drive,
frequency of sexual fantasies, and desire to have sex increased significantly
on bupropion compared to placebo, but increases in sexual activity frequency and sexual response were not significantly different from placebo.
When the treatments were crossed over, 74 per cent of patients improved on
changing from placebo to buproprion while 41 per cent lost their improved
sexual functioning when bupropion was changed to placebo.

REVERSAL OF DRUG-INDUCED SEXUAL
DYSFUNCTION

The most appropriate treatment of a drug-induced sexual dysfunction is
withdrawal of the offending medication and replacement by another agent.
Occasionally this approach is not possible on account of the clinical condition of the patient. In this situation it is sometimes possible to reverse the
sexual dysfunction without loss of the desired therapeutic response. Most
experience has come from reversing sexual dysfunction induced by psychotropic medication. For example, cyproheptadine has successfully reversed
orgasmic dysfunction induced by antidepressants (De Castro 1985; Steele
and Howell 1986; Riley and Riley 1986; McCormick *et al.* 1990; Sovner

1984), as have yohimbine (Price and Grunhaus 1990; Hollander and McCarley 1992) and bethanechol (Gross 1982). Yohimbine has also resolved ejaculatory dysfunction and reversed reduced libido induced by psychotropic medication (Hollander and McCarley 1992). Bethanechol has been reported to reverse erectile and ejaculatory dysfunction (Yager 1986), reverse orgasmic dysfunction (Gross 1982), and reverse ejaculatory dysfunction (Segraves 1987) induced by antidepressants.

CONCLUSION

As our understanding of the pathophysiology of sexual dysfunction increases and pharmaceutical chemists produce more selective pharmacological agents it should be possible to target drug treatment for specific sexual dysfunctions. It is important, however, to remember that for most people normal sexual activity depends on the interplay of two people. While drugs may restore sexual function they cannot directly improve a fragile, conflict-ridden relationship. We believe that, with only a few exceptions, drugs should only be used as an adjunct to counselling and other behavioural approaches and not used as the sole treatment for sexual dysfunction.

REFERENCES

Aboseif, S.R., Breza, J., Bosch, R.J.L.H., Bernard, F., Stief, C.G., *et al.* (1989). Local and systemic effects of chronic intracavernous injection of papaverine, prostaglandin E_1 and saline in primates. *Journal of Urology*, **142**, 403–8.

Allenby, K.S., Burris, J.F., and Mroczek, W.J. (1991). Pentoxifylline in the treatment of vascular impotence—case reports. *Angiology*, **42**, 418–20.

Ahmad, S. (1990). Scleroderma and impotence: response to nitroglycerine applied to the fingers and penis. *Southern Medical Journal*, **83**, 1495.

Aycock, J. (1942). The medical management of premature ejaculation. *Journal of Urology*, **62**, 361–2.

Bennett, D. (1961). MAOI for premature ejaculation. *Lancet*, **ii**, 1309.

Brindley, G.S. (1983). Cavernosal alpha-blockade: a new technique for investigating and treating erectile impotence. *British Journal of Psychiatry*, **143**, 332–7.

Brindley, G.S. (1986). Pilot experiments on the actions of drugs injected into the human corpus cavernosum penis. *British Journal of Pharmacology*, **87**, 495–500.

Buvat, J., Buvat Herbaut, M., Dehaene, J.L., and Lemaire, A. (1986). Is intracavernous injection of papaverine a reliable screening test for vascular impotence? *Journal of Urology*, **135**, 476–8.

Buvat, J., Lemaire, A., Buvat-Herbaut, M., and Marcolin, G. (1989). Safety of intracavernous injections using an alpha-blocking agent. *Journal of Urology*, **141**, 1364–7.

Claes, H. and Baert, L. (1989). Transcutaneous nitroglycerin therapy in the treatment of impotence. *Urology International*, **44**, 309–12.

Clark, J.T., Smith, E.R., and Davidson, J.M. (1985). Testosterone is not required for the enhancement of sexual motivation by yohimbine. *Physiology of Behaviour,* **35,** 517–21.

Colpi, G.M., Fanciullacci, F., Aydos, K., and Grugnetti, C. (1991). Effectiveness mechanism of clomipramine by neurophysiological tests in subjects with true premature ejaculation. *Andrologia,* **23,** 45–7.

Cooper, A.J. and Magnus, R.V. (1984). A clinical trial of the beta blocker propranolol in premature ejaculation. *Journal of Psychosomatic Research,* **28,** 331–6.

Corriere, J.N., Fishman, I.J., Benson, G.S., and Carlton, C.E. (1988). Development of fibrotic penile lesions secondary to the intracorporal injection of vasoactive agents. *Journal of Urology,* **140,** 615–17.

Crenshaw, T.L., Goldberg, J.P., and Stern, W.C. (1987). Pharmacological modification of psychosexual dysfunction. *Journal of Sex and Marital Therapy,* **13,** 239–52.

Crowe, M.J. and Qureshi, M.J.H. (1991). Pharmacologically induced penile erection (PIPE) as a maintenance treatment for erectile impotence: a report of 41 cases. *Sexual and Marital Therapy,* **6,** 273–85.

Damrau, F. (1963). Premature ejaculation: use of ethyl aminobenzoate to prolong coitus. *Journal of Urology,* **89,** 936–9.

De Castro, R.M. (1985). Reversal of MAOI-induced anorgasmia with cyproheptadine. *American Journal of Psychiatry,* **142,** 783.

Eaton, H. (1973). Clomipramine (Anafranil) in the treatment of premature ejaculation. *Journal of International Medical Research,* **1,** 432–4.

Fabbri, A., Jannini, E.A., Gnessi, L., Moretti, C., Ulisse, S., Franzese, A. *et al.* (1989). Endorphines in male impotence: evidence for naltrexone stimulation of erectile activity in patient therapy. *Psychoneuroendocrinology,* **14,** 103–11.

Federal Register (1982). **47** (113), 39412.

Gilbert, H.W. and Gingell, J.C. (1991). The results of an intracorporal papaverine clinic. *Sexual and Marital Therapy,* **6,** 49–56.

Gilbert, H.W., Gillatt, D.A., Desai, K.M., and Gingell, J.C. (1990). Intracorporeal papaverine injection in androgen deprived men. *Journal of the Royal Society of Medicine,* **83,** 161.

Goldberg, J.P. and Crenshaw, T.L. (1992). Bupropion treatment of sexual dysfunction. *Journal of Psychopharmacology,* Abstract Book of International Meeting of British Association of Psychopharmacology, Cambridge, 1992. A11.

Goldberg, M.R. and Robertson, D. (1983). Yohimbine: a pharmacological probe for study of the α_2 adrenoceptor. *Pharmacology Review,* **35,** 143–80.

Goldstein, J.A. (1986). Erectile function and naltrexone. *Annals of Internal Medicine,* **105,** 799.

Goodman, R.E. (1986). How to treat premature ejaculation. *British Journal of Sexual Medicine,* **13,** 178–9.

Gross, M. (1982). Reversal of sexual dysfunction by antidepressants. *American Journal of Psychiatry,* **139,** 1193–4.

Hashmat, A.I. and Abraham, J. (1987). Papaverine induced priapism. A lethal complication. *Journal of Urology,* **137,** 201.

Haslam, M. (1992). A trial of idazoxan and yohimbine in erectile dysfunction. *Sexual and Marital Therapy,* **7,** 261–6.

Heaton, J.P.W. (1989). Synthetic nitrovasodilators are effective *in vitro* in relaxing penile tissue from impotent men: the findings and their implications. *Canadian Journal of Physiology and Pharmacology,* **67,** 78–81.

Heaton, J.P.W., Morales, A., Owen, J., Saunders, F.W., and Fenemore, J. (1990). Topical glyceryltrinitrin causes measurable penile arterial dilatation in impotent men. *Journal of Urology*, **143**, 1099–102.

Helmy, A.M. (1991). Gluteal device for penile injection. *British Journal of Urology*, **68**, 400–3.

Hollander, E. and McCarley, A. (1992). Yohimbine treatment of sexual side effects induced by serotonin reuptake blockers. *Journal of Clinical Psychiatry*, **53**, 207–9.

Hunner, M. (1926). *A practical treatise on disorders of the sexual function of the male and female*. F.A. Davis, Philadelphia.

Jonas, D., Linzbach, P., and Weber, W. (1979). The use of midodrine in the treatment of ejaculation disorders following retroperitoneal lymphadenectomy. *European Urology*, **5**, 184–7.

Kattan, S., Collins, J.P., and Mohr, D. (1991). Double blind, cross-over study comparing prostaglandin E_1 and papaverine in patients with vasculogenic impotence. *Urology*, **37**, 516–18.

Keogh, E.J., Watters, G.R., Earle, C.M., Carati, C.J., Wisniewski, Z.S., Tulloch, A.G., et al. (1989). Treatment of impotence by intrapenile injections. Comparisons of papaverine versus papaverine and phentolamine: double blind cross-over trial. *Journal of Urology*, **142**, 726–8.

Kiely, E.A., Ignotus, P., and Williams, G. (1987). Penile function following intracavernosal injection of vasoactive agents or saline. *British Journal of Urology*, **57**, 473–6.

Kiely, E.A., Bloom, S.R., and Williams, G. (1989). Penile response to intracavernosal vasoactive intestinal polypeptide alone and in combination with other vasoactive agents. *British Journal of Urology*, **64**, 191–4.

Korenman, S.G., Moorandian, A.D., and Kaisser, F.E. (1988). Treatment of vasculogenic sexual dysfunction with pentoxifylline. *Clinical Research*, **36**, 123A.

Kromann-Andersen, B. and Nielsen, K.K. (1989). Intracavernosal self-injection with injection pen. *International Journal of Impotence Research*, **1**, 127–30.

Larsen, E.H., Gasser, T.C., and Bruskewitz, R.C. (1987). Fibrosis of the corpus cavernosum after intracavernous injection of phentolamine/papaverine. *Journal of Urology*, **137**, 292–3.

Lue, T.F. and Tanagho, E.A. (1987). Physiology of erection and pharmacological management of impotence. *Journal of Urology*, **137**, 829–35.

McCormick, S., Olin, J., and Brotman, A.W. (1990). Reversal of fluoxetine-induced anorgasmia by cyproheptadine in two patients. *Journal of Clinical Psychiatry*, **51**, 383–4.

Madden, J., Akil, H., Patrick, R.L., and Barchas, J. (1977). Stress induced parallel changes in central opioid levels and pain responsiveness in the rat. *Nature*, **265**, 358–60.

Mellgren, A. (1967). Treatment of ejaculation praecox with thioridazine. *Psychotherapy and Psychosomatics*, **15**, 454–8.

Michal, V., Kramar, R., Pospichal, J., and Hejal, L. (1977). Arterial cavernous anastomosis for the treatment of sexual impotence. *World Journal of Surgery*, **1**, 515.

Morales, A., Surridge, D.H.C., Marshall, P.G., and Fenemore, J. (1982). Non-hormonal pharmacological treatment of organic impotence. *Journal of Urology*, **12**, 45–7.

Morales, A., Condra, M., Owen, J.A., Surridge, D.H.C., Fenemore, J., and Harris, C. (1987). Is yohimbine effective in the treatment of organic impotence? Results of a controlled trial. *Journal of Urology*, **137**, 1168–72.

Mudd, J.W. (1977). Impotence responsive to gyceryl trinitrate. *American Journal of Psychiatry*, **134**, 922–5.

Ottesen, B., Wagner, G., Virag, R., and Fahrenkrug, J. (1984). Penile erection: possible role for vasoactive intestinal polypeptide as a neurotransmitter. *British Medical Journal*, **288**, 9–11.

Owen, J.A., Saunders, F., Harris, C., et al. (1989). Topical nitroglycerine: a potential treatment for impotence. *Urology International*, **141**, 546–8.

Price, J. and Grunhaus, L.J. (1990). Treatment of clomipramine-induced anorgasmia with yohimbine: a case report. *Journal of Clinical Psychiatry*, **51**, 32–3.

Puppo, P., De Rose, A.F., and Pittaluga, P. (1988). Office and home protocols for intracavernous injections: results of 101 cases. In *Proc. Sixth Biennial Int. Symp. Corpus Cavernosum Revascularization. Third Biennial World Meeting on Impotence*. International Society for Impotence Research, p. 170.

Reid, K., Morales, A., Harris, C., Surridge, D.H.C., Condra, M., Owen, J., et al. (1987). Double blind trial of yohimbine in treatment of psychogenic impotence. *Lancet*, **i**, 421–3.

Riley, A.J. and Riley, E.J. (1979). Amitriptyline-perphenazine and the squeeze technique in premature ejaculation. *Journal of Pharmacotherapy*, **2**, 136–40.

Riley, A.J. and Riley, E.J. (1982). Partial ejaculatory incompetence: the therapeutic effect of midodrine, an orally active selective alpha adrenoceptor agonist. *European Urology*, **8**, 155–60.

Riley, A.J. and Riley, E.J. (1986). Cyproheptadine and antidepressant-induced anorgasmia. *British Journal of Psychiatry*, **148**, 127–8.

Riley, A.J., Riley, E.J., and Davies, H.J. (1982). A method for monitoring drug effects on male sexual response. The effect of single dose labetalol. *British Journal of Clinical Pharmacology*, **14**, 695–700.

Riley, A.J., Goodman, R.E., Kellett, J.M., and Orr, R. (1989). Double blind trial of yohimbine hydrochloride in the treatment of erection inadequacy. *Sexual and Marital Therapy*, **4**, 17–26.

Sandler, B. (1979). Idiopathic retrograde ejaculation. *Fertility and Sterility*, **32**, 474–5.

Schapiro, B. (1943). Premature ejaculation: a review of 1130 cases. *Journal of Urology (Baltimore)*, **50**, 374–9.

Schramek, P. and Waldhauser, M. (1989). Dose-dependent effect and side effect of prostaglandin E_1 in erectile dysfunction. *British Journal of Clinical Pharmacology*, **28**, 567–71.

Schwale, M., Frosch, P., Tolle, E., and Niermann, H. (1980). Treatment of retrograde ejaculation and anorgasmy with an alpha-sympathomimetic drug (Midodrine). *Zeitschrift fur Hautkrankheiten*, **55**, 756–9.

Segraves, R.T. (1987). Reversal by bethanecol of imipramine-induced ejaculatory dysfunction. *American Journal of Psychiatry*, **144**, 1243.

Shilon, M., Paz, G.F., and Homonnai, Z.T. (1984). The use of phenoxybenzamine treatment in premature ejaculation. *Fertility and Sterility*, **42**, 659–61.

Sidi, A.A. and Chen, K.-K. (1987). Clinical experience with vasoactive intracavernous pharmacotherapy for treatment of impotence. *World Journal of Urology*, **5**, 156–9.

Sidi, A.A., Cameron, J.S., Duffy, L.M., and Lange, P. (1986). Intracavernous drug-induced erections in the management of male erectile dysfunction: experience with 100 patients. *Journal of Urology*, **135**, 704–6.

Sonda, L.P., Mazo, R., and Chancellor, M.B. (1990). The role of yohimbine for the treatment of erectile impotence. *Journal of Sex and Marital Therapy*, **16**, 15–21.

Sovner, R. (1984). Treatment of tricyclic antidepressant-induced anorgasmic inhibition with cyproheptadine. *Journal of Clinical Pharmacology*, **4**, 169.

Stackl, W., Hasun, R., and Marberger, M. (1988). Intracavernous injection of prostaglandin E₁ in impotent men. *Journal of Urology*, **140**, 66–8.

Steele, T.E. and Howell, E.F. (1986). Cyproheptadine for imipramine-induced anorgasmia. *Journal of Clinical Psychopharmacology*, **6**, 326–7.

Stewart, B.H. and Bergant, J.A. (1974). Correction of retrograde ejaculation by sympathomimetic medication; preliminary report. *Fertility and Sterility*, **25**, 1073–4.

Stief, C.G., Wetterauer, U., Schaebsdau, F., and Jonas, U. (1991). Calcitonin-gene-related peptide: a possible role in human penile erection and its therapeutic application in impotent patients. *Journal of Urology*, **143**, 392–7.

Susset, J.G., Tesser, C.D., Wincze, J., Bansal, S., Malhotra, C., and Schwacha, M.G. (1989). Effect of yohimbine hydrochloride on erectile impotence: a double blind study. *Journal of Urology*, **141**, 1360–3.

Szasz, G., Stevenson, R.W.D., Lee, L., and Sanders, H.D. (1987). Induction of penile erection by intracavernosal injection: a double-blind comparison of phenoxybenzamine v. papaverine–phentolamine v. saline. *Archives of Sexual Behaviour*, **16**, 371–8.

Virag, R. (1982). Intracavernous injection of papaverine for erectile failure. *Lancet*, **ii**, 938.

Virag, R. and Adaikan, P.G. (1987). Effects of prostaglandin E₁ on penile erection and erectile failure. *Journal of Urology*, **137**, 1010.

Wagner, G. and Gerstenberg, T. (1988). Vasoactive intestinal polypeptide facilitates normal erection. In *Proc. Sixth Biennial Int. Symp. Corpus Cavernosum Revascularization. Third Biennial World Meeting on Impotence*, p. 146. International Society for Impotence Research, Boston.

Waldhauser, M. and Schramek, P. (1988). Efficiency and side effects of prostaglandin E₁ in the treatment of erectile dysfunction. *Journal of Urology*, **140**, 525–7.

Williams, G., Mulcahy, M.J., and Kiely, E.A. (1987). Impotence: treatment by autoinjection of vasoactive drugs. *British Medical Journal*, **295**, 595–6.

Yager, J. (1986). Bethanechol chloride can reverse erectile and ejaculatory dysfunction induced by tricyclic antidepressants and mazinodol: case report. *Journal of Clinical Psychiatry*, **44**, 210–11.

Zorgniotti, A.W. and Lefleur, R.S. (1985). Auto-injection of the corpus cavernosum with a vasoactive drug combination for vasculogenic impotence. *Journal of Urology*, **133**, 39–41.

Index